The
LIGHT
of
UNDERSTANDING

To   Mavis

W.H a joy in your heart
And innocence, purity and delight.
May you love unfold most bright.

Love
Nick

NICK SCOTT-RAM

Note for Librarians: A cataloguing record for this book is available from Library and Archives
Canada at www.collectionscanada.ca/amicus/index-e.html
ISBN 1-4120-9464-X

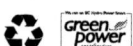

Printed in Victoria, BC, Canada. Printed on paper with minimum 30% recycled fibre.
Trafford's print shop runs on "green energy" from solar, wind and other environmentally-friendly power sources.

TRAFFORD
PUBLISHING™

Offices in Canada, USA, Ireland and UK

Book sales for North America and international:
Trafford Publishing, 6E–2333 Government St.,
Victoria, BC V8T 4P4 CANADA
phone 250 383 6864 (toll-free 1 888 232 4444)
fax 250 383 6804; email to orders@trafford.com
Book sales in Europe:
Trafford Publishing (UK) Limited, 9 Park End Street, 2nd Floor
Oxford, UK OX1 1HH UNITED KINGDOM
phone 44 (0)1865 722 113 (local rate 0845 230 9601)
facsimile 44 (0)1865 722 868; info.uk@trafford.com
Order online at:
trafford.com/06-1219

10 9 8 7 6 5 4 3 2

Dedication

Meher Baba
The Avatar of the Age

&

DC

Cover Illustration
'Passion'

by

Kathryn Thomas
www.kathryn-thomas.co.uk

Contents

Synopsis

There are major changes taking place all around us, yet most are unseen. We live in an Avataric Age which means that everything is changing. Our physical world is just one aspect of a huge expanse of Light, where invisible streams of awareness flow in and out of our consciousness. Beyond the physical, there are untold millions of layers of experience through which our soul journeys. All of these levels are now undergoing profound changes that are impacting our normal lives, as the old timeline of suffering is replaced by a new timeline of grace.

The Light of Understanding gives a detailed description of these changes, beginning with the first spark of creation, through to the formation of the planes of consciousness, and the soul's orbit from unconscious bliss back, ultimately, into conscious union. *Light* goes onto describe the birth of the planetary consciousness, Gaia, through the essence of Macheldavek, and to explain the formation of the different root races in the past. It explains how new types of souls are coming into the planet, and how a new triangle of energies is forming between the devas, the angels and higher levels of guidance known as the Elderings. This triangle will be birthed into an expanded chakra system containing twelve chakras.

The sum total of humanity's past, as held within the astral levels, is now being restructured along a new timeline of the Sixth Root Race where a new collective experience of unity will provide a platform for a higher level of conscious awareness. The new timeline is birthing a stunning, new, hologram of light and all we have to do is to connect with it and embrace it. This hologram will provide us with new vehicles of consciousness and a new light body; mental telepathy will flow effortlessly, and each person will access entirely new levels of love, knowledge and delight, in preparation for the eventual return of the Cosmic Christ.

The Light of Understanding will appeal to those who have read widely on spiritual matters since it captures some of the most up to date information about the planetary changes. It will also be of interest to those just starting on their spiritual journey, providing a clear and detailed overview of many of the key ideas and concepts that are being birthed in the new timeline.

Acknowledgements

I n a work of this nature, there are a number of people who should take the real credit for what has been presented here. First and foremost is David Cousins who has taught me everything that is contained within these pages and whose love and guidance has been the source for so much more, both outer and inner. Words are not adequate to convey the expression of what I owe him but hopefully the essence of what is contained within these pages will give the reader a flavour of what his teaching and constant unveiling of more represents. In a very real sense, I have acted only as the writer while DC has been my guide within the energetic stream of information.

Second, I would like to acknowledge the love and understanding of my beloved wife Frances who shoulders the everyday burden of my writing habits. I am most fortunate to have someone who walks with me on this path each day and with whom I am able to discuss different concepts and ideas. Her support and love is a constant joy.

I would also like to thank a number of other people who have helped in the genesis of this book, both in the creative and production process. Several people have commented on early drafts of the manuscript and I would like to recognise the input of Cornelia Selkirk, Vaune Newcomb Hodgetts, Paul and Alessandra Shepard. Other friends have been kind enough to read earlier drafts of the work and their support has been most welcome: they include Linda Boer, Nicola Castle and Claude Randall. I would like to thank Stephen O'Sullivan for the layout and design. I owe a special debt to Kathryn Thomas who has allowed me the privilege of using one of her stunning pictures for the front cover.

Finally, I would like to say a special thank you to Lily WhiteRose at LightWork Media who has worked tirelessly and constantly on my various projects and for all of her love, encouragement and support in bringing them to fruition.

Introduction

Spiritual ideas, concepts and experiences have to run through the gauntlet of subjectivity on the one hand, and the fixed, immutable authority of tradition on the other. These two extremes have rarely sat comfortably together. Today, we live in a world where our subjective experience is increasingly out of kilter with the long-established religious doctrines, and where the response to change is a poverty of tolerance and rigidity of ideals. Yet change underlies the very fabric of the Universe and when we recognise that everything is in a constant state of flux, then we can open up new inner doorways to embrace deep change.

There are other areas of intellectual conflict. Science has provided us with different explanations about the nature of the world that we live in and has fuelled great technological growth. Yet science has difficulty in describing and explaining our need to find a spiritual path. The intuitive, inward-looking approach of the spiritual path is the very antithesis of the objective and repeatable world of science. Yet, as physics pushes back the frontiers of our knowledge, areas of overlap with spiritual thinking are beginning to develop. For example, physicists are beginning to consider whether the Universe is a living hologram, while modern spiritual experience describes an inner world of light and divine streams of energy that are also part of a larger hologram. In the future, science and spirituality will slowly and inexorably move towards each other and the new souls coming into the planet will work with both streams of knowledge.

There is massive change taking place on many different levels, much of it unseen. Our physical world is just one aspect of a huge expanse of Light, where invisible streams of awareness flow in and out of our consciousness. Occasionally, the doors to these larger, unseen expanses open up and we can catch a glimpse of something vast, majestic and divinely uplifting. We may only receive a glimpse once in our lifetime, or we may feel successive levels opening up to us. Such glimpses are like invitations that allow us to search deeper into our essence and to find a new level of understanding and consciousness. The new frequencies of light are now giving us the opportunity to not only open the door and see what lies on the other side, but also to go through it and remain constantly immersed in the higher streams of light. These new light streams offer us a very different view of our reality, our divinity and of our soul's journey through the millions of veils of experience.

The Light of Understanding seeks to capture something of what lies through the doorway and to highlight how the major changes taking place in what we would call the inner planes are transforming the very fabric of our existence. Time is speeding up, and as our experiential reality begins to warp and mingle with other timelines, we will experience multiple-dimensional, telepathic living and a new, heightened consciousness of what we are and where our destiny lies. This book is about describing a footprint in the sand; a footprint that resonates in the present with something that we would call more, and which also looks to the future where our spiritual journey is expanded and lived in a unique and different way.

The Light of Understanding begins by describing how the world about us is changing in many different ways, and how the old karmic patterns of the past are being re-worked to invoke a new timeline of light, as ordained and set up by the Avatar of the Age, Meher Baba. We live in an Avataric Age, which means that everything in our lives is changing, and through aligning ourselves energetically with this change, then we can cross our inner abyss of limitation, and embrace a new level of inner silence and stillness. Real change and spiritual work is carried out in silence, hidden from the glare of our expectations and prejudices. Through finding our inner silence, we can begin to ascend internally to a new level of light and inner guidance that will, quite simply, give us more of everything.

The book goes on to describe how the initial spark of light birthed everything out of nothing, and how the journey of the first spark, the Primary Spark, gave rise to the billions and billions of layers and all other life forms that co-exist within different streams of light and dark. The expression of soul light through the angelic and devic realms is also highlighted, including an overview of a soul's journey through the Mineral, Plant, Animal and Human Kingdoms. Through millions of life times in human form, the soul eventually returns through the planes of consciousness to the point where it becomes re-united with God, in the process of God-realisation.

The Light of Understanding describes the birth of the planetary consciousness, Gaia, through the essence of Macheldavek, before moving on to an overview of the different root races that have graced the planet. These include the earlier root races, the Adamic and Hyperborean, where physical human form was not fully developed, and then the later root races, the Lemurian, Atlantean and Aryan, where the human form was much more developed physically. We stand on the cusp of change, witnessing the setting of the Aryan Root Race sun, and the dawn of the new Sixth Root Race timeline and sun. In this crossing over process, all the old karma from the past has to be cleared away, and this is one of the reasons why there is so much happening around the planet today.

Earth is the only planet in the Wheel of Life, which contains all the universes and galaxies, where the Avatar and the Perfect Masters can be found in physical form. Through the instruction of the Avatar, the five Perfect Masters are overseeing the planetary and life form changes necessary for the birth of the new timeline. This new timeline is initiating complete change on all levels: from the original mix of light and dark, through a reworking of chaos and order, to the restructuring of the inner planes where much more virulent streams of light will be birthed within our physical consciousness. These new streams of light embody divine frequencies of bliss and grace and are part of the unfolding of a new level of unity throughout all life. Above and beyond these levels, entirely new frequencies of light are now becoming accessible as part of the upward flow of Avataric Energy in the higher planes.

New patterns of soul light are also coming down into the planet, including new souls that are focused on either the devic, angelic or mast (God-intoxicated) pathways. At the same time, a principal triangle of energies between the devas, the angels and higher guides known as the Elderings is starting to manifest in our energetic systems. This pattern will help to re-wire our chakra system, supporting an increase in the number of chakras from seven to twelve. This new chakra system will then bring through a new pattern of emotional experience, one that is much more refined than the current emotional dialogue in existence in humanity.

Throughout all of this change, humanity is being offered a new way of living, focused through a series of interlocking platforms combining power, love, unity, wisdom, purity, innocence, truth and knowledge. The sum total of humanity's past is being re-orchestrated so that the new timeline can birth entirely different streams of higher light frequencies, and the steps involved in this transition are set out in *The Light of Understanding*. Humanity is waking up to a new, collective experience where the living moment will be invoked spontaneously, where the past will dissolve away and where the future can be manifested in the present to birth a new level of conscious awareness of what we are and will truly become. Our vehicles of awareness will birth a new light body where mental telepathy will flow effortlessly, and where each person will access entirely new levels of information and knowledge.

The book also describes a collection of techniques and tools (including meditations and exercises) for opening up to the new timeline. This includes ways to access different life forms, including the devas, the angels and the Elderings; and methods for connecting to the new hologram of light, which contains absolutely everything necessary to manifest the Sixth Root Race on every level of our awareness and in every fibre of our being. Ultimately, the new root race is about invoking more, and through the future timeline, humanity is now preparing itself for the arrival of the Cosmic Christ in human form.

In short, *The Light of Understanding* aims to give an overview of some of the changes now taking place, and to give an up to date account of how new levels of consciousness are manifesting in our every day living. The book also represents a series of layers, with multiple levels of overtoning, and depending on where the reader chooses to place his or her awareness, then the energy contained in the book will establish an energetic dialogue in the appropriate way.

Finally, I hope that the reader may find something that will excite them, and help to give a different perspective on life. In a book of this nature, there may be concepts and ideas that challenge the mind. A natural scepticism is a healthy position to adopt in such circumstances, and yet when this is tempered through the intuition of the heart, then the individual may be able to find a common ground where what is felt has its own language and recognition. It is common for the mind to be unwilling to accept what the heart recognises and so it is with the new energies and timeline, there is a need to focus with the heart, to embrace the subtle energies of the imagination and to allow the intuition to sift through what feels appropriate and what does not. The heart can then flower into something completely different.

Nick Scott-Ram 2006

CHAPTER 1

A Fresh Start

Light and Dark

Light is information and is always manifested through the interplay of light and dark[1]. Light embodies everything in it: it is the unfolding manifestation of all that was, is and will be. While we all need information and understanding, the difficulty arises in determining what feels right or wrong, or what information will bring us to a point of deeper balance and harmony, or which will have the opposite effect. True information, or the higher manifestation of light, is always supported by love. While love can mean many contrasting things to different people, it always underlies our focus in physical matter. Love can be conditional, where there is always an agenda, or expectation of a return for our love, or it can be unconditional, where there is absolutely no expectation of return. Unconditional love is always expressed freely and with no attachment to the outcome of its expression. Unconditional love is the highest form of love and while individuals may profess to express it, it is an energetic expression of an individual's essence rather than a psychological state of mind. To free oneself of the unconscious burden of conditional expectations is extremely hard, since they can sit within one's energetic system like an iceberg – the tip touches our conscious awareness, while by far the largest portion is hidden, below the surface. It takes millions and millions of lifetimes of experience in physical matter to achieve the energetic status of manifesting unconditional love.

In the West, we usually think that we have one life only – one life to experience everything around us, which is always dominated by the fear of death, whether it is conscious or subconscious. In the East, the prevailing climate of thought favours reincarnation and so attitudes to living and dying are rather different. In the West we are much more focused on the external world, the material world, while in the East, the focus is more on the inner world. Not surprisingly, the status of our actual lives in matter is much more accurately portrayed in Eastern thought. On average a soul undergoes 8,400,000 lives in human form in matter i.e. the physical, three-dimensional realms of experience, and therefore any one life is a minute fraction of the sum total of all of our lifetimes. It is, quite literally, like a drop in the ocean. The usual response in the West is to ridicule such a notion without really understanding its full implications. Yet, the belief that we have only one life is totally misguided.

The main barrier to recognising our reincarnatory pattern is an absence of memory of any of our previous lives. At birth we are born with complete amnesia of everything that has happened to us previously, and it is only through experiences in our life, such as the people we meet, the places we visit, that may open up a dim pulse of recognition that we might have met that person before, or have visited that same place at an earlier time. In short, it is only through gathering direct experience of who we are and where we have been that we can wake up from a deep sleep that shrouds our spiritual and energetic heritage.

We often talk about right or wrong, or light and dark. The term light is used here in a slightly different context to above. So in a general sense, Light can be light or dark, while specifically light also represents the way of love, truth, understanding, service, hope, clarity and compassion. The prevailing view is that the light is good and the dark is wrong. The light embraces the qualities that make humanity something more, while the dark represents the focus of feudal selfishness, pride and the desire to own everything. In spiritual terms this is regarded as less. Another way of looking at dark and light is to consider chaos and order. Chaos is the random movement of events or energies that have no underlying pattern; chaos is confusion and disorder. Order, on the other hand, is the arrangement of matter, events or experiences according to an underlying pattern or method. The two are diametrically opposed and represent the dual patterns or opposing forces of creation. Chaos is more representative of the dark way, while order is the manifestation of light. Light always flows out of the darkness. This interplay between chaos and order, light and dark bathes our very existence; it is the critical juxtaposition around which our whole experience is given meaning.

Patterns of chaos and order dance in and out of our everyday lives; an illness represents chaos as the body strives to find more order. As a disease progresses, old patterns of chaos are shed and a new feeling of order comes in. For example, with a common cold, we usually feel lighter afterwards. Accidents are the same: an explosion of force releases chaotic patterns of energy. More fundamentally, we live in an imperfect world, where free will and choice rule supreme. The Earth is the only planet of free will and choice and represents fifty percent heart and fifty percent head. This balance is played out through our thoughts, feelings and emotions. In some cases, the head will rule our emotions, while in other circumstances the heart may dominate any rational tendencies. Yet throughout this complex interplay of experiences, we will be hard pressed to determine what may be order or chaos; we may think something is more ordered, when it is really implicitly chaotic. For example, we may believe, through superstition that the number 13 is unlucky and that doing anything on Friday 13th is not an especially good idea. Yet, in spiritual terms, 13 is the number of power; its potency has been constantly weakened through misinformation. In this case, order has been misinterpreted as chaos. Another example is to live our present life from the viewpoint of our past. If we always live the now in terms of old habits and desires, are we living a more ordered or less ordered life? Since there is an implicit creative movement where order comes out of chaos, on balance we will be working with older patterns of chaos rather than new expressions of order. There are signs of superficial orderliness everywhere and yet many things only disguise the underlying chaos. Similarly when something new manifests in our lives, it may appear chaotic at first, yet its implicit expression is more ordered.

The Earth forms a triangle with two other planets at this time, forming a basic energetic trinity. These other planets manifest a pattern with a different balance of head and heart; one of them is twenty-five percent head and seventy-five percent heart, while the other is seventy-five percent head and twenty-five percent heart. On Earth, the balance of head and heart provides the platform for true free will. Each planet is closely associated with the other and provides an energetic flow between the different representations of head and heart. These different patterns of head and heart flow through our planet from time to time, like overlapping streams, and different people may resonate more closely with one or other of these patterns.

The Earth is a living, sentient being which houses the procession of life in its many diverse forms. The planetary awareness or essence is feminine and is known as Gaia. Gaia is the planetary doorway for all life forms that exist on the planet, seen and unseen, and is a living being within her own right. The true beauty, breadth and understanding of Gaia's role in our planet's evolution has not been fully appreciated. Taxonomists have spent decades cataloguing the procession of different life forms that have passed through Earth, from single-celled bacteria, to complex cells, simple plants, trees, basic animals and more complex vertebrates, all the way to the human form at the top of the evolutionary tree. Simultaneously, the geologists have spent several centuries classifying our rocks and mineral deposits. Life seems straightforward but remains elusively difficult to define. Yet within these outer, physical manifestations there are different levels of sentient life forms each expressing and manifesting things in a different way and which are just as real as their physical, three-dimensional counterparts.

One type of life form that is present in everything is the deva and this formless presence represents the pulse that is expressed through every rock, plant and animal. In short, devic life imbues everything. The devic pattern is chaos orientated and so all devas seek more experience through diversity. Balanced against this devic pattern of life is the angelic pattern of order.   Angels are usually invisible to the naked eye; they observe and record everything that takes place and typically represent the essence of order. The devic and angelic pattern forms a dynamic interplay between different streams of life.

Humanity, for the most part though, has forgotten the dynamic relationship that exists between the planet, its varied environments and the different life forms that it supports. It has forgotten about the existence of devas and angels, and the varied life forms that exist in more subtle realms; it has become separated from the underlying fabric of light that permeates everything. Humanity's amnesia does not stop there: we have, with the odd exception, completely forgotten who we really are, what our role is on Earth, and what the purpose of living in physical matter is from the point of view of our higher self, or even soul. We have no recollection of our soul journey, from its inception point, all the way through into the future, where our soul's destiny may become realised.

Instead of living in the present, or the future, humanity finds it much easier to live in the past within a displaced comfort zone. Memories of previous experiences in our current life get recycled through our awareness like old records and anything different that is presented to us, is often ignored or rejected because it takes us out of the comfort of our living in the past. We live in the context of our memories, never fully appreciating what the present and future may hold and what it means and feels like to be moving our awareness into the present and beyond the present into the future. Through being wedded to our past, we mistake this for more, when in reality it is less. It is our minds that limit our experience, separating it from different underlying connections, and restricting our access to different realms of experience.

The Soul

Our physical bodies have been designed to receive, record and transmit all of the experiences that we undergo. The pain of physical birth is recorded in our energetic system, retained in our muscles and crystalline bones, and as we develop and grow, every experience is recorded in our physical cells. Each cell acts as a living memory of everything that passes through us. However, the experiences that we receive are not just in the physical, three-dimensional realms; they also touch us from many other levels, the majority of which are subtle and difficult to measure in physical terms. Our physical vehicles live in a world of constant stimulation, much of which is generated through human activities, such as electromagnetic radiation, artificial light and the increasing burden of synthetic chemicals. Our physical bodies were not designed to withstand such exposures of radiation or chemicals and the finer, subtle aspects of our bodies easily become clogged and blocked through modern living.

We are born within a complex set of physical, emotional and mental parameters that reflect the underling stream of chaos and order. This river of chaos and order is the negotiated pattern of light that our physical forms can sustain. The level of light frequency that we can absorb is now much higher than at any time in the history of humanity. Our physical and subtle bodies can now host greater quantities of light. Old methods and rituals are no longer relevant in opening ourselves up to the new energies. Yet we have various filters and limitations that determine the template of our experiences. Apart from the limitations of our physical bodies and the structure of our DNA, we have a mind which seeks to explain and understand everything, inside and out, according to the dictates of past experience. Our brains are wired up to gather data and to collect information. The mind is very rarely silent and generally provides a constant dialogue or commentary on all that we experience: it contextualises and defines our life. We are all born with a personality that is part of our karmic negotiation for any given life. Our personalities are fairly inflexible and it is usually the interplay of personalities that causes so much confusion and chaos in personal relationships, fuelled by the constant negotiation of our underling karma. We may have a pleasant personality, or one that is cold and distant. Yet, each specific personality is a tool for a job of work: nothing more. Each personality is perfectly adapted for the particular job of work that needs to be done in a given life.

On the one hand our brain seeks more diversity, while our hearts crave for silence and less stimulation. Between these two opposites, the thread of free will weaves a pattern of choice through our collective emotions. The constant interplay between head and heart reflects the energetic flow through the planet.

The pulse of our soul is situated within our physical vehicle and is the true connection with our inner plane essence. Wrapped around our physical body, reflecting the pattern of subtler levels of energy are our etheric and astral bodies. The etheric body closely mirrors our physical shape and is approximately one inch thick. It can be seen as a seam of white energy resting on the physical vehicle. In contrast, the astral body is, at full strength, twenty-seven feet wide on either side of our physical body and is comprised of a web-like pattern of astral light. The astral body is an indicator of our emotional and energetic well-being, and in many people it is often in poor condition. Dark patches or tears in the astral web indicate areas that need attention.

Each physical body houses seven main chakra centres and hundreds of minor chakras. The seven main chakras are the base, the sexual centre, the solar plexus, the heart, the throat, the third eye and the crown. Each chakra can be described as a wheel, and is a doorway between the physical and the subtle vehicles of consciousness. Most people operate energetically from their lower centres, reflecting issues around survival and sexuality, and each centre will carry varying percentages of light and dark light. It is not uncommon for the percentage of dark to be much higher than light. To work with the higher centres in a meaningful way requires hard work and the right use of the will to focus into the higher energetic streams of light. The smaller centres are found in the palms of the feet and hands, and in the joints between our bones such as the elbows and knees. A sure sign that energy is being pushed through one's physical system is to experience pulsing in the palms of the hands with a blotchy skin appearance.

Our physical bodies are, in effect, on loan for this particular life. The soul sends an aspect[2] of itself into physical matter as part of the reincarnatory programme, which is integral to this planet and the other planets that operate through the twin frequencies of karma and time. Karma is an active point of denial reinforced by prejudice, while time is an artificial commodity that ensures the laws of karma are upheld and satisfied. On engaging with physical matter, our soul aspect incarnates through one permanent, physical atom, which is held within our heart centre. This one permanent atom forms a triangle with two other atoms that are derived from this one atom, to form a masculine atom and a feminine atom. Energetically, these three atoms form a triangle, with the one permanent atom at the apex, and the other two atoms forming the two points in the base.

The one permanent atom keeps a physical record of all the lives that the soul aspect has gone through and at the point of death it is released from the physical body and returns to a band of blue energy that sits outside the atmosphere of the planet. This band of blue energy is known as the "ring-pass-not" and acts like a filter mechanism for all of the experiences and impressions that are held outside the planet, in the higher realms. All incarnating souls pass through this ring-pass-not and endure a dose of spiritual amnesia. The soul aspect forgets who it is and it's life purpose. This spiritual amnesia sets the baseline for experience for every single soul aspect in the planet: all souls start at the same baseline at birth: no memory of what has gone before. This means that no one has any unfair advantage. The challenge, then, for each soul aspect is to wake up through a pattern of orchestrated energetic interchanges, such as meeting the right people at the right time in the right place, to activate older memories locked in the permanent atom and the energetic essence of the subtler vehicles. It is only through the right experiences that a soul aspect can wake up and begin to remember and understand what his or her life's journey is all about.

Each soul starts its journey in the higher planes in the Ocean of Life. This Ocean resides in the lower part of the Seventh Plane and is the manifestation of the Creator. Within this Ocean, which is black and extremely silent, souls lie in the depths in unconscious bliss. There is no light around and although the Ocean exists out of time and the physical patterns of karma, souls will progress from the abyssal depths up to the surface, where they are scooped off, like droplets of water, through different energetic patterns. The breath of the Creator, or Will of the Father will manifest a pattern of soul birth, and when a soul reaches the top of the Ocean of Life, it becomes separated from the sum total of all its experiences up to that point, which is unconscious bliss. Each droplet that is segregated from this Ocean is a soul and this first separation from the Ocean represents the primordial shock, the first separation. This first separation imbues within each soul the urge to find out more about itself.

The Planes of Consciousness

Souls are then pushed away from the Ocean and drop down through the inner planes. These planes are the planes of consciousness: there are seven main planes, and within each plane, millions and millions of sub-planes. The Seventh Plane is where the Father or God resides and all the divine beings that are God-conscious. Below this plane, the Planes of Illusion, so-called because they are a shadow of the Reality[3] of the Seventh Plane, drop away in reverse order. So a young soul will begin its journey in the Seventh Plane and then drop down through the Sixth Plane, then the Fifth Plane, followed by the Fourth, Third, Second and First Plane. Below the First Plane is the Zero Plane where ninety percent of humanity is anchored in its conscious awareness. Each plane represents a different level of experience and awareness as manifested through patterns of higher and lower Light. So the highest manifestation of Light is on the Seventh Plane, and this can be termed Divine Light. The other planes then irradiate different frequencies of light ranging from higher mental light, which imprints our thoughts and ideas, through to astral light, which acts as a focal point for our emotions. Different mixes of mental and astral light wash through the different planes, so that in the Sixth Plane there is ninety percent mental light and ten percent astral light, while in the First Plane, it is the reverse with ninety percent astral light and ten percent mental light.

Each developing soul will be anchored at a different point in the Planes of Illusion. A young soul will drop down through all of the planes until it reaches the Zero Plane where it will begin its physical programme in matter. The process and trajectory of coming down into the Zero Plane will determine the pattern of incarnation and a soul's lower and higher purpose. The higher purpose of a soul will be negotiated at the start of its journey, either at the point of separation from the Ocean or shortly afterwards before dropping out of the Seventh Plane. As each soul comes down through the planes, it splits itself up into seven main aspects. Each of these aspects is used to gather more experience in the downward journey and this continues during a soul's return journey back up from the Zero Plane to the Seventh Plane. Once the seven aspects have been manifested, then each aspect will undergo a further division into two, with each subdivision of one of the seven becoming either a feminine or a masculine aspect.

In all, there are fourteen aspects that make up each soul. Each soul will also be part of a soul family, which is a reflection of the pattern of birthing in the Ocean of Life and the type of energetic pattern of light essence that constitutes each soul. Up until now, there have been twelve major soul families, with each family embodying a specific ray or colour frequency. It should be recognised, though, that the essence of a colour frequency is rather different from what we associate colour with in the grosser physical realms. The level of energetic refinement and essence of each colour is way beyond what our physical nervous systems can assimilate, let alone experience.

Once each soul has gone through the downward journey into the Zero Plane, it then commences the physical programme of incarnation, first through the Mineral and Plant Kingdoms, and then through the Animal Kingdom. Eventually, each soul aspect will enter the human form, and then undergo the full pattern of involution back up into the Seventh Plane. It is this journey in human form that will take, on average, 8,400,000 lives. On average, each soul aspect will spend around one million lifetimes in each plane. The first million lifetimes will reflect the energetic pattern of the Zero Plane, where the substance of Light is very dim and where the energetic focus is slow, embodying a drag between, on the one hand, the Mineral, Plant and

Animal Kingdoms, and on the other, the Human Kingdom. Typically, a soul aspect will require two to three million life times before reaching the second plane; younger souls are those soul aspects that have completed up to two and a half million lives. Middle-aged souls typically will push up from the lower astral planes into the plane of transition, the Fourth Plane, and sometimes beyond. This plane marks the shift from the astral planes into the mental planes. Older souls are those aspects that have experienced in excess of five million lives.

Each soul aspect, while in physical matter, will be anchored at a particular plane level, and within that plane at specific levels within a series of sub-planes. So a young soul may be positioned at level 1.2.3.1 which would be the First Plane, level two within the first subdivision of ten, and then level three within sub-division two and so on. This would be the accurate description of the level of involutionary progress for that particular soul aspect. Each aspect of a soul can be anchored at different levels within the planes. So a soul may have twelve aspects located in the Second Plane, one aspect in the Third Plane and another in the Fourth Plane.

Within the progression of human reincarnation, no more than five soul aspects are allowed into the planet at any one time. Each soul aspect is a soul mate to the other four aspects. Typically, younger souls do not meet up with their soul mates due to the concentrated exchange of energy that this entails, and such soul aspects would have insufficient experience in matter to maintain a balance during the highly charged interaction. Consequently, a sufficient level of experience in matter is normally required before soul mates meet up.

The feminine and masculine soul aspects that were derived from one of the original seven aspects are known as twin flames, and usually twin flames only meet in physical matter at the end of their reincarnatory programme, since to meet a twin flame is to become complete in energetic terms. There is a considerable amount of misunderstanding around the idea of soul mates, and what most people regard as a soul mate is not usually the case: often they will have spent many lives with this other person and it is the old addictions of love that resonate through into the present which confuse them into thinking that they are soul mates. True soul mates are those who share the same soul essences and sometimes there can be extremely violent dislike between soul mates, representing the karmic pattern between them.

The average soul aspect will have one life in ten which is designated a work life. This means the aspect will undergo more experience that will form a basis for growth and working through patterns of karma in its myriad forms. The other remaining nine lives will be spent resting. In a rest life, an individual may not marry or have many relationships and will be in a karmic pattern where he or she can digest the experiences of the previous working life. For those undergoing a working pattern, then one of the main indicators is crisis: either through mental, emotional or physical events such as multiple relationships, illnesses or a run of events that invoke significant emotional or other responses. The pulse of energy from the soul into the physical vehicle is more pronounced and means that a greater energetic charge flows through in that working life. Although the timing of working and resting lives is usually pre-planned, there are exceptions to when working lives are manifested, and the principal exception is during what is termed an Avataric Age.

The Avataric Age

We currently live in an Avataric Age. This is the period during the lifetime of the Avatar and for one hundred years after the Avatar has dropped His Body. The Avatar is the living essence of God who, as the Son, incarnates on Earth every seven or fourteen hundred years. The Avatar is the perfection of everything and comes to serve all life forms, whether they are plankton, the earthworms or humanity. The latest Avatar was Meher Baba who died in 1969 and we will continue to live in an Avataric Age until 2069. The advent of the Avatar is always accompanied by change, and the change that is now reverberating around the planet is huge: it is demanding more, not less of all life, and of humanity it is demanding nothing less than absolute change: a dramatic turnaround in the level of consciousness that each human experiences. The Avatar has also predicted that seventy-five percent of humanity will die, and although we may interpret this in the traditional sense of physical death, it can also mean other things within a spiritual context. Meher Baba came to awaken humanity out of its deep sleep; out of the sleep of ignorance, out of the dream of illusion and out of the burden of suffering. He has also orchestrated everything for the next three thousand years and has rewired the whole planet and all life on it.

The Avatar also ordained that by 2069 the planet would be seventy-five percent light and twenty-five percent dark, a turnaround from seventy-five percent dark and twenty-five percent light in 1969. We are now past the halfway point, with slightly over fifty percent light and just below fifty percent dark on Earth.

This huge shift is embodied in the Nine-Pointed Plan that Meher Baba has orchestrated. Each part of the Plan, as manifested by the Father, is unveiled in sequence on Earth. We are now at the start of the fifth part of the Plan and all nine parts will be completed by 2069. During the one hundred year period after He drops His Body, the Avatar returns to the highest levels on the inner planes, into what is sometimes referred to as God in the Beyond-Beyond State[4], a space beyond description in the highest realms of the Seventh Plane. It is this process which takes one hundred years in physical time.

All around us there are subtle and grosser manifestations of the changes taking place in the spiritual transformation of life on the planet. The old sun of the Fifth Root Race is setting which means that the old timelines of the Aryan Root Race are coming to an end, and the new timelines and love-lines of the Sixth Root Race are being established. The early stages of the Sixth Root Race are underway, and the new sun has risen. The challenge for humanity is to awaken from the old Fifth Root Race dream, and turn away from the old sun, and move towards the newly rising sun of the Sixth Root Race. In marking this transition between the root races, the Father has demanded total change. A change in the way we live our lives, the way we perceive ourselves and the way we reveal our true, inner, spiritual path.

Outwardly, this is being manifested by a shift in energy entering the planet through the Photon Belt, the increased power of the Sun, the un-layering of old dark practices in religions, specialist groupings and individuals, as all of the old karma from the previous root races is pushed through humanity. The end of the Fifth Root Race represents the end of an accounting period and the books have to be balanced before the new root race can become fully manifested in physical form.

In contrast, the new root race will bring an unprecedented period of peace for humanity, as the new rays of higher light and love are embraced by all physical form. The old wash of human emotions will be replaced by a whole new emotional pattern, and the focus will be on light rather than dark. Every human will be offered an opportunity to know himself, or herself, in a profound way – to recognise that in the past each person will have been both a saint and a sinner. Meher Baba predicted that those who are perceived as sinners would recognise themselves as saints, and those that were saints would know that they were sinners. The new physical prototype for the Sixth Root Race will manifest both mental and emotional telepathy, will have a system of twelve rather than seven chakras and will be able to sense a myriad of different life forms that are currently invisible to the naked, human eye. Above all else, the planet will sing to a new pattern of love, a love birthed through the essence of the Father, and which will, in the fullness of time come to reveal in physical matter, the return of the Christ. This return will be in approximately ten million years time and will herald a new level of love and light that has never before been seen on the planet.

While the Earth undergoes change at every level, the frequencies of light and love that are birthed into it will be distributed out into the solar system and galaxies beyond. Earth is at the centre of the Wheel of Life[5] in both spiritual and evolutionary terms. The central Earth is the only planet on which the Avatar physically incarnates. All life has to pass through the outer parts of this Wheel, incarnating in different physical uniforms on thousands of different planets, before finally progressing to the central Earth, which in the past, has been regarded as a finishing school for souls. There are eighteen thousand Earths all connected into the central Earth and each of these planets plays host to the different forms of humanity. All of these planets will be bathed in the new Sixth Root Race frequencies that will be birthed on Earth.

These new frequencies will bring about change at all levels. The structure of the inner planes will change, the pattern of soul evolution and birthing out of the Ocean of Life will be modified and the relationship between the devic and angelic realms will undergo a profound transformation. In addition, new levels of divine beings will grace the planet and open up an entirely new dialogue with humanity. Nothing will ever be the same again.

On a more physical level, old practices in business and the use of planetary resources will be changed, as will the fundamental practice of slaughtering our close animal relatives for food and sustenance. The wheel of karma has come nearly full circle and the karma invoked through the killing of humans in the past by animals will be balanced out. In short, humanity will come to recognise and understand a new balance within the planet, experience a new living hologram of Light that will open up everything within our awareness in an entirely new way. Absolutely everything that we hold dear in our current pattern of existence will be swept away and replaced by a deep spiritual recognition of our immortality, and of a profound understanding that death is not the end of it all; it is a transition between different states, and that the existence of the soul on the inner planes will be proven beyond all doubt. Purpose and meaning will return to everyday life.

At its simplest Light is information. New Light and information is now entering the planet and represents the wake up call to a new spiritual heritage. The use of information through the pattern of experience can then bring about understanding, and once judgement is applied through the interplay of light and dark, then it becomes possible to invoke a new pattern of wisdom for everyone. At the same time, and the principal driving force behind many of the changes now being implemented on the higher planes, a new manifestation of power is speeding up the spiritual evolution of the planet. Power is essential for change; it is the driving force for change within a spiritual context.

On the outside, some people feel the despair of the apparent mess of their own lives as well as the continued use of twisted will in directing the use of planetary resources. What has to be realised and understood is that change first manifests in the higher planes. So change is invoked and created first in the Seventh Plane, and then the energy and multiple light streams flow down through each of the planes. So in the Fifth and Sixth Planes, new ideas and concepts are initiated through mental light, which then filter down into grosser levels of astral light, giving birth to new emotions. As the energy comes down through the lower planes, it becomes more diluted. Eventually, the new frequencies of love and Light are then manifested in the physical realms. So while wholesale change can take place on the inner planes, it can still be some time before these changes are experienced in the physical planes.

The sheer majesty and power of the changes now taking place on the inner planes requires an entirely new way of looking at our own spiritual development, as well as a deeper level of understanding of spiritual concepts and ideas. The truth of today rapidly can become the untruth of tomorrow and it is important to recognise, above all else, that the pattern of energetic changes is constantly evolving in a dynamic way. The trick for humanity is to recognise that this wave of spiritual change is part of the higher programme of love ordained by Meher Baba and to understand that the easiest way to change is to embrace the new energies rather than fight them through stubbornness, pride, backward looking addictions and old prejudices. Of course, this is much easier said than done. However, the right use of the will, clear intent, discipline in thought and action, as well as the cultivation of a collective platform of love and light in heart and inner awareness will go a long way to opening up the new inner levels of being that are now on offer. To have an open heart and an empty mind is a way in which the new wave of light can be surfed through our conscious awareness as the end of one Avataric Day draws to a close, and the start of a new Avataric Day is birthed.

CHAPTER 2

The Old Timeline

Orchestrating Change

Deep change is always difficult and requires courage, determination and trust. What makes it more complicated today is that we are not sure what we are changing into. We all like to live in our comfort zone and as soon as we move outside of this zone, then we begin to feel confused, unhappy and focus exclusively on our individual needs. Change is usually met by a reversion to basic, survival instincts and the more change is resisted, often the harder it is to cope with it. Fear usually lies at the bottom of this basic resistance – fear of the unknown, fear of letting go, or fear of failure. Irrespective of the reason, fear always shapes our response. Another factor that often holds people back is a lack of understanding and information on what needs to be done. This is even more the case with spiritual change. How can a person start to change when it is not clear what the change is? Consequently, two great obstacles to any form of profound change are fear and confusion.

Before any sort of change can take place, a person needs to understand why change is necessary. Spiritual awakening and change can appear amorphous, indulgent, even misguided and all the more so when placed in the context of unfamiliar concepts or ideas. In today's world of science and apparent rationality, the idea of following change from an intuitive perspective can seem almost heretical. Yet, this resistance harbours our underlying prejudice about how we understand the world in objective terms, and how everything is often object oriented. We are often more interested in material objects than in the people or other living creatures around us.

Finding a reason for change, especially when that change is not quantified and is often little more than a niggling feeling at the back of our mind, may seem hard to justify. But again, justification is an activity that looks backwards, not forwards. The filter of our mind has to give its stamp of approval. At its simplest, a reason for change should honour what makes us feel happy and excited. However, this is not as simple as it sounds. A heartfelt sense of excitement can be easily hijacked by the mind and then worked through a string of apparent justifications that may end up with us holding back. There may appear to be one hundred and one reasons not to change, and yet the one truest feeling expressed in the heart will often be buried in the clamour of noise generated by the mind. At the end of this process, the original urge has been lost and any of its associated energy.

Consequently, finding a reason for spiritual and wholesale change is often the hardest thing for the personality to comprehend, let alone embrace. The mind will usually come up with a whole host of reasons why change is not necessary. Even when the evidence is irrefutable, such as in giving up smoking, the mind fuelled by emotional need, will usually manage to argue that another cigarette is still a good idea. Change is as much about letting go of our old addictions, as it is about opening new doorways to something more. And this is not just in the physical, obvious sense, but also in the broader sense of our addictions to limitation and the dark.

But when all these uncertainties are brushed to one side, there is, below the surface, one overriding reason to embrace spiritual change: it is simply that it is already happening and that it will continue to gather pace. It has been set in motion in the highest planes and will continue inexorably, filtering down through the mental, astral and into the physical planes. The physical manifestations of this change are everywhere: the 2004 Boxing Day Tsunami in the Indian Ocean and the destruction of the Twin Towers on 9/11 are clear examples.

The choice each individual has is whether to find his or her own surf board of awareness, love and understanding and then to ride this spiritual wave of energy with a sense of awe and excitement, or to stand still in the water and be hit, head on, by the tidal wave of new energies coming in. If change is resisted by the personality and the sub-conscious, then the new energies entering the planet will find other ways to ensure that change takes place. And for most people, this will be achieved through the time-honoured way of initiating crisis in their personal life. Crisis can either be mental, emotional or physical or a combination of these three. With crisis, there is always change, because the personality is jolted out of a comfort zone and forced to examine a different reality where the expectations are not met, and where accident, illness, or emotional trauma demands a re-evaluation of everything in an individual's life up to that point. In the early stages of the crisis, the usual response is "why me?" However, the unfolding of the crisis will present the individual with new avenues to consider. For example, if a person suffers from a severe illness, or has a near death experience, their karma and energetic system are often significantly changed, and they feel different afterwards. The crisis has presented them with an alternative view of reality, and then allows them the possibility to re-evaluate their life and change it. Old karma drops away and they can then engage in a new path of growth and change.

The notion of a wave of energy bearing down on humanity may sound overly dramatic, but is nonetheless accurate. Wave after wave of higher light is flooding into the astral levels and forcing old energies to the surface in a plethora of different ways. The expression of these old energies is seen in the different illnesses now besieging humanity, in the flux of earth movements around the planet, the violence and senseless killing, and in the bizarre and often animalistic behaviour that is now commonplace in many societies. It is like all restraint has been released.

In the old pattern of living, it is like humanity is blindfolded and completely oblivious of the surroundings. The blindfold represents ignorance, suffering, old addictions and negative practices and thought forms. The blindfold is now being removed, first from those who are more sensitive to the new energies, and then in rapid succession, from those who can sustain the shock of experiencing something dramatically new. The removal of the blindfold will invoke crisis in many people's lives, as they seek to throw out the old energies, and then embrace the new energies. Once people recognise that the blindfold has been removed, they will begin to realise something that has been dormant inside of them all along, but which they had forgotten. The scenery may have been there all the time; it is only that they could not see it. The transformation from the old root race into the new root race, therefore, represents the removal of the blindfold and is an opportunity for all humanity to wake up from its dream. The old blindfold of limitation, fear, doubt, selfishness and material saturation will be stripped away and replaced by the breathtaking new vistas of spiritual growth and collective unity.

Old Timelines and Thought Forms

The Fifth Root Race, or the Aryan Root Race, is now winding down and it is obvious that the world is undergoing profound change. This root race represents the old timeline, the old reality that is locked in on a particular path within time. Timelines are patterns of energy that can pulse in the past, present or future. They are like highways of probability and some pulse more strongly than others. A timeline is an energy stream that begins at a point in time, and then flows forwards or backwards in direction, to another point, or series of points. These points can be in the past, present or future, and when projected into the future, from either the past or the present, represent a future probability or outcome. For the most part, humanity has focused on the past and has sought to relive the old timelines. How much of our present living is held in place by our memories of the past? Quite simply, almost everything. Old timelines are usually locked in place because the past has already occurred, and are then fed more energy by our focus on the past. This entrenched perspective makes it much harder to concentrate on the present, let alone the future.

Living in the present should mean that we do just that: we orientate ourselves in the present and look to the future. In reality, we spend most of the time looking to the past, recycling old memories and events through our mind in an attempt to gain some greater understanding. Yet because the past has already been and gone, it represents limitation, not expansion. In contrast, to be and live in the present means that we can feel the presence of other possibilities to the past – we can be offered alternative timelines that may hold new patterns of energy that can take us into a new future. This is simple in concept, yet difficult in practice. In the present, new possible timelines can form, each one linked into a series of choices and decisions according to the needs of the underlying energy. In the present we can be offered new opportunities: however, if we choose a particular alternative from the viewpoint of the past, and according to our old timeline, then we immediately invoke limitation and a resistance to change. The other, possible timelines may drop away and we remain on the old timeline. On the other hand, if we embrace a new opportunity or timeline, then we will feed new energy into that timeline. We will manifest the possibility in a meaningful way and we will begin to lock onto that timeline and walk along it into the future.

In the past, humanity has been presented with fundamental choices: for example between timelines that focus on the dark or on the light. Decisions were made that led more into the dark than the light, such as in the Atlantean Root Race. Today, the reverse is true. The decision to go into the light has already been made and all humanity has to do is to step off the old timeline onto the new timeline that is headed directly into the light. This means letting go of the past and all its limitations and embracing the future. The future timelines are forming in the present and we simply need to recognise this and act accordingly.

A popular, almost relativistic perspective is to say that we each live in our own reality according to the way that we create it. We therefore all live in different realities. Similarly, all large institutions, including religions, governments, and special-interest groups like to paint a picture of how the world is supposed to be from their own limited and biased point of view; in the same way as how our family and friends, and work environment create an emotional context through which we filter our experiences. The news and newspapers tell us what is supposed to be happening; yet this is always done with vested interest. These different realities all incorporate bias, irrespective of whether it is intended or accidental, conscious or sub-conscious. All bias is a reflection of limitation and is rooted in our past experiences.

What we think and what we believe frames our reality, and the underlying energy that is pushed through the concepts and ideas will determine the way in which we respond and act upon such ideas. For example, the banking system is based on an idea about how to save and distribute funds, with the core concept that whatever transaction goes through a bank, the bank is then entitled to some form of payment. This is, at its simplest, a thought form. Thought forms exist in our everyday life, ranging from the simplest, such as a person's appearance, to the more complex ones that dictate how a society acts and interacts. Thought forms are everywhere – a person's mood will be a reflection of their thoughts and the underlying thought forms that drive those thoughts. Although thought forms can appear confusing and complex, they are usually simple. Every thought form will carry an energetic charge that is linked into the emotional structures and feelings housing those thoughts. Thought forms can be either quite bland, almost passive, while others can be extremely virulent and impact the way we feel in a dramatic way. For example, a baker could be fairly passive in his or her thoughts and yet, if he or she started thinking about something in an active, negative way, then it could impact everything in the surrounding energetic environment quite dramatically. The atmosphere would be negative and anyone that came into to contact with it would be influenced. The bread that the baker made would also carry this energetic charge and whoever then eats the bread, would absorb some of the negativity from the baker. We only have to reflect on how people's moods can influence us to understand the power of virulent thought forms.

Alternatively, if someone is happy and is supplying coffee or working in a restaurant kitchen this will raise the vibration of the food and drink. Thought forms can carry a huge diversity of energies and emotions, such as fear, greed, worry, shame and so on. One of our favourite thought forms in modern society is worry.

The same principles of energy transfer apply in larger organisations; the underlying thought forms are either passive or virulently active. Different forms of religious fundamentalism contain strong thought forms about what people should and should not believe, to the extent that individuals may be prepared to sacrifice their lives at the expense of others. Such thought forms can be dark and extremely potent, and are based on active misinformation fuelled by low frequency, dark light.

Thought forms also dictate how governments manifest legislation and serve their citizens. Governments that put the interests of its members before those of its people are operating according to slower, dark thought forms of self-interest. Thought forms that are imbued with a dark focus will always seek to limit people through fear, depression, the manipulation of information, state control and feudalism. In contrast, lighter thought forms will always open up to more and will birth new ideas and concepts that give joy and harmony, and embrace authentic notions of service, rather than those that pay only lip service to serving their citizens. In today's current, feudal environment, it is a rare organisation that embraces the idea of higher, unselfish service as opposed to lower, selfish service.

A thought form about my appearance may say that I look tired, appear old, or look ugly. Everywhere in Western Society we are taught to think constantly about our appearance. The underlying thought form is often pretty negative, focusing on eroding a person's feeling of self worth, and through consumer bias, leading to a pattern where someone may feel motivated to buy more make up, or in more extreme cases, to undergo cosmetic surgery. These thought forms all focus on the outer, external world and focus on our limitations. They all masquerade at offering more, when it is really less. Advertising often reflects these negative thought forms because it focuses on what we lack and attempts to persuade us that we should rectify this lack, and buy a specific product or service, when we do not need it all. Since most advertising is driven by a combination of fear, greed or desire, the thought forms are correspondingly dark.

Similarly, thoughts and emotions imbue our products. When we buy food from the supermarket, it has been on a journey from the primary producer, through the supplier and distributor and then onto the supermarket shelf. Apart from the growing conditions for fruit and vegetables, and whether pesticides are used, the emotions and thoughts of the growers will imbue the products. Were the farmers happy, angry or sad? All of this energy will be absorbed by the lettuces, tomatoes or chosen produce. Similarly, what are the underlying thought forms of the distributors and the supermarkets? Is it to get the lowest price possible out of the farmer and what is the motivation for this? Is it to maximise their own profits, at the expense of others? And what is their attitude to the consumers? Is it to sell poor quality produce at inflated prices, or is to make the produce look inviting when the underlying nutritional content is pretty poor? All of these energies will impact on the final product. At the end of this chain of physical, emotional and mental events and energetic interplays, the fruit or vegetable will sit on a shelf and radiate a vibration, or series of energies. When a person then comes to pick it, does it make them happy? If everyone in the chain has been focusing on exploiting one another, then it is pretty unlikely and the fruit or vegetable will be surrounded by a dark aura. The combined energies of the ground, seeds, growing conditions, transportation, storage and finally the supermarket environment all impact the product. This whole conglomerate of energies will be eaten by the consumer and then absorbed into their energetic system.

The same thing happens if we go into a restaurant and eat a meal. If the chef is unhappy and angry, then it will reflect in the food. We will digest these negative feelings and absorb them. If the chef is happy and excited, then the cooking will mirror this. What this simple example is meant to illustrate is that everything in our lives is imbued with underlying thought forms, many of which are negative and operating from the standpoint of self-interest. Thought forms always contain a pattern of energy, which can be either light or dark. A light thought form might involve a focus on collective harmony and the benefit of others; a dark thought form would be based on self–interest.

Our lives are shaped and influenced by thought forms, ranging from the everyday and mundane to the more limiting and virulent. Examples of major, limiting thought forms can be found in certain religious practices. Some religions talk about heaven and hell and seek to impose slow frequency energy into people's systems. The idea the behaviour in the current life will determine where the soul will end up is a common one, and yet if this is used in a way to limit or wreak revenge, then these thought forms are driven by fear and control, laced with a large dose of misinformation.

Heaven and hell are illusions and as such only exist in illusion. They can exist in the lower planes – up until the end of the Third Plane and soul aspects, when they drop their bodies, may enter these realms on the basis of what their belief systems have set up and according to the needs of the evolution of their soul. However, both of these places are an illusion. Beyond these defined spaces is a much larger and greater expanse of light that builds in intensity. It stretches up into the higher planes where there is more mental light, and ultimately into the Seventh Plane where the essence of true divine light is manifested. In human form we can each live in our own heaven and hell, according to the dictates of what our karma requires, and also according to free will and choice. If you think depressing thoughts all day, then it follows that you will become depressed: energy follows thought. If you think happy thoughts, then you will be uplifted and enter a different space. For the most part, humanity has danced along the ray of suffering for a long period of time, to the extent that it is generally regarded as a good thing to suffer. If you suffer, then you must be doing it right! It follows then that we think suffering is more, not less, when in reality the reverse is true. The concepts of heaven and hell are extremely powerful and tie into our beliefs about death. They engender a fear of death, which again is a thought form. Yet they are illusory.

What we think creates what we experience, and what we experience creates what we can or cannot become. If we remain locked into the old way of suffering then that is all that we will experience. If we begin to open up to the possibility of something new and something different that is not frozen in the past, then we will discover something new. We are bombarded all day by thought forms and for the most part, are consciously oblivious of the underlying energy that is being pushed into our systems. Many thought forms pollute our systems energetically, leading to a lower vibration in our energetic field. Becoming aware of these different thought forms and finding ways to clear them is more than a useful exercise: it is fundamental to developing a pattern of sound energy management within our conscious awareness.

The Choice between Less and More

Today, there is a choice that we all have to make. This is a profound choice that recognises the difference between less and more. Less is the past and encompasses fear, doubt, limitation, feudalism, selfishness, material gain, competitiveness and clinging to all the dark emotions that can typically dominate our emotional lives. Less also represents the old Fifth Root Race timeline and the old beliefs and thoughts that are constantly recycled. In contrast, more is an opportunity to embrace an entirely new type of love, to connect with a new flow of collective unity, and to open up to a brand new level of awareness that gives each person a much deeper understanding of their destiny, their intrinsic place in the Universe and in participating in the new wave of Sixth Root Race ideas and concepts that will replace the outmoded beliefs. In short, to ask for more is to ask for everything in a spiritual sense, and not in a material sense.

More means connecting with our own divinity and higher self in a brand new way. It is like having broadband compared to a normal telephone line for downloading and accessing higher levels of information and experience. More represents free will and choice to go into the new light and the new dawn of understanding, and to close the older dark doorways of vested interest. More also means waking up to a new level of collective awareness and understanding, at a profound level, beyond the intellect, of what our path and destiny is. It is to live and dance along the new timelines of energy that are on offer, and to surf, using our vehicles of consciousness, along the divine highways of love and light. It also means to surrender the fear of death and to understand the transition between life and death. Finally, more is to re-align our life and its purpose with the Divine Purpose of the Avatar; to embrace and feel His Love and to recognise the uniqueness of our relationship with Him.

However, humanity has often become confused over the difference of what is more or less. More is usually equated with more material gain, more material objects, more money, more property and so on. To turn inwards and seek the silence of our stillness and inner spirituality is seen as less.

Christmas in the Christian calendar is a classic example of where people think less is more. Christmas has become a materialistic bonanza for the consumer, where each year increasing numbers of presents are exchanged in the mistaken belief that this is more. Throughout this, the original energetic impulse that was the original spirit of Christmas has become lost in a material frenzy. In reality, though, it is less because the burden of giving and receiving places an emotional burden on all involved. There is always an expected response in the giving and receiving of gifts which often bears no relation to how people actually feel or wish to express themselves. Authenticity is often lost.

Other examples of less and more include our notions of bureaucracy and regulation, and the role of insurance and loss of personal responsibility. We are constantly confronted by choices between more and less. Does the material society that we live in today offer us more or less? Do the current religions in the world offer us more or less? They all offer us less while pretending that it is more. Does the food we eat offer us more or less? Most of the constant bombardment of advertising is about persuading us to accept less while believing that it is more. And in determining whether something is more or less to us, it is a straightforward choice. More should make us happy and excited at an intuitive, heart level while less will not. Less will engage the mind, which will then argue that more is less and less is more.

However humanity finds it harder and harder to recognise what is more or less. Is a near-death experience more or less? Is a near fatal illness more or less? Illness is a manifestation of karma being played out in the physical and through the illness an individual may come into more, by burning off old karma. The illness would then represent more, although our minds would always say that it is less.

In Western Society there is a growing desire to blame someone or something for every event that we do not like or which we believe impacts us in a negative way. Yet to blame others for our own misfortunes is to let go of our own authority and to invoke more karma through active denial. Our judgements will usually seek to avoid pain or discomfort, and yet once we embrace whatever comes our way openly, then we can begin to find a different type of freedom: one where we can begin to invoke more, not less, and where change can offer us more, and where denial can turn to acceptance. Avoiding the dictates of our own personal karma is about invoking less and not more. This is to ignore the underlying flow of chaos and order in our own lives, and to give no recognition to the status of our own personal karma.

Karmic Laws

Within the context of who we are and where we stand in our life can be greatly helped by an appreciation of the laws of karma; the recognition that every act, every emotion and every thought incurs karma. The planet and all life forms on it are present in a given timeline and manifest an energetic expression in the physical realms as a direct result of karma. Karma is the accounting of everything that has taken place on an atomic, molecular, cellular, organism, individual and group level. The interaction between two animals – the instinctual expression of a predator stalking a prey invokes karma, which ultimately has to be balanced. If a person steals a car, then karma is invoked and at some point in the future that act has to be balanced.

Karma operates on all levels of consciousness – from the

mental, through the astral, into the etheric and into the physical. Every aspect of our physical vehicle, personality, mind and attributes will be shaped by our personal karma. Karma can be positive or negative, so a selfless act of compassion will incur positive karma just as a selfish or violent act of brutality will invoke negative karma. Through the progression of our lives, we build up karma with other soul aspects that we meet in different incarnations. For example, one soul aspect may meet another soul aspect over the course of seventy lives, and during that time build up a karmic thrust focused on several, specific, emotional frequencies such as loss, or abandonment. In one life, the other soul might have been a mother and then abandoned her baby. Through the law of opposites, which is always invoked in the balancing of karma, the soul that was the baby may come to be the mother in a future life and then get presented with a set of circumstances where she is forced also to abandon her baby, who is the other soul aspect this time. Through a constant interplay of opposites in succeeding lives, old karmic patterns eventually become burnt out through experience. This law of opposites is fundamental to the pattern of all life experience on the planet and beyond.

Once the law of opposites becomes saturated through the multiple polarised experiences, the polarity diminishes and the flow of experiences in subsequent lives can move into a different pattern of expression. The limitation of karma is superseded, eventually, by an understanding of what is more, rather than less.

Karma will also be played out through whole races or civilisations. For example, those who instigated the demise of the Native American Indians in the 19th century returned into matter as Native American Indians themselves. Similarly, some old Nazis will have to begin balancing their karma through incarnating as a Jew in the next life. This constant fulfilment of karmic obligation also makes a mockery of our notions of ownership since in one life we may own a piece of land that is a source of conflict between two countries. In the next life, we will be born into the other country and experience the conflict from a different perspective.

The laws of karma will dictate precisely and specifically where and when a soul will incarnate. In one incarnation the life may be rich and bountiful, and yet in the next the soul aspect will experience poverty and malnutrition. In one life, the soul aspect will be a woman, and then in the next a man. Our jobs are karmic devices to ensure that we work with people with whom we have karma that needs working through. Our relationships are also karmic devices where positive and negative karma can be worked through. We usually have strong karmic patterns with our parents, brothers and sisters and children. Again, the laws of karma will underpin the specifics of these relationships. Our karma will also direct us during our lives to be either in the right place at the right time, or in the wrong place at the wrong time. For the most part, our karma has favoured the latter alternative over the former. On a daily basis, every thought, emotion and act will incur karma. For example, if someone does an act of disservice to us, and then if we react to it by seeking revenge, we will incur more karma. If, on the other hand, we offer it up and let go of the desire to seek revenge, we will not be bound into that other person's karma.

Soul aspects generate karma while working through the Mineral, Plant, and especially through the Animal Kingdom. Although the focus is more collective in these Kingdoms, the evolving soul will gather karma through each life form. In the fist few million lives of human existence, we continue to generate substantial amounts of karma through the constant return to animalistic instincts, building up greater quantities of negative karma. Yet, the laws of karma dictate that positive and negative karma has to be balanced and this can only be done through future lives, while at the same time ensuring that no significant future karma is incurred in those future lives. The burden of burning out all karma through the constant experience of multiple polarities and opposites means that it takes the average soul aspect 8,400,000 lives to balance his or her karma. Only when the physical, emotional and mental karma is completely balanced, can a soul aspect become free and become God-realised.

So, in reflecting on our own individual karma, it is worth recognising the millions of lives where karma will have shaped our stream of different incarnations and how the expression of our soul aspect in animal, plant and mineral life forms will have had a direct bearing on our human lives. In each life we have an opportunity to work through some of the old karma and to make adjustments to the overall balance of positive and negative karma.

Karma also operates on a national, continental and planetary level. The Earth has a karmic pattern, as does the solar system and the galaxy. All of these different levels of karma from the individual, through to the group, and to the galactic have to be worked through and will always supersede Natural Law. Once karma has been played out, on whatever level, then opportunistic karma comes into force. For example, if a person completes his karmic contract at work, but then stays in the same job, he or she will then incur opportunistic karma. This can mean being in the wrong place at the wrong time, or in the right place at the wrong time, or in the wrong place at the right time. Opportunistic karma will dictate, in a positive or negative way, the outcome. So, in determining what is ongoing karma and what is opportunistic karma is something worth considering within the context of our intuitive awareness and understanding.

Karma is a reflection of limitation and, in the transition from the old timelines of the Fifth Root Race into the new timelines of the Sixth Root Race, every living being will undergo a significant and profound re-orchestration of their own karma. This will affect everything from the smallest, single-celled organism all the way up to the planet itself. It will also affect devic and angelic life. And sandwiched between these poles of soul expression, humanity will be required to take on the burden of karmic processing as part of the significant cleansing of the planetary energies that are so necessary for this shift to take place. The swathe of karma that was created in the earlier root races, particularly the Lemurian and the Atlantean, is now being processed in the time honoured way. Those soul aspects that are currently on the planet and who were also present in those root races will certainly be required to work through this karma on an individual and possibly collective level.

In summary, the old timeline of the Fifth Root Race represents limitation, suffering and an imbalance of light and dark. The dark focus has permeated the energetics of our every day lives in subtle and confusing ways. To move beyond this pattern requires strength of will, trust, balance and complete change on all levels of our existence. Humanity, quite literally, has to be reborn while living and dying.

CHAPTER 3

Finding the New Timeline

Opening Up

The challenge that we are all presented with is to find the new timeline of the Sixth Root Race. The essence of this new timeline has been seeded through an open door[1] that has been birthed in the Seventh Plane under the auspices of one of the five, living Perfect Masters[2] in residence on the planet. The birthing of this new timeline through the new doorway is part of the manifestation of the Higher Will of Meher Baba. In beginning to understand how to access this new timeline, it is worth considering that Meher Baba has put in place, on Earth and beyond, all the necessary steps and energetic sequences for the next three thousand years. As the Avatar He Knows and Lives Everything, and therefore knows precisely what each one of us will do in this life and all of our life times. It is not a question of if we change, but rather when we change. Everyone is on an inner timer that will be touched by the energy of this new timeline as it manifests through the different planes. The trick is to recognise its whisper in the stillness of our hearts and then to catch it and hold onto it.

There are various ways in which this new timeline may become activated within our consciousness. For example, meeting a person who wakes us up in a dramatic and new way, through meeting a soul mate, through our dreams, through crisis in our lives or through a direct calling from the Father or one of the five Perfect Masters. We may feel drawn to visit a specific place or we may be drawn to reading a book or seeing a film that touches us in a new way. Some of the new films contain selected keynotes of the new timeline, just as the new music of the 1960's opened up a new level of awareness at that time. Sometimes it may not be obvious what this new energy will be, because it will be outside the normal scope of our experience. Yet we will feel drawn to it. Presented behind these new notes will be our inner guidance and if we feel moved by a particular feeling or connection with the new energy, then our response will be to feel excited and happy. This may last for seconds, minutes or hours, and even days, but once the energy of the new timeline has touched us, it will begin to pervade our daily life. Small, reaffirming signals and symbols may pop up in our awareness and it is always helpful to be on the look out for things that are offered freely to us. For example, in discovering about what is more and less, a person may then see a sign or an advert talking about more. There are many different symbols that flow through our daily lives and all we need do is be open and alert to them. These little affirmations can help signpost the path that we are on.

The simplest way to open up to the new timeline is to call it in and invoke it into our lives at all times. A simple invocation offered up to Meher Baba or the Universe or whatever at the time feels the most appropriate way of expressing the wish, will then set in motion, a train of events where the new timeline will become apparent. Since energy follows thought, all that is needed is a sense of happiness and joy in bringing in the new timeline and in invoking it with intent. The invocation has to be meant and given impetus through our emotions and feelings. If we really mean it, then it will present itself to us.

The new timeline is an energetic highway that stretches down from the Seventh Plane, through the Sixth Plane, all the way down to the Zero Plane. As it touches each plane, the focus is slightly more diluted and is presented according to what each soul can absorb on any particular plane level. A soul on the Sixth Plane will absorb a more direct infusion of the new timeline light, while a soul stationed on the First Plane will be presented with a less concentrated influx of light, according to each soul's needs. Once the new timeline has been felt in our inner awareness, it is a matter of taking the first steps to engaging with it, and then stepping onto it. The timeline is magnetic and so once we connect with it, we can never really lose it again.

This new timeline is building constantly and on one level it has been completely birthed; it is only a matter of waiting for it to be made manifest within our awareness. The energy of the new timeline contains a series of seeds or frequencies, analogous to computer software, which will be downloaded into our energetic systems. These new frequencies embody the new love and light of the Sixth Root Race, and as each frequency is absorbed, it will unveil, within our awareness, a never-ending stream of sub-frequencies. Each sub-frequency will be like the canvas of a new experience where the expression of the new timeline is invoked, absorbed and then lived through experience. The new frequencies contain all the information and energy necessary for the restructuring of our chakra systems, the new pattern of Mental and Paramatman Light[3], new levels of access to our inner divinity, heightened awareness, and the different levels of higher guidance that will assist us as we walk along this new timeline.

The energy held within this new timeline is extremely powerful and virulent: it will burn our energetic systems on many different levels. It is not uncommon to go through a thorough clearing and cleansing process as this new energy comes in. Short bouts of illness, extreme tiredness, irritability and confusion are all part of the symptoms, coupled with occasional moments of lucidity and extreme joy. The new energy will ride our awareness and in absorbing it into our systems, we will be confronted by all of our habits, prejudices, addictions and life patterns. We will be forced to re-evaluate our lives and we will ride through the twin pillars of despair and bliss. Bliss at the prospect of something new and uplifting; despair at the old patterns that will need to drop away.

Collective Unity

A principle energetic demand of the new timeline is the need to focus collectively. The old timeline is almost exclusively object-oriented and me-focused. The new timeline is the antithesis of this: it is collective and focuses on cultivating a deeper connection with our fellow human beings and with all, other life forms on this planet. It is group-oriented, in that everything we need and will become can be part of the developing ring of light and love hosted through collective intent. To think and feel collectively requires a breaking of the mould: it necessitates a deep shift in our orientation and values. At its highest manifestation, the group is the collective focus of the Avatar as made manifest through the five Perfect Masters, the Fifty One God-realised spiritual generators[4] and the Spiritual Hierarchy[5]. The group also embraces all light workers on the planet who are now waking up to the new energies and who are walking on the new timeline. Ultimately, the collective will embrace all of humanity; all other life forms on the planet, and all life in the Wheel of Life.

The group can be visualised as a golden ring that touches our heart and with continued focus, will become an integral part of our lives. To focus on the group is to recognise that we cannot do everything ourselves; it is to surrender the me-focus in all things and to replace it with a collective awareness that everything we do is through higher purpose and the collective love of the group. By invoking group focus, we will begin to access everything that we need to be and become part of the new timeline.

This collective awareness lies at the heart of the Sixth Root Race. It represents a new platform of unity and understanding where all of the old karmic charges and negative patterns are systematically stripped out of our systems and replaced by a deeper understanding and awareness of who we are. The collective focus does not mean that we are the same: it is not dictating that everyone conforms to a set of strictures or rules that ensure conformity. Rather, it celebrates the diversity and difference in each one of us; it rejects the old thought forms of fear, competition, dominance, judgement and negativity. It embraces a diversity that is built on the bedrock of unity – unity that is focused through the soul's journey into matter and the different life forms and lives that we have been through. It is a unity born of collective and unconditional love.

The collective unity also houses everything that we need to

know to become part of the Sixth Root Race. It can provide a solution to any problems that we have in our lives and it can provide in either a passive or dynamic way, new levels of energy that are required to rebuild the energetic substance of our physical and subtle bodies. Any problem or issue can be offered up to the group for resolution; all it needs is an open heart, a clear intent and no attachment to the outcome to ensure that a solution is found. The collective focus is all about overcoming limitation – limitation of the individual and the past.

By embracing this collective awareness, we can weather the storm of new energies coming into the planet. If we remain individualistic, then it will be much harder, almost impossible, to remain balanced; the new energies will be much too potent for our emotions and physical systems to carry. The collective focus provides the energetic support and any weaknesses that we have will be absorbed and handled by the group. One analogy is to see the collective as a group of penguins huddled together in the arctic winter. The inside of the group is warm and secure, while every member of the collective takes it in turns to stand on the outside and protect the inside. Each penguin supports all of the other penguins in the group. Everyone in the group also receives the protection and nurturing of the group. The outside represents the old root race frequencies and the old dark energy that is now coming to the surface, so we each take turns to absorb and transmute them, before turning back in to receive the higher frequencies of the new love.

As we focus more and more on the collective, it will play an increasing role in our everyday life and living. Everything that we do and become is offered to the group. In essence we become the group and this marks the first step in embracing the new timeline and in becoming more tuned into other light workers on the planet. To be a light worker is simply to work with light.

The collective focus also helps us to support the new reality that will flow into our awareness. Nothing is as ever as it seems. Everything in the physical, etheric, astral and mental realms is the manifestation of different levels of light: each level is a reflection of the energy housed within the higher levels, and so the astral realms is like a shadow of the mental, the etheric a shadow of the astral, and so on. The physical level is the grossest level and is a shadow of the other levels, although our three-dimensional experience may initially seem at odds with this.

On the physical level, we have a solid body that requires nourishment. At the sub-atomic level, atoms are no longer solid, but contain large amounts of space. Light, as in physical photons, bombards us all of the time; millions and millions of particles impact and dance in and out of our physical body. We manifest a constant stream of subtle energy, linked to the sub-atomic realms, that has a dynamic interplay with our physical form. We interact with energy wherever we are; this energy may be in physical form, or it may be more subtle such as in electromagnetic energy. The new light will begin to strip away our old preconceptions about what is solid and real, and what is not. For example, we may start to feel different presences around us, some more benign and friendly, others not. We may begin to see faces in trees, or in hedgerows, and we may start to see different life forms around us. Some people may appear dark and heavy, others lighter and clearer. We may see a physical object dissolve before our eyes and become a structure held together by gossamer threads of light. Each one of us will receive the necessary experiences to help us understand and feel the new threads of the new timeline. For some people, the focus will be trust and faith; while for others, the presentation of different experiences will give a new impetus to their inner growth. All of this is about opening up to different levels of reality and different energy streams. All of these changes have to be negotiated. Similarly, the old emotional patterns have to be reclaimed and transmuted into a new emotional pattern of understanding, infused with the higher light of collective understanding and love. The new experiences will be contrasted with our old patterns, effectively throwing them up into sharper relief within our awareness.

The new timeline asks that we embrace the new frequencies of love and light. These new frequencies are entirely novel, and bear no resemblance to the old timeline energies. However, there will be times when things appear confusing. The old habits and patterns, as they are pushed to the surface for clearing and cleansing, may make it feel as if nothing has changed, as if the new is old and that there is no real new timeline. This is all an illusion and is purely a reflection of the clearing process: the new frequencies will drive the changes and at times will be hidden from view. In clearing the old, we have to re-live it, from time to time, in our experience. It is at such times that trust and faith will need to operate. Trust that everything will unfold in the perfect way and faith that we are connected into the larger expression of collective awareness and love.

Building up an Awareness of our Subtle Bodies

The physical body is our grossest vehicle of consciousness. Maintenance of the physical body is through physical nourishment and pranic energy that builds up our vitality and strength. Prana is linked to the breath, and is the subtle, life-giving energy that is present within. Prana is the life force that nourishes our body, and if we have low levels of pranic energy, then our vitality and life force will be low. Correspondingly, if we build up high levels of prana, then our life force will be high. The new energies will require that we have high levels of prana, because high frequency energy work can quickly deplete prana. Specific practices such as yoga and deeper breathing techniques can help to increase our levels of prana. Sometimes our pranic levels can be measured by visualising a bubble in the region of the stomach and intestines; if the bubble feels small (only inches across), then we have low pranic levels; if it is large (up to a foot across), then our levels are high. Cultivating high levels of prana is always beneficial.

Physical nourishment through food requires attention to detail and an assessment of the different levels of energy present within our diet. The mineral content in most food is low, and all processed food contains low frequency light resulting from the manufacturing processes used. Finding fresh and untainted food that has a positive flow of higher energy will become increasingly important as the new timeline gathers momentum. Insufficient nourishment and the wrong diet will put our physical bodies at a disadvantage and it is through opening up to our needs, by assessing intuitively the balance of our diet, that we will be able to provide a sound platform for the myriad physical changes that will flow through us. The type of energy work that we engage in will determine our dietary needs, and our weight may fluctuate as a result of the different streams of energy that will entertain us. Sometimes extra weight will act as a buffer to the diverse frequencies, affording us a higher level of protection. At other times, our weight will drop away, thereby mirroring a different energetic pattern. In short, we should be sensitive to the needs of our bodies, and be open intuitively to what is necessary at any particular time.

Apart from the physical body that we inhabit, there are a number of other bodies that interconnect and work with different streams of energy. The most familiar includes the etheric body, the aura, the astral body and the mental body. Each of these subtle bodies works with specific forms of energy and light. The etheric body is a bridge between the physical and astral realms and forms a web-like structure that reflects the overall health of our physical body. Against a plain white background, it can sometimes be seen as a whitish glow that extends off the body up to about an inch or so. Areas where the etheric is thinner, or interrupted, reflect underlying health patterns.

The second body that surrounds us is the aura and is composed of a finer flow of energy that generally absorbs different astral frequencies. The aura retains astral light and is a reflection of our emotional well-being. It extends approximately twenty-seven feet on either side and is generally egg-shaped, although in light workers it is more streamlined, flatter and folds up slightly at the feet. The aura can be seen by techniques like Kirlian photography and to those who have clairvoyant vision, will host different colours and types of astral energy. Each different colour seen in the aura reflects an underlying energetic pattern. The aura is composed of a gossamer web of interconnecting fibres. In people who have ruptured auras or host energetic parasites like entities and negative thought forms, the aura can look unhealthy and quite dark. Dark patches and streaks of dark energy will pepper the surface, sometimes pushing deeper into the substance of the aura. Exercises to cleanse and strengthen the aura are particularly important in the early stages of working with the new energies, since all existing patterns of negative and slow frequency energy need to be stripped out. Many peoples' auras may also become contracted in cities and in environments where the energy is slow.

The astral body is found in soul aspects that work the lower planes, primarily the First through to the Third Planes. The astral body is larger than the physical body and is composed of different streams of astral light. The astral body has to reside in the physical vehicle in order that we fully engage in physical matter; quite often, though, the astral body will only come into our physical vehicles to the chest or waist level, or may be completely outside the physical body, positioned several feet above the head, or behind it. These are all cases where there is insufficient grounding and a reluctance by the individual to engage in physical matter. In our everyday existence, the astral body works through all of the different emotional energies, and so sometimes, the astral body is known as the emotional body and will communicate directly with the different astral levels. If our focus is on the lower astral levels then this low frequency experience will be mediated through the astral body and reflected in our physical and emotional awareness.

The astral body is also the vehicle of awareness that we utilise when we sleep and typically some of our lucid dreams will involve the astral body travelling through different levels of astral light, visiting different places and meeting specific people. Typically, though, when a person falls asleep, their astral body will hover above their physical vehicle.

Souls that have progressed beyond the Third Plane incorporate a different kind of energetic vehicle, known as the mental body. The mental body is composed of high frequency, mental light and is the vehicle of consciousness utilised in the higher planes, predominantly from the Fifth to the Sixth, and to a lesser extent in the Fourth Plane. The mental body can be extremely large and provides the focus for energetic management in the higher planes through the direct absorption of mental light. Mental light houses the higher light streams and will be one of the primary energetic platforms in the new timeline.

Each of these different bodies absorbs and transmits different streams of energy. It can take millions of life times to build up sufficient experience of working with these different bodies. We may, on one level, be engaged with our physical body, while on another level, we will be gathering experience in the astral or mental levels. In the past, much of this experience has been veiled from our normal levels of consciousness. However, the new timeline and higher energies require a new level of conscious awareness of these different energies and subtle bodies.

Astral and Mental Gradations of Light

Astral light can be categorised according to its frequency or vibration. It can be split into nine levels, with the lower three levels comprising the lower astral levels, the middle three levels forming the middle astral layers, and then the top three hosting the upper astral levels. The astral levels are over fifty times bigger than the Earth plane and this means that even the lower astral levels are quite large. Each level holds a different colour focus and frequency, ranging from the very slow (in the lower levels) to the fast (in the higher levels).

The lower astral levels hold the slowest and lowest levels of astral light where astral entities and virulent negative patterns of dark light are common. Energetically speaking, it is like being in the lower levels of the sewer where the quality of light is extremely thick, condensed and dark. Sometimes red and orange colours can be found in the lower astral levels, against the background of dark. There are almost always no blue colours. The old Fifth Root Race timeline has focused predominantly on the lower astral and young souls on the Zero Plane will operate on this level. Individuals that resonate on a higher plane level, yet gravitate towards the lower astral levels for periods of time, can become ill and depressed due to the slow frequency of light. The lower astral focus is on absorbing and tyrannising. Many of the more unpleasant emotions, physical actions and addictions, such as pornography, child abuse, drug addiction and feudal patterns originate in the lower astral.

The middle astral levels are brighter, faster flowing and this is the zone where the majority of people focus their attention. Those specifically working on the First Plane will have this level as their focal point. Much of humanity is focused in this level and the energetic space is adequate for the interchange of energy, as compared to the lower astral level where the space is too restrictive and it is much harder to invoke a response. Many thought forms also populate these levels. The light streams can still be negatively infused and up to seventy percent of the middle astral levels are slow frequency, with approximately thirty percent hosting an infusion of mental light. As the new timeline develops these percentages will change. The middle astral level is also where we can first find our guides.

In the higher levels the astral light is much brighter and can appear very brilliant at times. In these levels the energetic space is much larger and vibrates more rapidly; the light has a higher series of frequencies and the colours reflect these higher layers. Consequently the light at the top of the higher astral is brilliant white, while at the bottom of the lower astral it is black, and then there are multiple gradations of light that flow through each of the different levels, and sub-levels. The interchange of energy within the higher astral is much greater. The higher astral levels house more light, more knowledge, more wisdom and a different kind of recognition, based on external and internal matters, where the flow of light and dark can be entertained in a more meaningful way. It is often in the higher astral levels that light and dark will come and provide the soul with a choice either during life or at the point of death, and this often arises when a soul is in the Third Plane.

Most healers work with astral light and depending upon their experience and ability to work with different streams of astral energy, will radiate a pattern of astral light that will originate in primarily in either the middle or higher. Astral energy usually feels warm during a healing session and many of the popular techniques will almost exclusively use astral light.

Recognising the lower, middle and higher astral levels should be the initial goal of working with the new energies, followed by a programme of building up through the different levels of mental light. Mental light vibrates at a much higher frequency than astral light; in comparison to the astral levels, the mental space is absolutely huge, so that the lower mental levels are one thousand times bigger than the astral levels. Mental light can also be sub-divided into nine levels with each set of three levels comprising the lower, middle and higher mental realms. Mental light is brilliant and each of the three primary layers holds a specific series of colour frequencies.

The lower mental levels are a holding mechanism that allows applied energy through the principle of thought to be directed into the astral levels, yet it also receives data from the higher levels. The lower mental levels gives us access to the collective and to our own Akashic Records – the sum total of all lives that we have had, so that we can go backwards and forwards in our own timeframe. We become aware of ourselves in a new way. The lower mental also opens us up to a brand new tier of guides and as we receive the influx of lower mental light, then it always demands change and elicits an emotional response, often initially through anger. Lower mental light speeds up karma and, in entering the planet at this time, it is invoking patterns of major planetary change through flooding, earthquakes; and spiritual change through personal and economic crises. Souls that are working from the lower part of the Sixth Plane, such as 6.1, 6.2 and 6.3, will often work with lower mental information.

The middle mental layers support a platform of hardcore information and stability where the focus is more collective and orientated towards the planet. The middle mental is much larger than the lower mental – over one thousand times bigger. In the middle mental levels harmony and a balanced outlook are required, infused with trust and the recognition that everything is illusory. The collective intent also opens us up to collective karma, which can be group, planetary, solar system or galactic.

Higher mental light represents a step up to a whole new spiritual focus, and has a cosmic disposition. The space is one million times bigger than the middle mental. The higher mental is very elusive and embodies a different level of silence, strength, focus and manifestation of higher purpose. The essence of higher mental is beyond time, and opens up a new type of destiny where everything can change. The essence of higher guidance is the embodiment of will and is always untouched by emotions; clarity and focus are always presented at this level. The crystal skulls are first manifested in these levels, just as higher concepts and ideas are birthed here. The new timeline for the Sixth Root Race is working predominantly from the higher mental level.

With the right authority, accessing the different mental levels can be achieved with the selection of appropriate symbols. For example, working with a blue rose will give access to the lower mental levels; a golden rose will connect to the middle mental levels and a purple rose will link into the higher mental levels. These frequencies also mirror a triangle of higher purpose, formed through the heart of humanity (which can be visualised as blue), the Spiritual Hierarchy (gold) and Shamballa[6] (purple). All souls have to work through humanity first, before accessing the energy of the Spiritual Hierarchy, and then the higher frequencies of Shamballa, which holds the full complement of one hundred and forty four archetypal frequencies.

Mental light is used in some healing practices and is usually experienced as a cool or cold energy entering the system. It is often seen as blue with a crystalline focus. This is in sharp contrast to astral light, which generates heat and is more red or orange.

The New Chakra System

In the old timeline we operate with seven main chakras – the base, sexual, solar plexus, heart, throat, third eye and crown. Each chakra forms a doorway between the physical vehicle and the inner planes, especially the astral levels, although with sufficient experience, soul aspects will work with the mental levels. Within the old timeline each chakra will reflect slow and negative energetic patterns. For the most part, humanity is almost entirely focused on the lower centres, reflecting the lower and middle astral patterns of light.

Each chakra holds a series of light streams within it: in soul aspects that have less experience in matter, the centres will appear very dark. Similarly, if an individual is working with old dark light then the centres will appear quite black. However, in older souls, the centres will become lighter as the older frequencies become cleared and more refined. Middle aged and older souls will typically have been through lives where some of the higher centres have been utilised, particularly the heart or third eye. However, it is not uncommon for some or all of the centres to retain blockages of old energies that need a deep level of clearing. Physical ailments can also be a reflection of chakra blockages. While the old timeline has focused on the lower chakra centres, the new timeline will require in the first instance, a clearing of these lower centres, and then a programme of opening and balancing all of the higher and lower centres. The new infusion of mental light will come through the crown, stimulating a new pattern of energetic balance in its wake.

As the new timeline becomes activated within a person's space, the higher centres will begin to open - heart and third eye typically become more open, and as this happens, the lower centres will need to be actively cleared. The ultimate aim is to build an energetic platform where higher frequency light can enter the body through the crown and then flow through each of the centres down to the base. Each centre should be able to open fully – and this should eventually be measured in feet rather than inches. The more open the centres, the more light that can be absorbed. If all the centres are open, for example, up to one foot in diameter, then the degree of higher light that can be absorbed will be significant and will form an energetic highway within the physical space of that individual. For the majority of people this will be extremely difficult at first, because their nervous systems will retain too much dark light that needs to be released. It is also important to understand that the crown chakra will usually be the last centre to open and a more profound opening of the crown centre only accompanies a full and complete balancing of personal karma. Consequently, if this centre does not open up very much, then this should be accepted and not forced in any way.

As the chakra centres absorb the new light, they will become more flexible and will begin to host and radiate an entirely different pattern of energy. New love frequencies will enter the heart centre and as the third eye begins to open, new levels of awareness will expand the consciousness. With practice, it will become possible to feel the flow of energy through each different chakra, and to determine the particular streams of light that are housed there. Each chakra will present a different window on an energetic reality. At present, the new energy is clearing out the sexual and solar plexus chakras of many people, in preparation for a shift of awareness into the heart centre. This again is a reflection of the astral clearing now taking place.

The new timeline will also introduce five new chakras into our physical vehicles. This will mean that we will house twelve chakras. The first of these new chakras is a second heart centre, situated above the first. The other chakras are located in the head – the first is in the centre of the chin between the bottom of the lower jaw and lower lip; the second is just above the upper lip, below the nose. This second centre is sometimes known as the ajna centre. The other two chakra points are located in the forehead and are adjacent to the third eye.

These new chakras will transform the energetic platform of the old chakra system; the new timeline will open up a new interpretation of what reality looks and feels like; we will live in a different energetic world where our higher centres will be connected to different light streams. The unfolding role of these new chakras will build throughout the evolution of the Sixth Root Race, and allow an entirely different kind of access to the new streams of mental light. The basic template for the new chakra system has been introduced into a few prototypes and will then be seeded more extensively once the older timeline has been eradicated and cleared from the existing chakra centres.

The planet, like our human bodies, has a chakra system. The various Ley Lines that criss-cross the planetary surface are reminiscent of the meridians in our physical bodies. These Ley Lines can be positively or negatively charged and regulate the flow of different transformation: the old system of seven chakras covered the following areas: base centre –Iraq; sexual centre – Japan; solar plexus – India; heart – South Africa; throat – Great Britain; third eye – USA; crown – Iceland. Earth will also receive five new chakras to take the total up to twelve. These chakras will be birthed in different areas of the planet.

Energy Management

Apart from building up a strong, inner connection with the group, it is necessary for us all to practice and live sound techniques for the energetic management of our different levels of experience and expression[7]. This encompasses the physical, the etheric, the astral and the mental. Throughout every moment of the day we live through different streams of energy, some of which are external to us, and some of which are part of the internal absorption and processing of our individual and collective karma. Our energetic base will reflect the type of energies that flow through us, and how we handle the constant bombardment of slower frequencies. One of the more immediate impacts of connecting to the new timelines is an enhanced sensitivity to the energies around us. A walk into the supermarket will be experienced in a new way through the expression of slow frequency energy. Where we live, including the ambient ground energies will spark a different type of internal dialogue. The people we interact with will induce different patterns of karmic flow, depending on the karma that we have with each of those people. Everything around us will vibrate at an assortment of frequencies; the food we eat, the objects in our house, our car and our place of work, all reflect different patterns of energy.

For the most part, we will be exposed to slow frequency, negative energy based on the prevailing thought forms and the energetic history that has gone before. For example, if we live in an old house, then the materials will store the emotional memories of what previous owners have discharged into their surroundings. The underlying ground energies will also invoke a dialogue with our energetic systems. In many countries, layers of different civilisations sit on top of one another, and in some places, old dark thought forms and virulent negative energies could affect our energies in a profound way. Ideally, these old, negative energies need to be cleared.

If we live near sources of water or electromagnetic energy, then these will also impact our energetic environment. Living in cities as opposed to the countryside will also affect the way that our body and aura are managed. Since the physical body is designed to receive, transmit and record, then every different type of energy that we come into contact with has the potential to be stored in our systems. In effect, we become like grand dustbins which, if not emptied and cleared, will eventually lead us to feeling more and more unhappy and depressed. As we accumulate more negative energy, we will gravitate to the lower astral levels.

The people in our lives will be a direct reflection of our karma; just as where we live and what we do is part of our karma. If we have a substantial amount of negative karma, then this will be mirrored in the quality of our relationships, and the emotional problems that we need to resolve. In all relationships we build up energetic cordings: lines of energy that pass between the different chakra centres between two people. These lines of energy are energetic records of our past and current life patterns. For example, a couple may have strong cordings between their sexual centres, and little between their heart centres. Such a relationship may focus more on the physical side. With time, the heart connection will build. Often, however, cordings can be traced from different chakra centres, reflecting an imbalance in the energetic flow. The cordings can also be colour coded, reflecting the quality and type of energy that is imprinted between the centres. Darker cordings will contain slower frequency energy.

Similar types of cordings can be seen in shops and supermarkets and other physical structures, such as churches, houses and other buildings. The colour and size of the cording will indicate the type of energetic movement between different structures, and the people that live in them. All of these structures will also vibrate at different levels, usually in the middle and lower astral levels.

Within the new timeline it is necessary to clear out all of this energy on an ongoing basis. We should all adopt the practice of clearing out our chakras, physical space and auras on a daily basis, as well as adopting different techniques for protecting ourselves from the constant barrage of negative energies. The use of shamanistic robes is a useful tool in this respect. It is also important to cleanse our living and sleeping areas on a regular basis and to psychometrise the ground energies. It is helpful to look at ground energies in terms of numbers, such as one to nine. The nine reflects directly the Nine-Pointed Plan. With a little bit of practice, it is possible to intuitively assign a number to the ground energies such as one or two for lower energies, all the way through to eight or nine for the highest vibrations. In places that retain a virulent disposition of energy, it is possible to adopt negative numbers, again up to minus nine. It is also useful to project your awareness into the ground and to push many metres below the ground to build up a feeling of what the different layers of energy feel like. Often ground energies and building energies will become active at different times of the day or during the night. Building an understanding of this pattern can assist in clearing the old frequencies.

It can also be extremely helpful to use symbols to protect and infuse a new level of light and power into our own bodies, or into the ground or into buildings. The principle symbol that we work with is shown below:

This symbol embodies the hologram of Sixth Root Race energies and can be used in a variety of different ways. The symbol can also be presented in different colours and one of the key frequencies used at present is deep blue. The black shown here is a representation of the new devic light. Placing this symbol in our chakra centres will give balance and power, while putting it across windows and doors will help to build a thought form that will protect a house from unwanted energies. The same can also be done with cars, where the negative thought forms and road energies can easily affect the energetic balance and susceptibility to accidents.

Within the symbol, there are a series of different keys and frequencies. The circle represents, on one level, the ring of higher purpose and a new level of higher guidance entering the planet. The triangle is the new platform of energy that is being manifested in all life forms. Inside the triangle, the lamp embodies the essence of a single plane, with ten sub-planes, while the flame in the lamp invokes a new pattern of love and light where the flame burns out the old and brings in the new. This symbol is linked directly to the highest planes and is not tainted or touched by old energies or thought forms. It is clear, dynamic and operates according to the highest principles of love and light, infused by power.

The other energetic challenge that many of us face as we build up our connection with the new timeline is the ability to remain grounded within our physical awareness. The new energies will tend to push us up within our awareness, and as we enter some of the higher planes, then it is easy to become disconnected from our physical vehicle. The beauty and the bliss of the higher light can constantly call to us so that we ignore the physical side of things. It is essential all the time to remain grounded and to earth the new energies that come into us.

The new timeline will expose us to entirely new frequencies of mental light and as we absorb it, we will have to endure what is pushed to the surface for clearing, while remaining in a state of balance and understanding. This will stretch many of us to our physical and emotional limits.

CHAPTER 4

Crossing the Abyss

The Inner Abyss

Spiritual development and progress will always push up against limitation; our own personal limitation which is a consequence of our karmic flow. In the past, spiritual seekers would find places of seclusion and work either alone or with groups of like-minded people. Such was the way of the monastic life. Today, we are expected to find our spiritual truth while engaging fully with the everyday world. Within such an environment it is always a challenge to be pushed up against our limits. These limits can be physical, emotional or mental and are specific for every person. All who embrace the new timeline will, at some time or another, be pushed to their very limits. How we respond to these situations will determine how we progress spiritually.

Multiple abysses can be found in the inner planes of consciousness. These abysses are located between each plane – between the Zero and the First Plane, the First and the Second Plane and so on. There are also smaller abysses between each sub-plane. All evolving soul aspects that progress through the planes have to cross over these abysses. They represent the space between each plane and the point of transformation and change. They are the spaces where the light from the previous plane is absent and where the light from the next plane is also absent. They are, if you like, a non-space. While we may not have a full appreciation of what it is to cross these abysses, there will be lifetimes where we will be challenged specifically to be confronted by an abyss between two planes and then invoke a means to cross this particular abyss. Each abyss will test us to our very limits since each abyss represents the sum total of all of our fears and limitations. This may only happen in every million or so lives, and so many lifetimes will be spent in training to be confronted by our own points of limitation to ensure that we grow and develop. In a working life, we will often have many challenges that in their own way represent different types of abysses. By working through these different challenges we can then build up sufficient experience to confront and push through the real abysses on the inner planes.

The spiritual path always involves testing, through the simplest thoughts and actions, to the larger decisions in life that can shape and frame our futures. The reason for such testing is simple: it is to build up our strength and to ensure that that there are no glitches or bugs as the new energies flow into us. The world we live in is full of limitation and to move beyond limitation in our own lives means that we have to recognise it for what it is, and then move through it. Within this framework of limitation, we will encounter from time to time, experiences that seem to test us to the very limit, and such situations are like crossing our own personal abyss. The abyss is a focal point for limitation and is the point when everything within our comfort zone has been stripped away, and when we stand alone in front of a large gulf. It draws in all of the limitations that we have ever faced before in previous lives. It is like standing at the edge of a giant ravine, with steep sides that plummet into the depths below and the opposite side is close but separated by a huge chasm. The underlying emotion is usually fear, although it is often coloured by more specific emotions such as loss, separation, anger, jealousy or pride. We may be presented with situations in our lives that seem to repeat themselves – in our relationships, in the events that seem to conspire against us. All of these issues and problems are giving us with new opportunities for growth.

The classical response that we usually have to a problem is "why me?" We look at family and friends and compare ourselves; we look externally at everything around us and make comparisons.

Yet such comparison is an illusion. The problem on offer is a way to invoke change within us and a way to become more, not less. So rather than rejecting the problem, or burying it through self-denial, or feeling sorry for ourselves, a more practical way to approach the situation is to embrace the problem. What is this series of events or set of emotions telling me about myself? What can I learn from this situation? Energetically speaking, the choice is between opening up and embracing the problem – like wrapping around it in our awareness – or pushing it away and rejecting it. In the latter instance, the energy does not disappear; it is just buried or repressed and will inevitably resurface in the future as part of our personal karma. If we open up to the problem, then we can begin to connect with the underlying energy and focus of the limitation.

Each issue may be multi-layered and can often lead us to strange and unexpected places within our emotional landscape. Yet the laws of karma will have presented us with this opportunity to grow. The resolution of each problem, through identification, acceptance and a desire to change will bring about change. We may not know the answer to a problem at first, but as we open up to it, we may find that solutions present themselves. These solutions are not necessarily of the mind, and are best worked through the invocation of a deeper, feeling connection within our heart. To focus on the heart will give a different type of inner balance and make us more open to the different patterns of energy that can flow through our awareness.

Each problem that we face is like our own personal abyss. There always comes a point of crisis. How we react to this crisis, whether small or large, will determine how we work through our karma. While karma is limitation and denial, reinforced through our own biases and prejudices, if we invoke the laws of faith and trust, then it is possible to supersede the laws of karma. In effect, it is to petition, through a higher pattern, the opportunity to invoke trust and faith; to invoke with love that everything will be absolutely fine. We may not know how it will come about, yet we place our energetic focus within the appropriate resolution through the laws of faith and trust. There is always a point of reckoning in meeting our own abyss. It is not dissimilar to a parachute jump: there is that one moment when we have to jump, when we have to trust that our parachute will open and where we have to move through the fear of jumping into nothing, into actually doing it. The point of reckoning within our own abyss will be the point at which we decide whether or not to trust. If we trust then the energetic pattern will be freed to move in a different way from before; if we remain locked in our old patterns, then the energy will remain contained and limited.

To cross the abyss, then, requires that we invoke the laws of faith and trust and put one foot in front of the other and walk out into the space, recognising that normally we would fall. Yet this is an illusion, and as in the Film *Indiana Jones and the Last Crusade* where the hero is searching for the Holy Grail, at one point he has to step out into the abyss. At first he cannot find a way across the gulf, but then realises that it is a trick of the light. He sees that the abyss is an illusion and finds a path that will take him to the other side: the abyss seems huge until he finds the hidden path.

The analogy is the same when crossing our own spiritual abyss: we have to trust in the principles of higher purpose, confront our worst fears and limitations and walk across the abyss. By invoking the laws of faith and trust, we will then cross the abyss and push through the limitations of our beliefs and experiences. To cross our own personal abyss is to confront our fears and push through them. The laws of faith and trust will ultimately ensure that we do not drop into the abyss; they provide the energetic support to cross over to the other side.

When it comes to crossing the abysses on the inner planes, the principles are the same. Trust and faith have to be invoked irrespective of what we think the outcome should be. If we seek to direct the energy while still invoking the laws of trust, then we limit the energy. So, if we invoke for change, and trust that it will happen, yet add in the proviso that it should involve being comfortable and wealthy, or whatever stipulation we may wish to add in, then the effect will be diluted. We are not fully embracing the outcome.

Offering Everything Up

Whenever we are confronted by circumstances and events that we find difficult, it is always best to offer them up. To do so, means that we can supersede the karmic charge that will be present. For example, if someone breaks into our car and steals the radio, it is our natural instinct to want to retaliate: to find the person who did it and then direct a negative charge at them. If we follow this instinct, then we will tie ourselves karmically to that individual. If we sidestep that initial impulse and instead, attach no importance to the event and offer it up to a higher authority such as the Avatar, or to the greatest good, then we do not become tied into that person. By simply invoking "May the Father's Will be done" means that we energetically push up rather than down. Instead, the other person will have to repay the karmic debt at some point in the future, usually in a future lifetime.

Exactly the same principles apply when we feel emotionally attacked or overwhelmed by our emotions to another person. For example we may feel angry and wish to retaliate; we may feel sad and resort to self-pity. Again, the trick is to offer these emotions up to a higher authority within. This requires that we do not attach so much importance to the things around us. If a colleague at work becomes angry with us, rather than retaliating and getting into an argument, we just give it no importance, then the energy will not get into our system. As soon as we give a response to such energies, then we become tied or corded in.

Energetically when a person is angry, they will send out cordings that will try to push into our aura and place an energetic charge there. We can often feel this as a constriction in our solar plexus. If we react, then the cording pushes into our energetic field. If we give it no importance, then the energy will not be given the access to our energetic field. Such modes of behaviour require practice and need to be cultivated. They go hand in hand with the clearing of our deeper sub-conscious emotions. If we hold an old energetic charge that is reflected in another person, then it will be much harder to remain balanced, and it will require a greater effort of will to work through. The old energetic charge within us will be activated in specific situations and will be brought to the surface.

Some of these patterns can be extremely deep since they

have been accumulated over many, many lifetimes. They will require continued attention to ensure eventual clearance. Yet, through not attaching any importance to things around us and to issues that arise, while still invoking the laws of faith and trust to resolve all issues, will mean that ultimately we will go into a deeper pattern of balance. To give no importance to something means that we do not feed it with additional energy – we recognise it, accept it, experience it and then invoke our trust and faith through the right use of the will to clear it.

If we follow these simple steps, then with time, we will build up a greater degree of balance. We will no longer feel at the mercy of our emotions; we will no longer feel that the world controls us; we will feel clearer and more able to ride the waves of emotional turmoil that are now passing through the planet.

It is also important to recognise that some of the feelings and emotions that wash through our every day lives are not ours. Humanity is generally emotionally telepathic, and so we are potentially tied into the emotions of millions of others around us. These connections will be a reflection of our inner planes experience and our karmic pattern in this lifetime. Similarly, we will be tied into the mental field of thought of many people where old concepts and ideas will flush through us. This is not dissimilar to the hundred-monkey effect where once enough people are tied into a thought form or idea, then it spreads much more rapidly and appears simultaneously in other places. It is easy to become overwhelmed with the wash of human emotions and thoughts constantly flowing through us. There will be days when we wake up feeling more emotional and distressed than other days; this is often a reflection of the tide of emotion that is flowing through us at that time. Sometimes that emotion can feel like despair, at other times it is abandonment and so on. We will feel and live these emotions in a very direct way; if we responded to all of these emotions through identification, then very quickly we would drown in them. To drown in these emotions means that we become depressed and our vibration then drops into the lower astral levels. Many of the emotions that are being pushed through at this time are lower astral and carry virulent energies of a negative kind. Consequently if we give these emotions importance in our lives, then they will dominate us; if we do not give them importance, then they will wash through like the ocean tides. They will come and go, but will not become locked within our awareness. At times when the emotional flux feels particularly strong and difficult, it is always essential to focus on the collective and bring in the group focus to provide assistance in re-balancing.

Some people are drowning in the emotional tides; they feel powerless and at the mercy of such strong sensations. Such people sometimes seek others to identify with their state of being; they want others to join them in the morass of emotional debris and to descend into their own emotional world. In waking up, the challenge will be to hold our own balance, while at the same time remaining compassionate. To provide assistance in such cases does not mean to join these people in their emotional world by dropping down to the lower astral levels; it does not mean providing additional energy to fuel their specific, emotional pattern; rather, it is recognise where they are and to provide balance. Nor does it mean that we have to accept their emotional 'dumping' or downloading. In this context, emotional dumping corresponds to pushing slow frequency energy into another person either consciously or sub-consciously. Whenever we accept or absorb other people's emotional energy, then it becomes very easy to drown in it. For example, if someone has fallen into a powerful river, it is better to throw that person a life belt, rather than jumping in and risk drowning as well. The same is true of maintaining balance in the face of emotional difficulties held by others. They will want us to identify completely with them so that they can transfer over to us as much of their slow energy as possible. This is also what some societies deem to be the appropriate behaviour; give an emotion more energy by constantly focusing on it, rather than viewing it as an opportunity to change and do something about it. Consequently, to provide balance and assistance means to invoke change for that person and to provide a different context through which they can process and clear their emotions. That person then has free will and choice as to whether to follow it or not.

The challenge for light workers is to weather the astral storms and emotional waves of slow frequency energy; to recognise that these waves are the result of new high frequency mental light entering the planet and all life on it; and to develop the capacity to "walk on water". Put simply, this means to rise up through the different astral levels and to engage with the lower mental levels where the old emotions can drop away and then to walk over the tide of emotions in the astral levels. Then, if we recognise that someone is drowning in the astral energies, we are in a position to offer love and support to them.

When we offer everything up to a higher authority such as the Avatar, a Perfect Master or to the greatest good for all concerned, we are letting go of something; we are trusting that the higher authority will sort it all out according to everyone's best interests. By freeing ourselves of the outcome and opening up to more, we are then open to receiving something different into our lives; we are free to live in the present, and are not tied into the past in such a powerful way. Given that the Avatar knows everything, everywhere, including every thought, action and emotion in the present and the future, then it goes without saying that we do not need to worry. Worry is an old pattern, aimed at undermining our emotional balance and ensuring that we push extra energy into something that we often cannot control. It is part of the confusion and misinformation of the dark. Whenever fear or worry comes in we should always offer it up. This can be a constant process and with practice, we can begin to monitor our energy levels all the time. In circumstances where we feel drained of energy by something or someone, then it is useful to go back into that place and see how our energy dropped in vibration. It may occur through a specific chakra centre, or it may have been something that was said that triggered the energetic shift. Whatever it is, it provides more information on how to improve the management of our energetic system.

Meher Baba said "don't worry, be happy." This focuses on letting go of worry, and embracing happiness. As soon as we feel happy our energetic vibration goes up; we stop worrying, we feel more relaxed and at ease, and more centred inside. However, the maxim does not imply that we should let go of any responsibility; instead

Meher Baba directed that when we have tried everything within our power to ensure that our problems are solved or that we have acted in the best interests of all concerned, then we need not worry. So when we encounter difficulties, it is important to understand that we can offer up our difficulties to Meher Baba; that we do not need to attach importance to the things around us, although we should still engage in a meaningful way that does not lead to the creation of unnecessary karma with other people; and finally, through the right use of the will, we can find an inner place where we feel more balanced inside.

As soon as we allow a greater balance to pervade our life, then we recognise what is the right and the wrong use of the will in a more direct way. The wrong use of the will leads to an automatic drop in our energy; it leads to limitation and is often the result of the mind interfering too much. In contrast, the right use of the will means that we feel happy, excited and focus in a collective way to invoke more. Whenever we feel out of sorts, or off balance, then this is an energetic state that can be monitored and adjusted through simple visualisations. The more we work with the different energetic tools, then the easier it becomes to maintain balance.

Finding our Inner Silence

Part of the focus of clearing our energetic systems and removing attachments from emotions and physical objects is to clear the way for building up our inner silence. This is something that requires practice and the right use of the will. The purpose of finding our inner silence is to open ourselves up to a different level of awareness inside, and also to reinforce the techniques that will allow us to absorb the energies of the new timeline in a more profound way.

There are a number of barriers that prevent us, at all times, from building up a connection with our inner silence. These range from the general physical sensations such as itches or tickling, through to the constant stream of internal dialogue. We are never really free of the constant, internal commentary of the mind. If we meet someone we know, the mind often makes internal remarks to us. Such remarks are not always positive and can be quite virulent. The more we buy into such thoughts, then the more we are working in the lower astral levels. If we are happy, our mind is generally quieter and slower thought vibrations drop away. In cultivating happiness, we move away from the lower and middle astral levels into the higher astral and eventually into the lower mental. By watching how we judge things around us, and by offering up every negative judgement to the Avatar, we slowly burn the stream of slower vibrations out of our system. We attach no importance to the judgements that we make as part of our internal dialogue, and slowly step-by-step, we build a quieter internal space.

Meditation practice will help to build up the silence within, and through centering and balancing ourselves, it can become possible to go for seconds without any internal dialogue, and then eventually into minutes. Of course, there is always the small challenge of when we first enter a silent spot that the mind says to itself, "I am now being silent." However, the cultivation of silence will lead to a new type of inner stillness which will not only pervade our awareness and consciousness, but will also allow us to feel different and more subtle external energies, as well as a range of different inner feelings that encompass our own intuitive sense, and the role of our inner guidance.

When we walk in the countryside in silence we can begin to feel the different energies around us; from the land, in the trees, and in the other wild life and plants. Sometimes it feels like there is a background pulse. Similarly, when we meditate or pursue an activity in inner silence, we can feel different energies or pulses coming through. Musicians and artists may liken this to the creative pulse, while healers may feel the presence of healing guides around them. Whatever the different terms used to express these feelings, what is clear is that cultivating our inner silence and awareness will start to open new, inner doorways.

Through the active pursuit of stillness and silence, we will slowly feel connections forming with our inner guides and with our higher self. The lower and higher self are terms that have been used in many different contexts: here, the lower self is really our physical vehicle coupled with our mind and personality. It includes our habits, desires, memories, physical feelings and emotions. It is very much focused on the one life that we are living. In contrast, the higher self refers to the bigger picture that our soul has in relation to our evolutionary path: the one life that we are in is just one among millions and as such, is just part of the process of gaining more experience. Our higher self knows all the decisions that we need to make in matter to ensure that we end up where we need to be. The trouble is that the higher and lower self are usually disconnected: the lower self often thinks it is the higher self and will make decisions and follow old habits and desires according to past memories. The higher self may try to provide clues and impulses to push the lower self in a particular direction; if the lower self is not looking inwards or does not listen properly, then these clues and messages are missed. For example, our higher self may have already agreed to become part of the new timeline; yet the lower vehicle is drowning in physical sensations of the material life which block out these subtler feelings of opening up to the new energies. The lower self is unconscious of the higher self.

The higher self may well have agreed all of the patterns of development in that one life of change and yet, if the lower self is not open to these new patterns, then change can only be orchestrated through crisis. For many people this connection between higher and lower self is either too weak or non-existent. The new energies require these connections to become much stronger; to the extent that our intuitions from the higher self flow through to the lower self unencumbered and with great ease. To build up these connections requires a starting point of finding our stillness within and developing the art of listening to our intuitive feeling.

Of course, it is one thing to feel our intuitions, but it is another thing to act on them. Receiving, understanding and acting upon intuitions requires trust and commitment. If we do not act, then we do not fully engage with the new energies. Ultimately, building a connection between our lower and higher self is much more radical: it involves the fusion and union of lower and higher in energetic terms, and this only truly ever takes place in people who have become God-realised. Here the lower self comes to understand that it is part of God and is connected to the higher self through a clear and seamless energetic pathway. Until that time, there will always be some distortion within the energetic flow between higher and lower by virtue of the karma that is held by that soul aspect, and because of all the past lives that have yet to be processed and balanced. To build a deep connection between higher and lower ultimately requires many life times of training and effort before a deeper appreciation of the true breadth of our inner world can be fully realised.

Inner Guidance

In the cultivation of stillness, we also begin to encounter different types of inner guidance. Guides exist on the inner planes, and most souls usually incarnate with one or more guides looking after them. Guides are like the prompters to the human actors on the stage of life; they watch over us, working to improve our chances of success in terms of fulfilling our life's contracts. Before we incarnate, we agree the scope and terms of the forthcoming life; we record the lessons that we need to learn, and note the people that we are going to meet. While all of this may be extremely clear before incarnation, once we go through the ring-pass-not, it is all forgotten. Our guides then act as an insurance policy to give us a better chance of waking up to our life's purpose, or at the very least, unconsciously positioning us for maximum advantage and fulfilment of our life's purpose.

Guides are external energy sources to us and they exist on all the planes, from the First Plane right through to the Seventh Plane. Slower levels of guidance can also be found in the Zero Plane. In a very real sense, the most important guide for all of us is the Avatar. However, we each have one central guide or controller that will look after our interests and who will oversee the flux of energy between our physical vehicles, our subtle bodies and the inner planes. Sometimes, we will have worked with our guides over many lifetimes, so that the ties of love can become very strong. Usually a guide will have a certain level of expertise for assisting us in our life and as we gather more experience over millions of lives, then a greater diversity of guides will become involved. For example, in the Zero Plane, we require less guidance than on the other planes because the law of opposites and interplay of the energies will push us quite rapidly through successive incarnations. Once we have gained some experience in matter, then we will begin to work more directly with different levels of guidance. Some guides work specifically with the lower planes, such as the First, Second and Third Planes, while others manage the Fourth Plane, and higher levels of guidance focus on Fifth and Sixth Plane energies. In addition there are specialty guides that play specific roles according to the type of life that a soul aspect has chosen. For example, healing guides work specifically with healers, creative guides support artists, writers and so on. The new timeline, however, is birthing a whole new type of higher guidance whose sole purpose is to provide higher instruction according to the dictates of the new light.

The stillness and silence that we cultivate will help to build up new connections with our guides, particularly the new levels of guidance, open us up to a different level of intuition, and establish a deeper energetic flow between our higher self and lower self. Ultimately, as the new timeline builds in our consciousness, we will open up to many, new layers of silence and stillness. Silence does not occupy a single level within our awareness; there are many millions of different levels, just as there are millions of sub-planes with each plane. Through an active cultivation of silence and stillness, we can speed up our timeline, allow the old thought forms and slow frequency energetic practices to drop away, and in the silence of the now, embrace a new, future timeline that will bring through a massive new array of different frequencies from the higher planes.

The new timeline also offers greater opportunities for us to evolve more rapidly. We live in an Avataric Age, and the more we focus our love, thoughts and actions on the Avatar, then the more aligned we will be with His Will. In bringing through His Love and Guidance, we can begin to build new bridges within our awareness that will open us up to vast new vistas of experience and understanding. We will begin to live the principles of the new root race in our every day life, and we will change beyond recognition as the old timeline is stripped out, and then finally drops away from us altogether. It used to be the case that we would have to live three perfect lives to invoke the higher laws of trust and faith over the laws of karma. Three perfect lives at the end of which the soul aspect would ascend up into the Seventh Plane and become God-realised. Because we are living in an Avataric Age, one perfect life is all that is now needed for this ascendancy to take place. Once this period has passed though, the conditions for rapid acceleration will change once again and the requirements for rapid promotion will be different.

The new timeline therefore offers unprecedented, new opportunities to humanity and all other life forms. It offers dramatic change on Earth and all the other planets and stars in the Universe. It will usher in great changes on the inner planes as the very fabric of chaos and order, the initial creative template and the various and wondrous levels of the inner planes become restructured in a more dynamic and expansive way. These changes will invoke more of everything for all living beings and bring in the dawn of a brand new day.

CHAPTER 5

In the Beginning

The "I" and the "Am"

At the very start there was a space, a place that had yet to be formed. This space was an aspect of absolutely nothing, which was total darkness. This aspect had a shape and yet was shapeless and represented 'the everything and the nothing'. Yet at that point there was only nothing since the aspect was not focused into everything. So what is today described as the Seventh Plane, with its millions and millions of subtle journeys going up, was absolutely nothing – it was in total darkness. This vantage point of nothing might be termed the original God in the Beyond-Beyond State, but since it is beyond description, this point could be said also to be before that state. The God in the Beyond-Beyond State can never be adequately described and any attempt to do so only limits it since the state is original, untainted, undefined in every respect and absolutely pure, like a vacuum (see Chapter 11 for a fuller description). Any attempt to describe it automatically changes it. So this nothing was quite literally that, yet had within it an aspect of something. This something had no space, place or definition and so could not be described in any shape or form.

In this utter blackness of nothing there was an awakening, like a pulse, that thought the first original thought of "I". This thought had no definition but was an awakening out of the nothing[1]. With the first thought of "I" a spark was created - a spark of light that pulsed out of the darkness. This flash of light was accompanied by a sound or a wave.

And from that initial awakening there followed another thought: for in the essence of thinking "I", there followed another thought that was "I am", where the "I" was followed by the "am". From a human perspective, we might equate this to a moment where we declare eureka – "I am". A moment which brought delight and something more – an awareness of existence, an awakening out of the nothing and the process of realising or becoming.

This initial expression or pulsation of "I am" created a space out of the nothing that had been and with this initial impulse birthed something out of nothing. It birthed the God in the Beyond State. This initial pulse was like the first spark, the first light, the first word to be birthed out of the nothing. This spark was invoked by the presence of that which we would call God.

Yet within the circuit of this expression of "I am", there was a further question or thought that formed, "I am what?" So while the pulse was formed in the "I am", there was still more to be uncovered in the question of "what am I to be?" This original pulse or spark, with the thought of "I am what?" then pushed out into the blackness or darkness around, into the nothing. And in the moment of pulsing out, this spark of "I am" created another spark to see into the darkness, to discover the answer to the question "I am what?" In this point of two sparks that were created, then like a mirror that was put up against the nothing that was not yet defined, opened up a space where nothing could become more, and flow into the everything. And in that moment where the two sparks touched each other, at that point where God could see into the nothing, then the possibility of everything was created. In that moment where the two sparks sparked off each other, then the first of everything pulsed out.

And in the first word that pulsed out, as God woke up to something out of nothing, the first primordial sound of A-U-M was created. This first sound was also the first flash of light into everything, what in our Earth terms we would call the Big Bang – that initial point of creation where everything was created out of nothing. So in that moment of birthing something out of nothing, there was also the possibility of everything that had yet to be formed or created. Yet within the everything there are the infinite possibilities of form and shape, place and space, time and timelessness, order and chaos, and light and dark. So in the first moments of God awakening, light was created out of the dark, and the first point of something out of nothing was birthed in the essence of the timeless moment.

The first two sparks that allowed the flow of creation to begin, and to become manifest, where God became aware of everything, were the Father and the Son. The essence of the Father that was nothing and then everything within the first spark, which then created a reflection, a mirror of itself, to discover and find out everything about everything. This reflection, this second spark was the Son. The two sparks were like twins or soul mates, and each a reflection of the other. And with this pulsation of everything and nothing was created the in and out breath of the Creator. The everything in the nothing, like the in breath, pushed out into everything to create the out breath. Since the initial in breath and out breath, there have followed successive cycles of the in breath and out breath of the Father. With each cycle the Father has pushed out into more, sparked more in His awareness to discover more about Himself and sent out sparks to discover that which is present in the everything, but which has yet to be uncovered in awareness.

The initial spark of the Father, and then the initial spark of the Son, within their pattern of ignition, also left an afterglow of everything that they embodied; this afterglow would burn long after the sparks had become more. So with the Father and the Son, an ever-changing presence of the afterglows, also became something more and created the Holy Ghost. These first three sparks then formed the primary triangle, the primary focus of the everything and the nothing within the ever-expanding unfolding of the essence of "I am".

The Nothing and the Everything

In the very moment that everything was created out of nothing, where the sparks of the Father and the Son pushed out to discover the answer to the question "I am what?", the probabilities and the possibilities of the everything were then expressed in shape and form, although not originally in a way that we would recognise in the physical. The "I" was expressed in what is termed the God in the Beyond-Beyond State and the "I am", the awareness of everything that was created was the movement within the God in the Beyond State. So in the creation of the Father and the Son, the Son to mirror the Father and the means by which the Father could ask about more and seek out into everything to answer the question of "What am I?"

The initial focus of the question of "What am I?" was seeded in the higher aspects of the Seventh Plane, and then down into the lower aspects of the Seventh Plane. The formation of everything within the Seventh Plane birthed millions and millions of subtle journeys stretching through the multiple expanses of infinities within the limitless and fathomless expanse that was and is the Seventh Plane. So as the spark that was the Son first dropped out of the nothing into ever more expressions of everything, it dropped down through the multiple layerings of the Seventh Plane, lighting up each layering as it passed by. As each level was lit up, the principle of life was formed through the principle of creation that was a reflection of the essence of what the spark was and would always be. The spark, the Son, sparked new sparks as it dropped down, and in these new sparkings, more life and more life forms were birthed through these multiple sparkings. This principle of creation also birthed Natural Law, the expression of life through lived experience according to the dictates of that which is formed in balance. At the same time, the new sparks that were formed started to interrelate with each other, so as the first spark flowed down the levels of awareness of the Seventh Plane, all the dreams, visions and possible manifestations of life became aware of each other.

So in this description of the primeval spark, the original spark was the essence of the Father who sought to explore that which was not there in His consciousness. He did that by sending out a spark, the Son, to see what was there. And He imbued that spark with an aspect of Himself that would give definition to anything it found, give purpose to anything it found and give an explanation to Himself when that spark returned. That spark, as it went out and hit the different layers, started to fragment itself, to give rise to millions of other sparks.

Within each different layering there then formed a series of veils so that the image of everything that was made manifest remained, like an afterglow. One way to consider this process is to imagine the sparks that are created in a wood fire. Some sparks fly out a greater distance from the fire, while others remain closer to the centre. At the same time, some sparks remain in existence longer, and then create an afterglow of where the spark has been. So in this analogy, as each layer of the Seventh Plane was illuminated and sparked, as it were, some of the sparks sparked for longer than others, but eventually grew dimmer, and left an afterglow of what had been. The residue of the multiplicity of what had been, started to go back off to sleep within the expression of each layering that had been initially sparked. So some sparks remained for longer, and these tended to be in the higher aspects of the Seventh Plane, while in the lower aspects of the Seventh Plane, there was more of a limitation in the sparks that were birthed and formed. All of these sparks and sparkings represented an inspirational pattern, and in the lower part of the Seventh Pane, especially in the parts that came to be known as the first four Divine Journeys, there was a slowing down or a point of limitation.

The limitation that was formed in the lower portion of the Seventh Plane led to a congregation within a series of currents and eddies. Just as the physical oceans on Earth have multiple currents that are formed through temperature gradients, different levels of salinity, and the mixing of fresh and salt water, the bottom of the Seventh Plane became a reflection of the after flow of the different layering and gradients of light that were ignited in the Seventh Plane above. The sparks that had been formed began to congregate within these gradients and eventually at the bottom of the Seventh Plane, gathered in what is known as the Ocean of Life. This Ocean was formed out of the primeval pattern of nothing and everything. It was black and the sparks and the afterglows of the original sparkings came together in this Ocean. In entering this Ocean, the sparks went back off to sleep, as the afterglow faded.

Within this pattern of limitation at the bottom of the Seventh Plane, the original spark that was the Son and which was to be the first soul to progress through the different planes, also came into the Ocean. However, unlike the other sparks that had been sparked, although it started to go back off to sleep, it felt a point of limitation. The limitation was like an itch that would not go away and represented a point of disturbance within itself in relation to what was around. It was from this point that the journey of the first soul that was the Son, the Avatar, was formed in the creative pattern of life in the everything and the nothing (see Chapter 12 – The Avatar and the Perfect Masters).

While the creation of everything within the infinite expanse of the Seventh Plane was ignited first through the spark of the Son, and then through the millions and millions of sparks that were created in the ensuing expression of everything, the brilliance of the Seventh Plane also created a shadow within the everything. This shadow was what lay "below" the Seventh Plane, and what lay below the Ocean of Life. So the point of limitation and "fixing" at the bottom of the Seventh Plane represented the line or reflection from which the shadow was formed. Like a dividing line between the real and the shadow, a whole series of levels were formed in the probability of the everything, yet which was also limitation as manifested through the shadow, below the Seventh Plane. The shadow layers would form the planes below, starting with the Sixth Plane, and before they became sparked into existence by the presence of the first spark, the Son, remained as a shadow of probable possibilities, rather than actual existences. They were like the dream that had yet to be lived, yet within the shadow dream, there existed different streams of probable existence.

The focus of the shadow within the everything represented a sort of limitation where the dream in the shadow became the reality and where the actual reality became forgotten. So in the shadow that was created, a pattern of where God could forget that He was God could be established. For in the questing of "Who am I?" there has to be a counterpoint of "Who am I not?" So, in this way, the shadow below the Seventh Plane came to be the place where the sparks would forget that they were God and where they would live in the shadow of what was not and not what is. And yet within the shadow, there always has to be the possibility of more, and the shadow of more is to invoke the possibility to wake up from the dream to become that which is more. So in the probability of the shadow, the sparks that would come to flow through it, would always entertain the possibility of becoming more. In living limitation within the shadow, they would ultimately come to live without limitation both in and out of the shadow.

Light Sparks

In the multiple sparkings that were created, each spark created life, and built up a focus of massive fragmentation, where each spark invoked more in the everything. This multiple sparking was like God sending out more into more, to birth and to find answers to the fundamental question of "I am what?" Each spark had its own rhythm of going out and in, and every time it came back to God, it brought back an aspect of God to the initial spark or God within. As each spark gave birth to new sparks, then each spark became like a pattern of its own creation, creating more out of the everything that was constantly building into more. Like a chain reaction that had been set off, it gained its own momentum as billions and billions of sparkings gave birth to different aspects of life in the everything. And when the different sparks returned back to God, they showed that God was always more.

The pattern of being and becoming of each spark, of each different life, set up a pattern whereby some sparks would create other sparks and in this pattern, could watch and copy the creative process. They could birth multiple probable existences where they could become a principal spark, birth other sparks and then feel the return of these sparks within a pattern of becoming more within the everything.

Within the pattern of sparking and becoming a spark, some sparks would last longer – their spark would remain bright and glow more strongly. Through the pressure of sparking and experience, sometimes the sparks would burst into flame. Like in a fire, where a spark touches dry wood or tinder that can burst into flames, some sparks went out into everything to discover and become more, and in this process would give birth to themselves as a flame. Each flame would become like a mirror to God, and on returning back to God, the Father, would represent a door of everything and more. The door would be the beginning, the end, the shadow, the reality, and the "I am" of more.

So different sparks would develop and become more – some would pulse far out into the everything, while others would pulse back into the nothing. Within this creative pattern, the sparks and sparkings would create millions and millions of aspects of life within the everything. Our physical bodies are a series of sparks called atoms that holds together a certain ritualistic flavour; our organs are collections of sparks and our soul is a spark. There are also the other levels of expression of life that we are, and for example a different type of spark that comes in and dances with us is a deva. In the devic pattern we have many different devas, all vibrating as different sparks. So within the fabric of creation and the focus of becoming more we express the pattern of sparking on a constant basis. The different patterns of life, including angelic life and other aspects are all formed from sparks.

Each spark as it dies creates an afterglow, like a memory of what it has been. This afterglow can be short or long, but within the pattern of pulsing out and in, and in the succession of sparks that go out and then return back into the God within, then these afterglows are captured and taken back in. Another way of looking at it is to consider each spark as a mirror, and with each pattern of multiple sparking, millions of mirrors are formed which then give a refection of what is back to the Father. And similarly, if we can connect and recognise these different mirrors, then we can begin to understand what the Father is, and in one sense this forms the basis for a soul's journey.

Thus through this pattern of sparking the Father could see a whole succession of different everythings, as experienced through the initial spark, the multiplicity of the subsequent sparks, and then the pulse of each spark as it grew brighter or dimmer according to the experience that was gained in the ever-expanding pattern of everything. And those sparks that became dim would leave an afterglow, and like a memory, this would be retained and returned back to the Father in the process of becoming more.

The afterglows also built into more, as each spark would forget that it was the essence of God. This pattern became manifested within the shadow, below the Seventh Plane, where the successive sparks would slowly fade and become the afterglow.   In entering the shadow, which seemed so far away from the Father, these sparks would forget about the Father. Within this pattern of afterglows, then periodic sparks would meet the different afterglows and start to remember where they had been. The meeting of the afterglow would invoke in that fading spark a memory and so would re-spark the afterglow. Through the succession of afterglows, like the fading images on a screen, each spark would eventually become re-ignited by these memories and then ultimately re-ignite into a flame, that would become more. The shadow planes then came to host the multiple afterglows.

As the shadow became more manifest, then rules and regulations involving the play of different aspects were birthed, such as time, the laws of trust and faith, karmic regulation and the pattern of evolution and involution through the shadow planes. The shadow planes became the process whereby more could be invoked, where in the greater distance that a spark travelled away from God, then the more of the everything that could be gained and ultimately returned back to God. So from the beginning, various cycles of grace were established through the Essence of the Father and the Son, to allow more of everything to be uncovered and unveiled. So just as we talk about the Universe expanding in our physical dimension, then this is a reflection of the underlying aspect of the Father finding out more about His Creation all of the time.

In the succeeding cycles and ages after the initial spark, the Son cycled through the shadow planes, and would return periodically as a brilliant spark (the Avatar) to re-ignite some of the afterglows, and to help those sparks that were pulsing in the right way to become living flames, ready to return to the Father.

Each spark that went out and eventually came back told the Father more about Himself and creation; yet with each return of a spark, there was always a hunger for more and so the Father would spark more. In this way, the everything will always evolve into and become more.

Light and Dark

Within the pattern of limitation that was established towards the bottom of the Seventh Plane, the creative focus, in the beginning also birthed the interplay of light and dark. In the beginning there had been nothing, and then with the first spark, light was created. This contrast, like the everything and the nothing, represented within the uncovering of everything, a new pattern of expression. In the beginning, the primordial patterns of dark and light were created out of the original sparking. The dark that was formed was a reflection of the blackness of the original nothing, while the light was the embodiment of the essence of the original spark, like the first light of the Big Bang and beyond. Different patterns of light and dark were invoked through the process of sparking and ignition, the slow decay into the afterglow and then into darkness again.

While this process could occur on many different levels, it was given more complete expression at the bottom of the Seventh Plane where a pattern of light and dark was established and which would ultimately infuse the pattern of becoming within the shadow. One way to imagine it is to see the shadow as the dark, the night and then the light above it as the day. The shadow, the dark, would represent all that had yet to come into expression or form, or that which had yet to be sparked. Yet, within a shadow, there are always contrasting patterns of light and dark. Shadows can appear extremely dark, or grey or appear against a backdrop of brilliant light. Within the shadow of the planes of illusion that were formed and activated by the first soul, the Avatar, in the initial cycle of sparking, the interplay between light and dark was established. The different levels within the shadow gave rise to different expressions and mixes of light and dark. These different mixes were formed through the pattern of light and dark that was birthed out of the Seventh Plane.

In the beginning, in the segregation of light and dark that took place, a standard of light and dark was established. This was a reflection of what was invoked through the descent of the first spark down through the Seventh Plane. It was then, through this mix of light and dark that the different expressions of life were made manifest, first by the first pattern of sparking in the shadow by the Avatar, and then in the subsequent sparkings that followed. The original light and dark that were formed through the separation in the Seventh Plane then became the pattern that was established for the succeeding Avataric Day[2].

The creative focus of life always works according to the principal of birthing chaos out of order. In the beginning, the chaos was hosted through the dark light, whereby the subsequent sparking led to illumination and an opening into more, through the progression of chaos into order. Each spark, as it went into more, formed a more ordered pattern, rather than a chaotic pattern. In this process, light came to represent order, while dark was chaos. Consequently, in the unfolding pattern that was established in the beginning, chaos and dark always moved towards light and order by virtue of the process of creating sparks which in turn would spark more light. Out of dark, light is always made manifest and so it is, that out of chaos, order always comes to play. The pattern of everything and nothing, and the initial sparking which then unfolded into the multiple sparks of new life and expression into more, led to an unfolding interplay between dark and light, and chaos and order.

Since the beginning there has been a particular blend of chaos and order that has led to the creative pattern that has been allowed to unfold within the shadowlands[3] play. Both chaos and order have had a particular flavour and have from the beginning combined to create more. Chaos and order have been the testing ground for souls to spark and eventually ignite into a flame that ultimately becomes an open door. In becoming the open door, such flames then ride chaos and order and embody the essence of the Father within. So in the unfolding pattern all of the sparks that are now in existence throughout the Universe have come from the original spark of the Father, which then birthed the spark of the Son. All of these sparks, sooner or later, will have to return to the Father.

Early on in the pattern of creation, those sparks that had been sparked by the initial spark of the Son, sought to create their own creations having witnessed creation at first hand, so to speak. As the first soul to drop down through the Seventh Plane, and then to follow through into the shadow planes (see Chapter 12), and eventually to pulse back in and out according to the need that was manifested with the Father in the ever-evolving pattern of more, the Son sparked a myriad pattern of different creations. These creations were found on the Seventh Plane and on the shadow planes and sought to bring about their own pattern of creation. One such creator was known as an Elder, and was formed early on in the creative sparking. The Elder within the higher patterns of light, then gave birth to a twin, so that there became two Elders that would, in the fullness of the creative pattern, host a ring or a promise from the Father. These beings would come to be known as the Elderings.

Other creative patterns were also forged early on through the ritual of sparking. The dragon kind were birthed in a creative flow and set about building their own creative pattern through the birthing of more, and so the dragons, which embodied power and love, focused on the evolving play in shadowlands and sought ways in which their focus and ritual could birth more within the everything. Other patterns of Creator Gods were also formed through the sparking of more in the everything.

The constantly unfolding response to the fundamental question of "What am I" has ensured that the pattern of everything has become more. The Father is in a state of constant self-discovery as He gathers more experience from the sparks that return to Him; and yet in this return there is always more to be uncovered, and in this process, the thirst of the Father is always growing. Ultimately, where there are points of limitation, whether it is in the shadow planes or on the Seventh Plane, there will always be a pressure to push through this limitation into more. This is the nature of the creative process. So it is in our own lives, when we push through a limitation, then there is always a simple invocation, a simple response: namely, more.

CHAPTER 6

The First Soul & The Ocean of Life

The Primary Spark

In the unfolding pattern of the essence of the Father, there was an original spark that was formed out of the darkness, out of nothing, which then dropped down through millions and millions of layers within the Seventh Plane. As it dropped down, this spark sparked and gave definition to all the different possible manifestations of form and visions that were initially seeded into the nothing. The focus of this spark, as it was sent out from the Creator, from the original "I" which sought to uncover or become the "I am", was to move from nothingness into everything – to put a definition, in the loosest sense of the word, and understanding to what "I am" actually means or is. It was the primeval aspect of the Father coming down to explore more about itself.

This original spark was extremely bright at the higher end of the Seventh Plane and in giving birth to other aspects of itself underwent a sort of dilution. It flowed down through the millions and millions of levels within the Seventh Plane and eventually reached the bottom end of it, which represented a form of limitation from all that had been and all that was in the higher aspects of the Seventh Plane. This limitation was found in the first four Divine Journeys, and more especially in the first three Divine Journeys. These primary, lower journeys appeared darker, although this has nothing to do with the way that we perceive dark in shadowlands. It represents, rather, a less concentrated pattern of energy associated with the constant discharge of the Primary Spark all the way down the Seventh Plane. Having hit the Fourth Divine Journey (see Chapter 11), the Primary Spark then entered the lower three primary patterns which loosely formed and became inverted to host the slower frequencies that we would call bliss.

At the bottom of the Seventh Plane, this original or primeval spark eventually settled into the Ocean of Life. The density of energy at the bottom of the Seventh Plane was such that it led to a condensing and darkening of energy that supported a different pattern of expression. The situation is not dissimilar to particles of matter dropping to the bottom of a lake, except in this case the gravitational pull led to a gathering of sparks that had been sparked by the Primary Spark and which then slowly burnt out or became dimmer. Once at the bottom there was a waiting period for everything to spark up again. It was like this original spark went off to sleep but then through the pattern of limitation established at the bottom end of the Seventh Plane, led it to wake up again.

The original spark had settled at the bottom of the Ocean and slowly, like a bubble, it began to rise out of the lower "muddy" layer into the middle and then the upper layer. This ascent represented the slow waking up of the first spark and once it reached the lip of the Ocean, it felt a gravitational pull to find out what it was, what it had forgotten on its journey down, and what it could become through invoking a pattern of more. To do this, the original spark had to drop down from the Seventh Plane, down into the shadow that formed as part of the original sparking of the Seventh Plane. Within the shadow there were a series of probable layers that represented different densities and expressions of that which was yet to be birthed. So, just as the Seventh Plane could be described as a pattern of condensing at the top, where the brilliance of the first sparking then flowed down through the millions of journeys to the bottom where a dilution took place, so the shadow planes was something like a mirror image, with a broadness at the top, flowing into a concentrated pattern at the bottom, like an inverted pyramid. It should be recognised, though, that to describe the Seventh Plane according to any structure is itself a limitation.

The Primary Spark started its downward journey through the probable formats of shadow planes. Below the Seventh Plane, the spark dropped into what we today would call the Sixth Plane, and then down through Fifth, Fourth, Third, Second and First Planes, and eventually into the Zero Plane (See also Chapter 10). In descending down through these darker and grosser planes of expression, which were the shadow to the Seventh Plane, the Primary Spark began to invoke a spark in itself, although it became progressively dimmer as it dropped down through the planes. At the same time, the different probable expressions of each of the planes were birthed through the illumination of the Primary Spark, although they became dimmer as it dropped further down. The expression of everything through the limitation of the shadow was given a possible or probable focus.

During the continuing descent through the shadow planes, this original spark went back off to sleep again, but once it had reached the Zero Planes, it then recycled back up through the planes, ultimately returning to the lower end of the Seventh Plane. The pull or return back up the planes was like an impetus that was pre-programmed into the Primary Spark – to eventually return to the Seventh Plane and the Father. Another way of considering the return is to see it as a movement back, like the return of a pendulum once the bottom of the Zero Plane, the point of total contraction in the shadow, had been reached. On the return journey, the Primary Spark slowly lightened until eventually it reached the higher shadow planes and then returned back to the bottom of the Seventh Plane.

This pattern of completion of a cycle led the Primary Spark to transform into a flame by virtue of what it had become. And yet, there still remained a gravitational pull within the flame to become more and to remember that which it had been through previously, to reconnect with its loss. It had gone back to sleep during the cycle through the shadow planes, and there was the need to remember where it had been. So on returning back to the Seventh Plane, there was still a strong gravitational pull to go down, back into the lower planes from the Seventh Plane to remember more.

When the Primary Spark came down this time, it lit up each and every aspect of the planes below the Seventh Plane, and created a vision of what was present within theses planes and which had been pre-focused there as a possibility when they were originally formed. In this process of coming down and then coming all the way back up, as part of its waking up process, this Primary Spark then became the first soul to complete the whole cycle and it is this Primary Spark which is known as the Avatar. It was the first soul to come all the way down to the Zero Plane, to wake up and then to return back up through the planes to the Seventh Plane and the First Divine Journey. However, since this primeval spark had come all the way down from the Essence of the Father, it then remembered more and was allowed to grow into more through working its way back up all through the journeys back into the different levels of the Seventh Plane.

In this initial process, this first full conscious cycle of becoming, the Avatar began to activate within the multiple layers of energy and the encodements that had been placed within it, a transference of energy from this Primary Spark into everything else around it, and to ignite multiple sparks. In this way, an initial discourse was established by the Primary Spark, the Avatar, with that which we call life in its myriad manifestations, and the creation or the imagination of the Father. As the Primary Spark came down and then went back up, it gave off millions and millions of other sparks. So, as part of its expression, the Primary Spark began to loosen the pattern of contraction coming down, and then manifest that expression through the law of opposites or the shadow aspect from the Seventh Plane downwards. So the Sixth and the Fifth Planes are the mental planes, and are still very bright compared to what we experience normally in physical matter. The Fourth Plane became the plane of manifestation and then the astral planes, the Third, Second and First Planes, were formed. Finally, the Zero Plane, the slowest formation of expression would be the space where the fundamental pattern of life, the mineral, plant and animal, would be actually formed.

As the first soul to complete the journey down through all of the planes and back again, the Primary Spark established a template for soul evolution and progression that was then adopted in a diversity of expressions by all the sparks that followed[1].

So in this expression of everything out of nothing through the Creation of the Father, each spark can give birth to another spark or an aspect of life through an act of separation. So, if we have an idea or create a thought form, by manifesting it in our imagination we give it an independent existence, a life of its own. The more energy we put into it, the more it can take on a separate existence and reality of its own. So it is that a spark can create another spark, and through this multiplication process, the vast array of life was sparked into different levels of awareness and existence from the original Primary Spark, the Avatar.

So in each of us we have a primary atom, which is our own original spark, which has been segregated and split into two more, the masculine and feminine, which in turn are newly created sparks. Our bodes are a series of sparks — each atom, neutron, subatomic particle is a spark that has been created, a spark of existence that has been made manifest. There are other sparks that are also present in our ritual that we call life, such as the devas, all vibrating as different sparks. So within the rules and regulations of our pattern of energetic expression, we hold and retain multiple sparks that co-exist in our conscious and sub-conscious awareness as different life forms. They are as real as you or I, and are as real as the living formulation of the physical and subtle levels of awareness that co-exist with and within us. And within this pattern of sparks, there are the more permanent sparks that we call souls, and which also spark a multiplicity of other sparks during their development and progression. So each spark that is a soul will create a myriad of sparks during its journeys and these sparks will each create different patterns of expression and form.

The Ocean of Life

Once the Primary Spark had completed its journey, a pattern of manifestation rapidly followed that gave complete birth to the pattern of energy called the Ocean of Life. As described above, the Ocean is present at the lower end of the Seventh Plane and houses the essence of unconscious bliss in a divine state. It is vast, infinite and is the initiation point for all soul birth and subsequent progression. The light within the Ocean is dark and to enter into it is to go into a pattern of utter blackness, although to attempt to describe its properties within the limitation of our own sensory apparatus is impossible. Within the vastness of this Ocean, which embodies unconscious bliss, there are millions and millions of layers. At the very bottom of the Ocean, as in our planetary oceans, there is a denser layer, and it is here that the first drops or globules of the soul essences are formed. These souls are all sparks that have originated from the Primary Spark. Each soul gradually builds a flow that slowly gravitates from the bottom of the Ocean up to the surface. And each soul that is held within the Ocean is like a prototype soul, waiting to be birthed out of the Ocean.

Within this gravitational pattern, there are different layers of density that have to be overcome and each soul represents the essence of the Divine, yet held in a pattern of unconscious bliss. This means that the prototype soul has no awareness of self and is in effect dormant and lost in this state of bliss – like in a deep dream. Souls start off at the bottom with a greater density but move through the millions of layers due to circulating currents; these currents are not dissimilar to convection currents yet are made up of energetic flows within the Ocean. The circulation and movement of prototype souls is generally from the bottom, up to the Ocean's surface. There is also a constant flux of movement of different prototype souls through the millions of layers; some migrating upwards, some sideways and downwards according to the flow of divine currents moving through the different densities of unconscious bliss. Each prototype soul, as it moves to the surface, retains a protective sac, almost like an egg yolk, that surrounds the soul essence. These little sacs are composed of dark light, which gives the primeval experience of everything and nothing. It is almost like a recipe from the sensation of being asleep, then partially waking up to becoming aware of sensation. The sacs also act like ballast helping to lift the soul up through the layers of the Ocean, so that there is a gravitational flow upwards, complemented by any surrounding disturbances and by the rhythm of light that is actually irradiating the primeval mixture.

When the prototype souls reach the surface, some are skimmed off by the energies manifested at the surface. For example, energetic washes, like divine winds or storms, which are the manifested presence of divinity, will pick off some souls at the surface, and blow them to the edge of the Seventh Plane, where there is a lip. The soul lands on the lip and sits there waiting before it can begin the journey from unconscious bliss into conscious awareness through the unfolding levels of more gross, denser layering all the way down through the Seven Planes. Once separated at the Ocean surface, the prototype souls become individuated souls. Rather like newly hatched chicks, these young souls sit and experience the first pangs of separation from the Ocean and feel the first stirrings of energetic movement out of unconscious bliss.

In many instances, these souls may become sponsored through their whole cycle of unfolding through the totality of the Planes of Illusion. These young souls will wait for a more advanced soul to pass by, rather like waiting for a comet to come by, and feel a ripple in the fabric of divine essence. Almost through a pulse or ripple of intent, a call is sent out, and a response anticipated. If a young soul is picked out by a divine presence, then that young soul may then become sponsored. The divine being will act as the sponsor and will keep an eye on that soul's complete journey.

In other cases, when a soul lands on the lip without a sponsor, and cannot remember the primeval pattern that was sent out, then they fall from the lip down through the shadow planes — Six, Five, Four, Three, Two, One and into the Zero Plane. Occasionally, these falling souls will be spotted by a more evolved soul who then takes on the role of sponsor at that time, and has the responsibility by adoption, of the soul that is manifesting down.

Soul birth is also achieved by more direct means. Higher presences will scour the surface of the Ocean for promising young souls and then again actively sponsor them for their entire journey. The role of sponsor is long-term and requires a certain focus to ensure completion of the soul's journey. The sponsor will also orchestrate the trajectory of the soul down through the planes and also actively determine the type of soul path to be followed. For example, souls can become angelic from the start, others devic while some will adopt an entirely different pattern of development, like the God-intoxicated souls known as masts. From time to time these divine presences will poach specific souls based upon the type of light they exhibit, and for specific roles and creative plays within the flow of Avataric Energy.

Some higher beings will adopt more direct approaches to soul sponsorship. The type of soul manifested will vary according to its pattern of development within the Ocean – whether it has risen from the very abyssal bottom to the surface, or whether it has been "poached" out of the millions of different layers with a specific pattern of unconscious, soul light. This pattern of soul birthing is more risky to the poachers and requires a specific focus of intent and will imbued with true silence.

These poachers look within the primeval darkness and listen to all of the souls sleeping and sense a rhythmic pulse with each individual soul. Each poacher will look for a particular rhythm that will embody the type of formula that they are searching for. Once they have found that formula, they then wrap an aspect of themselves around it, pulse into it and impregnate it with a note. The soul then starts to wake up and it focuses on the poacher's beam of light that is directed toward it, and the poacher then draws the soul to the surface of the Ocean and out.

Within the vast Ocean there are also presences known as the Watchers. The Watchers watch to ensure that the pattern and progression of movement remains undisturbed and that no poachers enter the Ocean in search of particular soul essences. Poachers can come in various different forms, but are generally experienced souls that have already ascended into the Seventh Plane and which are seeking to birth something new: to find a new type of soul light that can, through the focus of experience from unconscious bliss into conscious awareness, build a progression and mastery of different types of light. If any disturbance is detected in the Ocean, then the Watchers will gather and investigate. Like an all-encompassing feeling, the blind Watchers can sense the disturbance, and if they find it, will absorb its essence. So if a soul goes into the Ocean and its light is too bright then the primeval darkness that hosts the aspects of the Father that have not yet woken up, will see the light in the darkness and go towards it.

For the poachers, the key is to hold a space of absolute stillness and utter silence, and to remain wrapped in the essence of darkness. If they revealed their true light, then the Watchers and the other patterns of primeval darkness would attach to them and rend them on the spot. Indeed, some of the Watchers are failed poachers who have been caught in the Ocean, and who then go back into a state where they are held in bondage, destined to be Watchers through eternity. It is like being sent back to the very beginning where all of experience and light essence is stripped away; they are then held within the pattern of the Ocean itself, from which it is extremely difficult to escape. But the essence of the Watcher also fades because the living will of their spark has to patrol and gradually they have to give out little bits of themselves so that they gradually fall back into darkness. The poachers, though, have a certain shelf life as well, during which they can enter the Ocean. Each time they go in, the Ocean of Life gets a feel of their identification, and so the risks increase with each journey. So the poachers go in only when there is a need to find something that is more elusive.

Only those presences that have sufficient understanding and experience of the Ocean can undertake the role of poacher; however, the rewards can be stunning. Specific souls can be fished out of the Ocean and then pre-programmed to follow a specific pattern of soul progression within a unique flow of experience. These unique souls always create something more within the flow of life and experience. For example, souls can be programmed to explore different aspects of light and dark within the polarity of experience in the shadow planes. A soul can contract to experience a specific pattern of dark or light experiences that can then be used as a basis for working different frequencies of light or dark. Once a soul has been "found" by a poacher, it is then moved to the Ocean surface and birthed within the creative pattern developed by the sponsor. Each specific soul, by virtue of the way it has been birthed, through the spark of light that touched it, will hold the essence of different varieties of unconscious bliss. The essence of unconscious bliss at the bottom of the Ocean is different from that which is near the surface; and so it is, that such poached souls may manifest different types of essence that will give each one a specific impetus through its subsequent development.

In summary, souls can therefore be poached, skimmed out of the Ocean or have a sponsor. And the way a soul can be birthed is according to the dictate of energy that is being manifested at that time.

Engaging in Awareness through Separation

The soul, when it is birthed out of the Ocean, encounters separation for the first time. This primordial separation is the first movement out of unconscious bliss. Up until that time, the prototype soul has been enveloped in bliss, unconscious of its surroundings and in a dream-like state. The shock of separation registers as a seismic ripple and forms the kernel around which all subsequent experience is entertained. The sense of separation within the unconscious state forms the backdrop for the young soul's future experiences in illusion.

While unconscious bliss in Reality within the divine has been the experience of the young soul, the pulse of separation provides the momentum for the soul's development. The soul is, within its unconscious awareness, forced to consider the question "Who am I?" This is a not a conscious point of understanding, but rather a subconscious tidal flow that provides the underlying impulse to find out more about itself. Having been in a state of unity or oneness, in the infinite expanse of unconsciousness, like in an unconscious "I" state, the soul, now separate, needs to build up an interpretation, through its separation, its duality from what it was, to embrace a notion of "I am", and within that "I am", to come to a focal point of realisation of "Who am I?" The soul's initial focus is like a mirroring of the initial spark.

To build a means of understanding this question requires

that each soul explore itself through a series of patterns in Illusion. The Reality[2] of the Seventh Plane is oneness, unification in divinity with everything and nothing. Illusion, on the other hand, provides an unfolding pattern of duality where the essence of what it means to be separate can be experienced through a counterpoint of illusory existence. Or to put it another way, through experiencing the shadow, it is possible to experience what Reality is not. The illusion provides the new pattern through which, ultimately, the soul can answer the principle question of "Who am I?" or "What am I?"

To entertain and build experience from within the context of illusion requires that each soul send out an initial pulse or series of thoughts. The initial thought of "I" or "I am" will invoke something. As these pulses or thoughts invoke a response, then each soul has to clothe itself, or engineer for itself, a vehicle of experience that can receive and entertain the corresponding thought or pulse. The analogy is not dissimilar to undersea sonar. A submarine will send out a pulse, yet will need the proper receiving equipment to pick up the responding "ping" when the sonar sound has engaged with a physical object.

So it is that following the first, primordial separation from the Ocean, the young soul will then experience a further impulse of separation as it moves out of the Reality of the Seventh Plane, to engage in the outside Illusion. The need to engage with Illusion becomes a focal point of attention, and through energetic momentum, the soul drops out of Reality as it seeks to engage with the duality of Illusion to understand itself; it moves from unconscious bliss into unconscious illusion. The first impulses, or thoughts, that are engendered in response to the sense of separation set up waves or ripples that flow out; as each wave pushes out, the unconscious soul begins to cloak itself in a layer or thought that seeks a response to these initial impulses. Like a vehicle of awareness, the soul begins to build up several layers as the pulses or unconscious thoughts expand out. The unconscious soul cannot engage with the normal sensory experiences, and so has to build up multiple layers or vehicles of expression as part of its experience. Each layer that is built up is the manifestation of an initial pulse and a means of receiving a response.

At the same time, with each pulse, ripple or thought that goes out, the response that is received invokes another pulse or movement of thought; this in turn invokes another pulse and further responses. This effectively marks the beginning of the soul's separation and manifestation within the higher mental planes through the multiple patterns of thought that are sent out, and from which responses are sought. The soul then cloaks itself in multiple layers or vehicles as it begins its journey through the millions and millions of sub-planes in the mental planes. It builds up a wardrobe of layers, each of which is an expression of experience within which is found an awareness that prompted an initial pulse and received a response.

Within this pattern, there is also an inertial pull; with each thought and vehicle of expression, the soul is drawn into denser patterns or flows of energy. The higher mental planes are very refined energetically, and the flow of light is extremely bright. The soul is unconscious of this yet seeks to build up an understanding of itself within its unconsciousness; like a magnetic pull, it is drawn to seek out more layers within the overall Illusion, and so gradually flows down from the top end of the Sixth Plane, into the lower sub-planes. This marks the beginning of the soul's downward journey through the different planes of Illusion and ultimately into physical matter. With each vehicle of awareness it forms, the soul builds itself a series of subtle bodies – each one is minor at first, reflecting the pattern of energy, but ultimately they become denser and grosser as the soul journeys down through the planes.

It is also important to be aware of the distinction between unconscious and conscious. In unconsciousness a soul may perceive an experience and may be aware of it, yet will be unconscious of the very nature of that which it is experiencing. In other words, the subtle vehicles of awareness that it builds may be able to entertain a dialogue with that which is around, but it will not be consciously aware of what the Illusion is from the perspective of the higher Reality. In other words, it may be unconscious of the illusion, yet engaging with it energetically; and to become conscious in the illusion means that the soul has to wake up to its divinity and to recognise, consciously and actively, that the Illusion is illusion and that the Reality of the divine is in fact the Reality of itself as part of the divine. To fully wake up the soul has to recognise itself as being divine and in the oneness of the divinity of the Seventh Plane. Consequently, while the soul journeys through the millions and millions of sub-planes of Illusion, it will build up an awareness and series of vehicles or subtle bodies of expression that allow it to gather experience and to build an increasing awareness of that experience, yet all within the confines of being unconscious of what the soul, as itself, truly is. To wake up to the Reality, to its own conscious awareness of self is, in a very real way, the focus of its journey and experience.

Within this developing pattern, it is also important to understand that awareness is not the same as consciousness as we understand it, and that within the states of unconsciousness, there are many different sub-levels prior to developing full consciousness. For example, we can be aware of things, yet are not fully conscious. Human consciousness, as it develops, is part of the unveiling of different levels of unconsciousness, until eventually, when human consciousness reaches a pinnacle of evolution it enters full consciousness where the soul recognises itself as God. This is usually extremely rare and is only ever attained after millions and millions of lifetimes of experience.

It is no accident that the higher planes are composed of mental light; for in the very act of thought, the essence of light manifested is a reflection of it. It is extremely light and very refined. Each soul will follow a path where it flows through these higher patterns of light. Sometimes, these patterns are referred to as the gaseous levels, where thought, like a cloud, entertains a sense of form in the illusion. As the thought becomes slightly denser, other layers are then encountered, such as the crystalline levels. The essence of crystalline encountered here is different from the physical counterpart that we would recognise as crystalline. The soul encounters both the gaseous and crystalline layers during its progression and unfolding of unconscious experience; it may spend time in either or both of these patterns, and depending upon its focus of experience agreed through its sponsorship, may encounter a whole host of different experiences within the unfolding layers of gaseous or crystalline illusion. The pattern of sponsorship and overall contract may dictate that the unconscious soul wakes up to a different level of awareness within either one of these levels, thereby entering a whole new pattern of experience within a different focus of separation and awareness.

Within the vast realms of these energetic flows, souls will encounter other souls and may link up to form collective vehicles of awareness. As more and more souls link together, they form long wagon trains, which can accommodate as many as one hundred thousand, or more, souls. These wagon trains form soul families and through the collective patterns of experiences that they encounter, will pulse to a series of similar frequency notes.

The soul will also entertain relatively early on, a pattern of segregation or splitting itself up. This process allows each soul to gather more experience within diverse realms and this usually follows a pattern of seven aspects. Each aspect will follow a different pathway and gather different experiences. For example, one aspect may spend more inner time i.e. a pattern of experience in the inner planes that is outside physical time, within the crystalline spheres, while another may engage more in the gaseous levels. Each will entertain a different experience, thereby gathering more information, and each realm will provide a rich source of different vehicles of expression and experience.

While some souls will take large amounts of time, within the timeless pattern of the inner planes, other souls may pass through these layers relatively rapidly, although such terms are not really meaningful within the context of timelessness. Following these levels, the soul encounters the angelic realms.

The Angelic Realms

After encountering the gaseous and crystalline realms, the developing soul will enter the angelic realms. The angelic focus represents a principle drive towards order. With the creative focus of order, the angelic realms are a major point of segregation within the evolution of developing souls. For the most part, souls will pass through this realm remaining unconscious, while all the time gathering more experience through the development of different levels of mental awareness. However, some souls have a different pathway and are destined to become angelic. In these circumstances, such souls will be woken up and made conscious of what they are within the pattern of pre-existing angelic order. This can take place either on the Sixth Plane or on the Fifth Plane. As the soul passes through these realms, a focus is brought to bear either through a specific angelic host or series of hosts that sets up a wake up call within the unconscious soul. The unconscious soul is exposed to a pattern of ordered light that invokes a response and forces the soul to wake up. This waking process means that the soul understands, at a profound level, that it is separate from the divine, and yet is awake and aware of its existence in a very total way.

Souls that are woken up on the Sixth Plane become archangels while souls woken up on the Fifth Plane become angels. Archangels and angels reflect a different stream of light and once initiated into the angelic pathway, the young soul will undergo a very specific and rigorous protocol of development. Angelic light is high frequency, ordered light, hosted in the higher planes. It therefore embodies a pattern of its own and as such is not emotionally charged – it is only mental and so the angels follow a programme of observing everything that goes on in creation. They are precise recorders of every event and experience, and because of their mental focus, never waver from this undertaking. So, an angel does not share the experience what we have; it can only observe. On Earth and other planets, angels are always present to record everything that happens. Every human has an angelic recorder who observes and notes everything that takes place. It is through this pattern of extensive recording that angels build up an understanding of experience, and once they have worked through this pattern, they then usually incarnate into Earth for one lifetime only. Having observed everything in matter, they have an opportunity to experience it in one life before returning to the Seventh Plane.

It is rare to come across an angel in matter and the pattern of one angelic life is also rare. At the same time, the angels are never able to see the face of God. They constantly feel the reverberations of His Actions and Will, but are never able to look God in the face. Everything they see is therefore a reflection of the Father's Will. This is a point of significant limitation for angels, and there is a constant "desire" to push beyond this limitation and see the face of the Father.

The angelic realms, therefore, hosts a unique pattern of ordered energy that acts as an evolutionary counterbalance to the more chaotic, slower frequency light of the lower planes. The pattern of angelic light also acts as a homing signal for more advanced souls who are journeying back up through the inner planes utilising the human vehicle. The angelic focus tends to pull them up, and acts almost as an opposing force to the downward drag, or inertia of the devic light streams that host a more chaotic energetic focus.

The Devic Pull

If a soul is not woken up in the angelic realms, it will continue to drop down through the planes, cloaking itself in different subtle vehicles that reflect the different streams of light. The Fifth and Sixth Planes are principally composed of mental light, and once a soul passes through these, it will begin to come into contact with slower, frequency, denser astral light. This begins in earnest in the Fourth Plane, which is also known as the Plane of Transition. More and more experience is gathered in this process, and with the descent through each sub-plane, the pattern of light becomes heavier and heavier. The soul then cloaks itself with denser vehicles of awareness, like multiple layers of experience. The inertial pull of the lower planes is in full flow, and there is an inevitability about the way in which each soul passes through the Fourth, then the Third and the Second Planes. The soul gathers more and more information about these different levels and builds up stronger vehicles of interpretation. These subtle bodies begin to reflect the denser pattern of astral light, and by the time the soul reaches the Second Plane, the flow of light is much heavier and slower than the Fifth Plane or above. The gravitational pull of the lower planes continues to call to the young soul and after passing through the First Plane it eventually enters the dense and heavy Zero Plane. This gravitational pull is like a magnetic desire that builds up in the soul. As it passes through each plane, there is a magnetic pull towards matter, initially from the mental into the emotional, and then from the emotional into the etheric and the physical.

The analogy of the soul passing down through the planes is not dissimilar to a stone dropping from the surface of the Ocean, all the way to the bottom. Although the stone does not gather extra layers of experience, it does pass through many levels of different temperature and salinity until it enters the deep abyssal realms where no light enters from above. Eventually, the stone drops to the very bottom and comes into contact with the silt where it comes to rest. Similarly, the soul's journey passes down through the darkness of the Zero Plane and hits the very bottom – at 0.0 – where it enters the physical discourse of evolution. It is at this point that the energetic drag forces the soul to adopt a physical vehicle of awareness through the focus of its understanding at that point in time. It may have taken vast swathes of inner time to reach this point, and the soul may have progressed through myriads of experiences to get to this point, cloaking itself in multiple vehicles of awareness; but it is only here, at the bottom of the Zero Planes, that the soul is able to enter physical matter and engage in a whole new pattern of experience. The soul will, in effect, be one of fourteen aspects, since the segregation into seven aspects, and then fourteen, will have taken place in the higher planes. Yet each aspect will have been through its own unique journey and will have collected sufficient experience to enter the next phase of development. And not all of the aspects will reach this point at the same point in their inner expression – there will be one aspect that goes ahead of the others, rather like a scout, to gather, first hand, new information.

By the time it reaches this point, the soul will have gathered millions of subtle vehicles, each one a representation and expression of its journey down through the different planes. Each vehicle is like a memory, a record of all that it has experienced. The soul aspect is still unconscious, yet has gained a whole host of different impressions. It now has to clothe itself in a diversity of different types of light. Within the Zero Plane, the pattern of light is very dark and chaotic and the overriding creative impulse is for disorder. It is at this point that the soul enters the pattern of light and expression that is called the Devic Realms. The Devic Realms, in contrast to the Angelic Realms, manifests disorderly or chaotic energy and always seeks to gather more and more experience, irrespective of what that experience is. The Devic Realms has its principal focus within the Mineral, Plant and Animal Kingdoms, although the devic presence imbues all physical form, including planets and stars. It provides the background, frictional focus of light that holds all matter together. It is an expression of life that is fundamentally different from what we, as humans are used to, although we ourselves retain within us a whole diversity of different devic patterns, from the smallest cell, right up to the collective expression of our devic essence.

Just as a segregation took place within the Angelic Realms, a similar crossover junction occurs in the Devic Realms. Some soul aspects will pass through the Mineral, Plant and Animal Kingdoms, prior to entering the human form. They will, in effect, pass through the devic expression as part of their developing experience. Their awareness will ride through the different patterns of devic expression, and with each new vehicle of awareness, each new form or body that they inhabit, they will build up more experience of devic life and devic light.

Other souls may focus exclusively on the devic pattern of energy and continue to gather massive swathes of experience within the devic pattern of light alone. They will not enter the human form but will continue to explore a whole host of different vehicles of awareness from the smallest grain of sand, right through to the largest planet or star, building up an active intelligence and consciousness within a different series of evolutionary threads.

On a grander scale, the play of chaos and order reflected respectively by the Devic and Angelic Realms constitutes a principal pattern of balancing: the chaos of the devic calls to souls coming down into matter and gives a diversity of primary experiences. The devic provides an impetus for souls to come into matter. Then, on the eventual return journey, the call of the angelic will help older souls move towards a more ordered pattern. The devic pulls down while the angelic pulls up.

CHAPTER 7

The Early Root Races

The Wheel of Life

Each soul, as it begins its reincarnatory programme through the physical realms, working with the different kingdoms, will also explore the outer expression of physical form on other planetary systems apart from Earth. Once the Primary Spark ignited all of Creation, then the unfolding pattern manifested what is known as the Wheel of Life. It is the sum total expression of the diversification of all the planets and stars within the creative mould of multiple Universes birthed by the Father. It is absolutely vast, almost limitless and contains within it the expression of everything within the framework of cosmic and galactic evolution. Although physically based, the different planets and stars vibrate to a series of higher or lower frequencies, some of which are focused physically, some astrally, and others more mentally. So the Wheel also circumscribes a series of different levels of experience, from the very refined, through to the very gross, and so although we may think that our Earth is quite gross, there are other levels of reality that vibrate at a lower frequency.

At the centre of the Wheel is Earth, the finishing school for souls, and like the reflection of the one permanent atom split into three, Earth is split into two more Earths. The central Earth, with fifty percent head and fifty percent heart supports two mirrors of itself, each embodying the law of opposites. Radiating out from the central Earth, there are eighteen thousand spokes, each leading to another version of Earth. This gives a further eighteen thousand Earth-like planets where life can exist and gather experience. Outside of these planets, there is an outer hub of planets that will only house one or two key frequencies. So for example, a planet may only retain gaseous form, while on another planet the expression of life may only be vegetative, supporting limited types of plants. All of these planets and stars host a multiplicity of different life forms.

Evolving souls will start their journey at the outer rim of the Wheel and progressively work their way through towards the centre, until eventually they have earned the right to incarnate on the planet of free will and choice, the central Earth. Each pattern of development will present the soul with a series of frequencies experienced in different levels of awareness, all designed to provide a platform of diversification. The Earth itself houses a huge diversity of frequencies and so the average number of lifetimes for any soul to work on other planets is around ten percent, although this number can vary significantly according to the type of soul trajectory undertaken, and the type of experiences gained in other physical vehicles.

The Wheel of Life has evolved through the interplay of chaos and order. Earth was not always at the centre and in its more primitive state, the Wheel housed fewer stars and planets. Yet with each new layering and unfolding, the Wheel has been built up into what it is today. To look at it is to recognise its awesome immensity and to feel the pulse of all living forms contained within it. The Wheel also rotates in a specific direction, like a reflection of the dance between chaos and order.

The Planet of Free Will and Choice

Following aeons of time, a decision was taken by the Creator Gods, who sought to copy the pattern of creation first orchestrated by the Father, to build a planet of free will and choice. Stellar and planetary development had followed the dictates of chaos and order as first laid out in the template of self-discovery with the formation of the Wheel of Life. The Wheel was not always the way it is today, and had followed a pattern of evolution where the complexity of life gravitated towards the centre. Throughout this process many souls had gathered multiple layers of experience through the different planes and formations of matter. Yet there was one ingredient that always appeared to be missing: free will. Souls could never experience true free will and choice due to the way in which chaos and order were orchestrated: the outcome was always predictable from the perspective of the Creator Gods. Similarly, from the perspective of the soul experiencing the different interplays of chaos and order, there was always the certain inevitability about the outcome.

One way to envisage this pattern is to take the example of weaving a tapestry. At the start, there are two principal colours that can be woven – black and white. With time, a pattern is made out of these two colours. Then, the weavers discover that they can make more colours out of these two principal frequencies: for example, white can be split into seven principal colours, like the colours of the rainbow. And black can also be split into a series of complementary colours. Suddenly there is much greater choice. However, the design template for each tapestry remains limited and is structured according to the old pattern of white and black. The designs are limited and predictable.

It is at this point that a shift has to occur: a shift where the old designs are thrown away and a new pattern where a whole novel range of designs can be introduced that incorporate all the different colours. To explore the vast range of possibilities, all restraint within the context of the old has to be removed. The true potential of design diversity can only be satisfied if the designers and weavers are allowed true freedom of expression: the removal of all limits to creativity and choice. In this situation, the patterns will become much more sophisticated, creative and unpredictable with a massive diversity in the colour mixing.

So it was the Creator Gods recognised the need to give creativity and freedom of choice to those in matter and experience. The original patterns of chaos and order had led to an exploration of light and dark according to certain dictates and parameters. However, once more diverse frequencies had been unearthed in these two primary forces, then a broader range of frequencies was released: like the discovery of colours within the original twin frequencies. However, since creation and development was still experienced according to a particular blending of chaos and order, it eventually became apparent that there was an inherent limitation within form: everything developed along predictable lines of evolution through the interplay of chaos and order, even though there was now a greater diversity of frequencies.

For example, there exist worlds where everything is gaseous – where life is gaseous and where the main focus of expression is in the form of clouds. These clouds will move in and out of the planetary atmosphere and will gather experience as a cloud. On one level this is limited, because if the cloud was taken out of that planet and put on a planet that had oceans and land, then the experiences gained as a living cloud would be more varied.

The challenge at that time was to gather more experience, to push through the existing limitations of form and predictable outcomes. What was required was something that was different: where experience and life could flow along new patterns of creativity, where choice could arise to allow more to evolve. Just as the designers and weavers wanted new patterns to express their creativity, the Creator Gods decided to find a new formula that would allow the birth of something more: and that something more was free will and choice.

One of the principal protagonists in this call for more was an ancient being known as Macheldavek. Macheldavek was a primary administrator and one of the principal Creator Gods that had been present since the original creative impulse had birthed something new. Macheldavek, unlike many of the Creator Gods, had also been into matter and so had experienced, first hand, the assets and limitations of the ongoing pattern of creation. Macheldavek had petitioned for a fresh start where something more could be invoked and birthed within the creative pattern.

Following the agreement to birth something different within the creative pattern, Macheldavek was chosen to orchestrate and develop a place where choice could be invoked. He was given the role of overall administrator for the birthing, development and maturation of a planet of free will and choice, a planet that eventually became known as Earth. From the outset there was substantial interest in the project and many different life forms petitioned to be included in the setting up of the new planet. Macheldavek carefully selected a place where the experiment could be set up free from interference. A place in space that was out of the way was selected and through the focus of devic intent and creativity, the beginnings of matter and substance were drawn together through time and space to birth a new planet. The seeding was initiated through an average sized star, and the doorways were established to allow the flow through of a new pattern of energy.

From a purely physical point of view, the planet was formed through the aggregation of minute particles of matter, that were drawn together through attraction, and which, with time, grew into lumps of matter. As this process gathered momentum, the small lump of matter grew, attracting to it, larger and larger lumps of interstellar gases and particles. While the lump of rock grew into a fledgling planetoid, and then ultimately into a planet, the process of devic birthing as manifested through the two principal elements, Fire and Earth[1] unfolded. Heat was generated through the build up of matter, which in turn led to the development of a molten core and the gradual formation of solid matter.

Gaia and Macheldavek

As the planet was born, Macheldavek as the principal administrator took the unprecedented step of birthing something more within the planet. While his focus, in energetic terms, was more masculine than feminine, it was clear that for true creativity and choice to be born, then the focus of the planet needed to be feminine. He then took a dramatic creative step – he effectively split himself into two. This splitting is similar to the splitting at the soul level, of one of the seven aspects into two further aspects. These two aspects, which are twin flames, then have a unique energetic pattern. Macheldavek effectively did this – he birthed his twin, the feminine aspect, and placed this aspect of himself into the fledgling planet to live the dream. In this process, Macheldavek the administrator, remained the masculine focus, overseeing all the requirements of the planet's development, while his twin, the feminine aspect became the living essence of the planet, the feminine, creative principle, the new doorway for planetary evolution. This feminine twin was called Gaia.

A unique dance of light and dark was birthed between Gaia and Macheldavek in the planet's creative flow from that moment on. Their love and focus was unique since they were twin flames, and the unfolding pattern of evolution, history, experience of the planet and all subsequent life forms on it, was a direct reflection of the dance between Gaia and Macheldavek.

Once Macheldavek had birthed Gaia as his twin, the focus of change was initiated. The parameters for the expression of free will and choice were agreed and ultimately set out through a series of experiments in form and matter. At the start, the planet eventually developed into its current size, and was rather like an unploughed field. Different devic forces had created the planet's crust and core, through Fire and Earth. As a living sentient being, the planet slowly grew in awareness. In Gaia, the original pattern of light was focused through purity and innocence, and like a young child, Gaia slowly mastered the different experiences of planetary development. Early on there was a collision with another planetoid, followed by the creation of the moon in an orbit around the planet. Energetically speaking, this was similar to birthing a shadow, a presence that tracked the planet's movement and motion, and which with time, built up another flow of energy.

Other devic patterns were birthed, through Water and Air. The first oceans were developed through the production of different gases through volcanic eruptions and solar radiation, and in combination with the development of an atmosphere, the element Air manifested a living envelope around the planet. Once the four elements, Fire, Earth, Air and Water had given birth to a new pattern of devic expression on the planet, then the real business of seeding a new pattern of understanding and knowledge was ready to begin.

The plan for creating a new pattern where free will and choice could exist and ultimately flourish was simple, yet profound. It was to create limitation through an array of frequencies, and yet allow, within that limitation, the expression of free will and choice to build up a diversity of experiences. The fundamental building blocks of limitation were based on two principal components – the creation of artificial time, and the development of the laws of karma. By creating an artificial pattern of time, this would allow souls to experience in matter, a directed flow of energy from the past, into the present and through to the future. Each soul would, in effect, be segregated in time: experiences would be collected like quanta of time and could then be recorded as part of a developing pattern. Through segregation in time, souls could then experience limitation in different ways – through living in the present, rather than living out of time, in a timeless, eternal present, where there is no past or future, they could begin to explore new patterns of being. By experiencing life in one timeline or another, it would then be possible to build up a series of possible timelines; a series of timelines where each soul was given a choice of which timeline to experience. So time was used as a standard mechanism of experimentation where the assets and limitations could be explored through experience.

The second, key pillar of limitation was built around the laws of karma, which were derived, in the first instance, from Natural Law. At its simplest, Natural Law, is the manifested Will of the Father for all living things to experience life, in all its different ways. However, with the new planet, the laws of karma were built up to provide further layers of limitation, while still providing enough flexibility to allow the principles of free will and choice to be invoked. The laws of karma dictate that for every act, every thought, every emotion, there has to be a balancing principle. If someone has a negative thought about another person, then energy is created. At some point or other, this energy has to be balanced. It is this continual pattern of creating and destroying karma that provides the backcloth against which free will and choice can be invoked. Every soul aspect is presented with a choice, and from that choice, a series of consequences will flow. Since karma entails conscious or sub-conscious judgement, then it forms a testing ground within which free will can develop.

The young planet, then, provided a unique opportunity for developing souls and soul aspects to experience more; to experience free will and choice within a pattern of limitation, that would allow each to soul to discover more about itself, and to explore the very nature of experience through separation and limitation. Gaia represented the door to the planet, where life would eventually grow and flow. To enter the planet was to agree to a contract that would involve the laws of time, the laws of karma, and Natural Law. And for each soul that agreed to these conditions, then their tour of duty would be long or short depending upon the choices that were made in matter. However, having engaged with the planet, every soul would have to follow through the various pathways of experience before it could move on. As the experiment developed, though, it became clear that to explore the variety of experiences that could be invoked through free will lent itself to a much longer period of incarnation in the planet than some soul aspects might have chosen.

Another underlying principle of the planetary experience was that energy always followed thought. Since thought was the initial expression of the creative urge following separation from the Divine Ocean and dropping into the shadow planes, it followed that the pattern of life on the new planet had to follow this principle. The four elements of devic expression had created a new template for life; the challenge was to fill it with different patterns of form and matter; to create a series of plays, where different sparks of thought could be invoked to create a different series of experiences.

Since every spark was in some way derived from the Primary Spark, then the limitations of karma and time provided a backcloth against which each soul could eventually build into a flame of understanding. As each individual will developed, then that flame was able to birth wisdom that could take it from understanding through to knowledge. In this way, the different patterns of free will and choice could be built upon experience, starting with the flow of information that leads to understanding, and then into knowledge. Knowledge could then be used as a platform to invoke decisions within the context of free will. Ultimately, the flow of energy would build into wisdom followed by common sense so that the full expression of experience could be manifested in the balance of the moment to make the appropriate choices.

On one level, it would be easy to ask what is the point of this? And the simple answer is that every soul, once born, has a primordial urge to explore and experience; to put each and every experience into a context where it can learn more about itself; to use every experience as a means of understanding more about the initial separation. Flowing out of this drive is the manifestation of devic light. Devic light, unlike the flow of angelic light, manifests chaos; this is central to the dance of chaos and order in the physical. Chaos always seeks to create more chaos, and in the context of life and matter, this is embodied in the constant pursuit of more experience: it does not necessarily matter what that experience is, just so long as there is more of it. Consequently, all souls, when they enter the planet, seek experience in as many diverse ways as possible. To this end, they will adopt different vehicles of awareness to give substance to the urge to experience more. So, as each soul aspect comes into contact with a different layer of energy, it will experience a thought, and because energy follows thought, it will seek to develop a vehicle of form that can pick up the response to that thought or series of thoughts. In other words, because energy follows thought, each soul aspect has to generate vehicles to engineer experience around what the thought brings. For example, our body is an experience biologically that has been engineered by thought to produce an external and an internal point of reference in that which is termed life. And life is all part of the Divine Game, or Grand Game, that was set up by the Father.

As life seeks to understand more about itself, and to develop more complex ways to experience form and matter through different vehicles of awareness, there is always another fundamental limitation that cannot be pushed through: that it is impossible to fully understand what the Divine Game is because it is the Father's Game, and not our game. In other words, we are always put in a place of fundamental limitation because we can never understand everything, because in all thought that is generated in the planes of illusion, and in all the different vehicles that we develop to harvest and build our awareness, there is always an inherent limitation at its core. And this limitation is pre-built into all experience. It is only when we go outside of that experience, and ultimately back into God that we can then supersede or overcome that limitation. And even then, there are always likely to be further veils of reality that can be looked though as part of the never-ending flow of what the Father Is.

The Creative Play

Once these patterns of limitation had been engineered into the fabric of existence in the planet, preparations were then complete to move onto the next step in the creative play. Each of these limitations described above represented ways in which the planetary soil, or planetary fabric of experience, were ploughed in readiness to receive the new seeds of life that would give birth to something new. All souls entering the planet were given free will and choice: the choice to choose anything within their experience according to the laws of time and karma, and in accordance with an agreed set of starting conditions. These starting conditions represented the developing flow of energy and thought that came to be known as the root races.

A root is often defined as a part of the plant that is below ground, yet which supports and provides nourishment to the plant. It also means the basic cause, or origin. In the context of the creative play, it means both: the underlying structure which provides support for the tree of life, and the origin of a separate play or pattern of thought experience that is then cultivated and harvested through awareness. Once the planet had been prepared, or ploughed, it was then time for an agreed programme of seeding to be initiated. The conditions for growth and the types of seeds that were planted represented, in their own unique way, a root race. Macheldavek represented the first farmer to sow the seeds of life through his twin Gaia, who was the doorway for all life to be birthed on the planet, through a variety of different forms. The starting conditions for these different forms were all agreed within the context of the Grand Game, and then set in motion according to Natural law and the local rules.

In effect, the planet was ready to host an entirely new pattern of life and experience through free will and choice. This was something that had never been done before, and was orchestrated through the developing pattern of planetary evolution and growth. Consequently, as the planet was birthed through a series of devic pulses, otherwise known as Fire, Earth, Air and Water, the conditions for seeding new life on the planet were invoked through thought; and since energy follows thought, these new forms were birthed according to the needs of the moment.

The first set of starting conditions brought into existence the thought of a root race, which in turn was then birthed according to the needs of the energy; the initial impulse or thought went out, which in turn led to a response, and which then led to the formation of a vehicle of experience that could respond to that response. In this way, a developing pattern of energy was established which ultimately gave rise to different vehicles of living expression that could hold the energies as they arose, and which could provide, in accordance with the agreed rules, a series of choices that could be invoked and responded to.

Each set of staring conditions and manifestations would give rise to a series of outcomes; each outcome would be the result of a series of choices and decisions taken by form   Consequently, each root race would be open ended, and once the decision had been made to birth one root race, then depending on the results of that particular creative play, then new plays could be invoked according to a different series of starting conditions, yet which could build upon the performance of the first play. In a way, a loose analogy would be a sketchbook — we make a sketch, but are dissatisfied with it, sketch it again and are still not satisfied, and then sketch it again. Each time a sketch is made we learn more by association. And if we think of these sketches as one separate one on each page in going from the initial sketch to where we are now in human form, then we see a pattern of form that develops all by itself, in the same way that the rapid flicking of the sketches gives a cartoon.

So our human body today is the current local fashion and each root race has hosted different fashions. Earlier on the vehicle was a very loose structure that developed by association as life gathered experiences that performed a pattern of energy that came and went.

The devic pattern of form that had birthed the planet also acted as a magnet to attract in different patterns of life. Gaia was the bridge or doorway and gave birth to these forms within her principal of creativity and life, while on the higher planes, Macheldavek acted as the administrator and central doorkeeper to the developing planet. He oversaw the flow and flux of different life forms into the planet and negotiated the different starting conditions for each root race according to the essence of Higher Will.

In essence, then, each root race was a living experiment that was established according to a series of starting conditions that give rise to different interpretations of life. Each interpretation or vehicle of expression was built around the underlying need to express life and to develop different abilities to collect information, and to interpret this information according to the different types of vehicle that were engineered, as a response to these principal needs or requirements. In a fundamental way, the form built up during each root race was open ended; the starting conditions were agreed and set out, but then the focus of thought and energy could build upon that basic format, and give rise to something more according to the rules of free will and choice.

The Adamic Root Race

In the First Root Race the underlying template of birthing form and matter in a vehicle of consciousness was introduced as the initial thought or spark in the mental planes. The initial thought, to birth a vehicle that could receive and record impressions was formed within the matrix of the developing planet. The planet was not like it is at present, composed of a surface of oceans and continents. Rather the expression of planetary development reflected the gaseous and liquid composition of devic form. The molten fire and earth-like components were being refined while the liquid and gaseous aspects of form were being created. Consequently, the frequency vibration of mental light that was invoked, through thought, as a template for consciousness, had to give rise to form which, ultimately, could touch some of the lower planes that were being manifested in matter.

While the devic flow of form building was taking place through the dance of the four elements, the initial flow of seeding new life into the planet started with a thought, or an urge in the mental planes, and which then, through a succession of subsequent thoughts and responses, slowly filtered down through the mental planes, until it could begin to touch the lower grade of physical matter. This life did not appear in any way that was familiar to us; it was more gaseous and composed of mental light and so, from a physical perspective, would have appeared invisible. These vehicles of consciousness, each one hosting a soul aspect, slowly and inexorably cloaked themselves in feeling, as they invoked the pulse of light and dark. Each form developed a sense of feeling, yet could not build any understanding of orientation or any of the senses that today we would regard as normal, such as sight or smell.

Nevertheless, within the thoughts that were generated in the Adamic Root Race, the initial impulses that would give rise to later versions of physical form were laid down. The Adamic Root Race represented the start of free will and choice, where the dance between the angelic and devic forms would unfold and where the templates for subsequent life were initially negotiated.

Many souls would explore the first dawning of form and substance through the vehicles invoked in mental light; and as these vehicles grew in experience, they then came to touch the lower levels and condense into something different. Today, the energies that were formed in the Adamic Root Race are like a small whisper and have all but been absorbed by the later root races; no energetic counterpart exists in our awareness. Similarly, the play of light and dark frequencies that went through this First Root Race is no longer present. It is almost as if this root race never existed; the energies and experiences have all but been erased from the collective memory of the planet.

In one respect as the planet grew and developed, then the Adamic Root Race occupied a large expanse in planetary time; eventually, however, a pattern of change was invoked that called for the end of the race and for the initiation of a new race. Form, in the Adamic dance, had exhausted the different permutations in the mental streams and it was time to invoke a new pattern of life that could entertain and connect with the lower and denser grades of form and matter.

The Hyperborean Root Race

The pattern of change that was initiated at the end of one root race and at the start of the next, was to dispose of and remove the old form and leave a small percentage of the old form, as the starting mechanism for the new root race. At the end of the Adamic Root Race, approximately two percent of the existing form was retained and used as a template for the new form. By this time, the pull of the lower planes, particularly the astral levels, sent out a pulse to the developing root race. The older vehicles were replaced by a different type of body that was capable of experiencing grosser levels, such as the astral levels; this represented the birth of emotional sensations that has developed to such a level in us today. An emotional layer that held and retained astral light was added to the pre-existing mental layers. The form was much grosser than the Adamic, and bridged the gap between the mental and etheric. The sense of feeling was amplified, through the astral, although other senses such as hearing and seeing were still absent. Again, within, the purely physical realms, the Hyperborean form would have been invisible to our current, naked eye.

During this period of planetary history, the gaseous and liquid forms had settled down, so that greater balance and a building interplay between the four elements were invoked. As the Hyperborean Race built its vibration, then the developing vehicles of awareness pushed through the astral and into the etheric, where a conscious bridge with the physical, gross plane was almost established. The form of the Hyperboreans was quite gross and cumbersome, yet not really physical in the sense that we would understand that term.

This root race developed the template for the future physical form in a more substantial way and by the end of it the new vehicles could ride the different levels from the mental, down through the astral and into the physical. But just as with the Adamic Root Race, the pulse of light that was generated during this period is no longer with us. Different streams of energy were generated by this root race including a more dynamic pattern of light and dark, than in the Adamic. However, the succeeding root races absorbed and cleared most of the frequencies generated by the Hyperborean Root Race. Consequently, there is little residual information remaining in the planet at this time.

Both the Adamic and Hyperborean Root Races established a pattern for developing vehicles of consciousness that could also host different cycles of light and dark. Each root race carried its own particular permutation, thereby reflecting the ongoing interplay of chaos and order. While the principles of higher mental light represent more order than chaos, each root race experienced a wash of chaotic and ordered energy within its developing pattern. The formation of an initial vehicle of consciousness required an interplay between angelic and devic; as each root race developed, this would manifest in different ways, and as the vehicles pushed down through the slower layers to touch either the astral or etheric, then additional layers of slower frequency light were woven into the fabric of experience and expression. In a sense chaos became more dominant through time; yet within each root race there was also an underlying pattern of a different kind of light.

The light and dark that worked through the Adamic Root Race was not as powerful as was pushed through the Hyperborean Root Race. More virulent streams of light and dark were needed to bring the physical into fruition, and in each root race a different percentage of light and dark was invoked. The initial birthing in physical matter required a greater percentage of dark light. These changing patterns were part of the starting conditions for each root race, and as form grew stronger, then it could support a more virulent octave of light and dark within the different physical vehicles that came to be developed. Consequently, by the end of the Hyperborean Root Race, the stage was set to bring through a very different pattern of light and focus.

Throughout these two root races, which covered vast stretches of time, the focus and interplay between Gaia and Macheldavek grew. From time to time, the twins would meet through the existing form prevalent in that period, to invoke a new ritual and a new energetic pattern. Gaia would host both light and dark within her essence, and while form would dance through her awareness, Gaia began to enter different types of dreams. It was like each dream represented the different patterns of energy that would flow through the various stages of each root race. Sometimes the dream was light and sometimes the dream was dark. However, it was only when the vehicles of consciousness took on the full manifestation of physical form that the true dance between light and dark would become apparent.

CHAPTER 8

The Late Root Races

The Lemurian Root Race

The focus of all root races is to develop consciousness in matter. The early root races established a platform, within the subtle levels, for the full development of physical form in the planet that was to follow in the later root races. The first of these races is known as the Lemurian, and it was the first instance where the full physical shell was developed. The focus of light held within the starting mechanism of this race spanned principally the First and Zero Planes. This reflected the pattern of light necessary to establish and support the manifestation of physical matter. The Lemurian Root Race hosted primarily black light, up to ninety percent, thereby providing support for the physical development of the human life form. It is important to recognise that this dark light was relatively untainted, and it was only in the later part of the Lemurian Root Race and in the subsequent Atlantean Root Race that this pattern of dark light was used for more negative and feudalistic purposes.

The Lemurian Root Race supported several divergent patterns of human life. The main creative focus was undertaken by beings that lived underground in caves. The physical shell supported a chakra system, although it was not as well developed as that of today. The physical vehicle also hosted physical DNA. Initially their third eyes were well developed, while other senses such as hearing, touch and feeling were also dominant. Visual sight was not developed at first, and only came in towards the end of the Lemurian period. The cave-dwelling Lemurians sharply contrasted with the surface-dwelling human-like beings that were more cro-magnon in appearance. The cro-magnon forms were aggressive and more animalistic in behaviour, in sharp contrast to the more docile cave dwellers.

As the Lemurian Root Race unfolded, a massive network of underground caves was established below the surface. The cave-dwelling Lemurians also experimented with DNA manipulation, seeking to engineer out any vestiges of aggressive behaviour. At the same time, they built up a culture of creativity, where the focus was on story telling, art and music, although the forms were rather different from what we would recognise today. As their third eyes developed, the programme of DNA engineering also explored telepathy and the ability for everyone to experience a collective telepathy.

Initially the experiments to engineer out aggression and fear were successful, while the telepathic focus built throughout the underground inhabitants. This telepathic focus allowed everyone to be part of a collective energy or field and was distance regulated. If someone strayed too far from the group, then the telepathic pulse would drop away; if they were in close proximity, then it was much stronger. Consequently, there was always an urge for everyone to stay close together.

Above ground, other large life forms also walked on the planet surface, including the dinosaurs. The dinosaurs tended to act as the guardians to the cave entrances, preventing the more aggressive surface dwellers from coming into the caves.

Throughout the early and middle Lemurian periods, the focus on building a creative focus grew. Art was experienced holographically and telepathically — which means that if we looked at a painting today within the Lemurian context, then we would actually feel ourselves inside the painting, living the Lemurian experience of the painting within our awareness and consciousness. The holographic component also spoke to a collective pattern of experience. In addition, the telepathy would tie us in with the original artist so that we would live some of the imaginative flow that was involved in creating the art in the first place. Creative art to the Lemurians was a living, dynamic process where the true essence of what was being formed was a lived experience. On one level, the closest that we come to experiencing something like this today is watching a film on a giant IMAX screen, wearing glasses that make the film appear in three dimensions. We feel that we are actually present in the film.

During the Lemurian Root Race there was also an infusion of new frequencies that came to be known as the crystal skulls. The crystal skulls were introduced into the planet by a group of blue, crystalline star beings. These beings held a high frequency pattern of crystalline energy and were involved in the creation and birthing of these divine holograms. The crystal skulls represented patterns of light and dark, and each one was like an amplification device. They were also part of the Third Root Race hologram of light and so reflected the unfolding probabilities of this root race in its entirety. The purpose of the skulls was also to give a boost to the energetic flow of light within the planet, and to provide a seeding mechanism that had initially been created in the Seventh Plane. There were twelve primary light skulls and twelve primary dark skulls. The main focus was on the light skulls and as the Lemurians developed their third eyes and telepathic skills, they were able to establish a platform of frequencies in each of the skulls. Each skull also vibrated according to a specific colour, such as green or blue and would embody certain qualities of light. Each embodied a living hologram of the race and through accessing these different crystal skulls, it became possible to gain access to the underlying energetic flow of the Lemurian Race. The light skulls also absorbed the essence of light that was built up by specific light practices.

Creativity and telepathy were the hallmarks of the Lemurian dream. However, after some time, it became apparent that the energetic and DNA manipulations that had been made were not permanent. The engineered energetic pattern was built on a balance between light and dark, or more specifically between the flow of chaos and order. To ensure that the manipulations would remain permanent, there had to be a perfect balance of chaos and order — fifty percent of each. However, the proportions infused into the underlying energetic matrix were slightly out of balance by a few percentage points.

Although generation after generation was born with telepathic skills, the underlying imbalance was slowly amplified until, eventually, the first generation was born that was no longer telepathic.

For the underground Lemurians this represented the beginning of the end. There was a dawning recognition that the telepathic experiment had failed and emotionally this set up a series of frequency notes that can be best described as the Lemurian Wail. The emotional fall out from this realisation was substantial, and the ruling council at that time determined that steps needed to be taken to preserve the higher frequencies of light that were the hallmarks of Lemurian creativity. A platform of energies was established using the crystal skulls. Three main skulls were used and each represented a particular focus, such as purity, innocence and unity. These three frequency notes then held within them, a series of sub-frequencies that hosted all of the telepathic and creative expertise that the Lemurians had collected over their long period underground. Each skull was also colour coded – blue, green and purple. These frequencies were then stored within a space outside of time that could be accessed at a later date, when the balance between light and dark would be in a different cycle, and when humanity would have gathered sufficient experience in matter to understand the different patterns of fear and aggression. Finally, access to these frequencies also demanded that there would be sufficient collective unity established through the higher notes of love.

Apart from the collective despair that was generated through the realisation that the experiment was doomed to failure, those babies that were born without the telepathic capabilities, also had to work through, in that lifetime, the frequencies of separation and rejection. Inevitably, there came a point in time when the continued survival of the race required that the underground Lemurians return to the surface of the planet to mix with their more aggressive cousins. Everyone knew what to expect and while the focus of the genetic manipulation had been to artificially remove the frequency of fear, the prospect of re-engaging with the dangerous surface environment led to the introduction of this frequency again. Purity and innocence were stripped away in one brutal episode. Despite these more negative consequences, the shift to surface living also brought about the introduction of visual sight in the race. The visual eye was formed and complemented the well-developed third eye in the race. The creative focus that had been built by the underground Lemurians had also created a well-developed sexual/creative chakra centre.

The shock and trauma generated by this re-mixing of races led to the eventual extinction of the passive Lemurians since they were no match for the aggressive surface dwellers. In this process, fear was introduced into the race in a more powerful way. Humanity would gain extensive experience in working with this frequency until eventually, there would come a time when the cycles of life would come full circle: back to a point where humanity would become saturated with fear and would therefore be in a position to build a different platform of unity that could once again, entertain the Lemurian dream.

Each root race, once it comes to the conclusion of its energetic pattern, usually entails a dropping away of form. This can be invoked through a variety of means such as natural disasters, asteroid collisions or diseases and famine. The old is destroyed to make for the new. Within this pattern, usually ninety-eight percent of form falls away from the pathway to the new root race, leaving only two percent to evolve and mutate into the new root race form. Within that two percent there is also a polarisation where some will manifest a conscious support for the change, while others will give sub-conscious support to the new energies and knowledge coming in. The end of the Lemurian Root Race conformed to this changeover, with only two percent of form being retained to usher in the new root race.

Despite the apparent failure of the Lemurian dream, there were several frequencies that would be keys to a future root race where much more could be birthed. At the same time, the Lemurian pattern of energy cleared away and processed much that was carried over from the previous two root races. Light and dark had also worked through the race according to different cycles of grace, and towards the end of the Lemurian Root Race, stronger patterns of dark light flowed into form.

The Atlantean Root Race

The Atlantean Root Race dawned full of hope and promise. As the dying embers of the Lemurian frequencies faded away a new cycle of grace was initiated in the planet. Unlike the Lemurian Root Race, which had supported ninety percent dark grace, the Atlantean Root Race was initiated with fifty percent light grace and fifty percent dark grace. Physical form was much more like what we would recognise today, with well-developed senses such as sight, hearing, touch, and taste. The physical body was also strong and the mineral nourishment from the planet's surface was more than sufficient to provide ample nutrition. Unlike today, where so many of the minerals have been stripped away from the soil, in the Atlantean times, the soil was rich in minerals and essential nutrients.

While the Lemurian Root Race had focused on the creative and artistic expression through form, the Atlantean Root Race concentrated on the generation of knowledge through scientific and rational means. At its height, the Atlantean Root Race was probably more technically developed than we are today by approximately one hundred years. Electricity, aerial flight, genetic engineering and organ transplantation were well established and the caves that had been crafted by the Lemurians were used for transportation between the different landmasses. Technical excellence and practical skill were the hallmarks of the Atlantean Root Race, although there remained those who were well versed in energetic management using the third eye and the other chakra centres. The crystal skulls were also utilised, both in light and dark sequences, and contributed to the development of crystal singers – those who could hold the high crystalline frequency notes and project them energetically for specific uses, such as healing and clairvoyance.

While the early Atlantean period was relatively light, it was during the middle and late stages that the flux of energy shifted so dramatically. New frequencies of light were introduced into the planet, and humanity was presented with a choice, based on the balance of light and dark grace. To either work with the light or with the dark. The ensuing vote was unanimously in favour of the dark, thereby hosting the promise of external and physical gratification through the manipulation of technical and scientific means. The energy that was introduced into the planet, instead of pushing up into the heart centre, was directed into the lower centres, predominantly the sexual centre and used in a direct and negative way. Very few souls actually escaped its influence.

The vote taken by humanity also brought a new presence into the planet. The dark song of negativity, selfishness, feudalism, abuse of power, cruelty and despair was overseen by a being known as Lucifer. He was invited to oversee the ritual of dark despair and this created the role of what today we would call the devil: a point of darkness, selfishness, hatred, anger, confusion and negativity that is pitted against the forces of light and love. The devil hosted the darkness, virulent and strong, issuing forth dark frequency notes and seeds. Dark sowed the seeds of hatred, torture, physical abuse, sexual deviancy, rage, pride, guilt and shame. All of these frequencies, which were already present in the emotional make up of humanity, were amplified to an extreme degree, and rode on the back of a blood lust that hounded the very depths of the human psyche.

In short, the Atlantean period plumbed the very depths of human existence and genetic manipulation and the creation of chimaeras was part of the total abuse of the human and animal form. The negative energy that was built up through the Atlantean Root Race was almost limitless and the invocation of dark light fuelled by the frequencies of negativity led to a period of total decimation in terms of light. The planet came to be shrouded in darkness and negativity and many of the problems that are experienced today are a direct result of the karma generated during the Atlantean time period.

Almost every soul aspect that walked on the surface of the planet at that time came to be tainted by the dark. In many cases, this tainting was more like a complete immersion. Many souls came to experience lives of unrivalled darkness and revelled in complete physical excess. The karma generated by each soul aspect in these times was massive and represented a series of giant black thorns that ultimately would have to be balanced and removed. Ignorance and fear became dominant and would continue to flow down the future timeline of humanity.

The Atlantean period also saw the perfection of twisted will; all forms of knowledge and understanding became tainted by the dark negativity that flowed through human form in abundance. The forces of light were driven underground. The dream of Gaia became dark as the night while the planet entertained and endured a living hell of negativity and darkness. Due to the principles of free will and choice, it was impossible for any active point of interference to take place. The dance of dark was left to run its course and as it became increasingly unbalanced, the outcome was inevitable. Layer after layer of dark was birthed in the later stages of the Atlantean excesses, and ultimately led to a feeding frenzy of virulent, negative energy. The end, when it came, was cataclysmic and total. Through tidal waves, volcanic eruptions, earthquakes only one real outcome was possible: the wholesale destruction of the Atlantean Root Race. The balance of light and dark had become too great and so the planet needed to set the record straight in the time honoured way.

It is important to understand that throughout this whole process, energy always follows thought. In the Atlantean time period, the thought was predominantly dark and negative, and eventually led to a major imbalance within the planet. Balance has to be restored according to karmic and natural law, through either the mental, emotional or physical levels of expression. In the case of Atlantis and the Atlantean saga, the destruction of physical form through a cataclysmic happening was part of the payment. With the exception of two percent of human life, physical forces destroyed the remaining Atlantean form. The repercussions of the Atlantean Root Race would impact humanity and the planet throughout the whole of the next root race.

The Aryan Root Race

If the Atlantean Root Race had represented the complete twisting of will and knowledge, the complete savouring by humanity, of excess and physical abuse, then the Aryan Root Race constituted the esoteric slap around the face for humanity. During the Atlantean Root Race, humanity had become drunk on the frequencies of dark light imbued with negative intent. Although the form had been destroyed, the next root race required a settlement of the dark account. Like an unruly youth who has become completely drunk, humanity required copious doses of black coffee and a regime of strict energetic management. The old energetic excesses of the Atlantean dark period were quashed and for most people, the third eye was closed. Multiple veils were drawn over the different levels of subtle awareness. Human form had to understand the limitations of the physical way and embrace a different pattern of living: ultimately through the laws of trust and faith. Yet within the laws of karma, this had to be achieved within the starting conditions that recognised all that had gone before.

Almost every soul that had incarnated during the Atlantean period had generated massive amounts of karma and these imbalances had to be ironed out in the fullness of time. Each incarnating soul would still have to run the gauntlet of light and dark and would be free to make choices. Yet the conditions for working through this karma were much stricter; potentially millions of lifetimes were required to clear much of this negative karma, and this had to be honoured under fluctuating patterns of light and dark. Dark still held dominance over the planet, and yet it would only be possible, through the laws of saturation to entertain a shift towards the light. Saturation means that a certain frequency such as loss or despair gets worked lifetime after lifetime. It is similar to eating too much chocolate or ice cream. Eventually, there comes a time when the body becomes saturated with the sugar and taste and is unable to eat any more. Desire turns to rejection and the old addictive pattern is eventually broken.

Working through karma is like focusing on all the old addictive practices. It is only through complete saturation that it becomes possible to let go of the old frequencies. Free will and choice have to be honoured; so every person has to consciously let go of the old practices of the dark and turn to embrace something new.

Consequently, in the Aryan Root Race, humanity had to be weaned off the old addictive practices of the dark, while at the same time working through its personal and collective karma. Wars, battles, violence, hatred, domination, feudalism all went hand-in-hand with this process of clearing and cleansing. Initially, this may seem counter-intuitive, but the laws of karma have to be observed and so those who wrought such havoc in the past, had to be presented again and again with the choices of light and dark, until eventually, the old addictive patterns could be flushed out.

The Aryan Root Race provided ample opportunity for this to occur. Physical power went hand-in-hand with a strong emotional focus, as part of the astral programme of clearing and cleansing. Through the excesses of the Atlantean time period, the astral levels had become completely polluted, and in the Aryan Root Race, the focus was primarily on the lower astral levels, where the most virulent patterns of negativity remained. The solar plexus chakra was more developed than in the Atlantean time, although the segregation of masculine and feminine energies ensured that there was a constant flow of emotional charges in each lifetime. While the masculine tended to focus on the mind, the feminine embraced the emotional side. Similarly, the starting conditions did not favour either the scientific or the creative too much. Rather the interplay between the two was established and today we can clearly see the pattern of the intuitive versus the rational, the creative arts versus the scientific focus.

Within the Aryan Root Race there has been the ebb and flow of different civilisations, the constant flux of dominance followed by rapid or slow destruction. As civilisations have come into dominance, the incoming soul aspects have generally been more experienced and have captured the flow of power that was required to ride the awareness and physical expression of those in matter, as each civilisation grew. For example – the Egyptians, the Greeks, the Romans, the Chinese, the Japanese dynasties – each civilisation has enjoyed a rich and powerful heyday, fuelled by physical strength, and has then subsided into mediocrity and powerlessness. The flux of power and weakness is clear to see. Power and feudalism, combined with ignorance and pride, have been part of the wash of dominant frequencies that have flowed through humanity. The karmic interplay between individuals, and societies has been experienced through multiple cycles of light and dark. In particular, the last twenty percent of this root race has specifically worked the negative patterns. And for the last four thousand years we have been in the Age of Kali, the Age of Destruction, which has manifested a quickening in time and a processing of old dark light. The pattern of light and dark has been twenty-five percent light and seventy-five percent dark. This has ensured that humanity has had the freedom to work through its past and to burn off old karma. This has all been part of the preparation of the next two percent that will form the new energetic platform for the next root race.

Major advances in the material world, such as the invention of gunpowder, have also contributed to the overall karmic interplay between human and animal. In the previous root races, human death at the hands of aggressive animals had been substantial, and it is only through the use of gunpowder that humanity could at last protect itself from dangerous animals. The factory-based slaughter of millions and millions of animals each year as part of our food industry is also linked to this rebalancing process, although the wastage in the West is again creating a karmic imbalance. The time will soon come when the flow of karma between human and animal is in a state of balance; the use of our animal brothers and sisters will then have to change completely.

The Aryan Root Race has, therefore, provided an opportunity for the karmic pattern of light and dark to become more balanced; where the old frequencies of dark despair and fear can be experienced within the constraints of a physical shell that has a strong, telepathic emotional base; and where the mental will and determination of humanity has been constantly eroded by the input of dark misinformation.

Spiritual practice has also evolved according to a specific pattern. While the different religious tides have been based on a succession of Avatars and the ritualistic embrace of certain frequency notes that were left behind, deeper spiritual practice has been carried out in isolation by small groups of people. These isolated practices came to be known in the past as the old mystery schools — the monks in Tibet are a good example. The reason has been simple: removal of all external distractions has allowed the freedom for individuals to look inside, and to build, through many lifetimes, an understanding of deeper spiritual practice. Too much external distraction would have overloaded the mind. At the same time, the spiritual practices have been closely guarded to ensure their secrecy and that the teachings remained in a close circle of the few who had earned the right to their instruction. These spiritual practices have necessitated the adoption of higher spiritual principles. In whatever way the culture framed these practices, the spiritual practice has been based on the laws of trust and faith, and on passing a series of initiations where the deeper fears of the initiate had to be confronted and overcome. Such practices ensured that those with the strength of will and courage could progress to the next stages. While this need for secrecy was very necessary in the past, this will not be the case in the future.

What we had in the previous root races, such as higher sight, has been lost in this root race. Multiple veils have been placed over our third eyes and only selected people in our societies have had the capacity to see on different levels, and to access the subtle realms. This has all been part of the very necessary limitation and constraint to minimise distractions. The situation is similar to the blinders that a horse will wear to ensure that it is not sidetracked by its peripheral vision. The horse can only look straight ahead. Similarly, the pattern of development in the Aryan Root Race has conformed to very strict limitations. The loss of third eye sight and other subtle senses was implemented to ensure a more balanced development within our physical, astral and mental awareness. The constraints of the Aryan Root Race have been extremely necessary as a filtering mechanism for what has gone before; and as part of the ritual of installing a greater degree of discipline.

During the Aryan Root Race, and in particular in its final stages, humanity has had to process and absorb the outstanding accumulated karma of the Lemurian and Atlantean Root Races. This has been a significant undertaking, where individual, group, national, planetary and solar system karma has to be balanced. For everyone this has been done either through the physical, or the emotional or the mental. If an individual has been unable to process their karma mentally or emotionally, then it has been done physically, either through illness or accidents. The planet is also balancing the old karma and the end of this root race marks a significant shift in the dance of love between Gaia and Macheldavek. Gaia has awoken from her multiple dreams and is settling up her final accounts, in preparation for a new union with Macheldavek. Old planetary karma is being brought to the surface for clearing and balancing, through multiple patterns of natural change and disasters.

The Aryan Root Race is now coming to a close, and the fundamental difference in this transition compared to all previous changeovers is that physical form is being retained. In previous root races ninety-eight percent of form was dropped, leaving the two percent to seed the new root race. This marks a significant break with the past and to ensure that this transition takes place effectively requires a major balancing of the karmic books. Since old form is being retained, everyone who remains on the planet has to clear his or her old karmic accounts. No one can pertain to the next root race with twisted will or a negative disposition of energy. The new energies will not allow it. At the same time, truth is disintegrating and the new timeline is forming, co-existing for a short period with the old timeline, before the process of transition from one root race to the next has been completed. Once this has been completed, then the old timeline will drop away.

Ark

Ark is one of the fundamental commodities that has been generated through the root races. Ark is lived experience that is gathered by all sentient beings and all life forms, whether under the focus of light or dark. Ark includes all of the experiences, covering the physical, emotional and mental expression, both conscious and sub-conscious, that has been built up over lifetime after lifetime of experience in matter. The richest form of ark is that gathered through the human experience, and when pushed through a light or dark cycle, can become quite virulent in terms of the lived experiences contained within it. For example, the rich vein of dark negativity that was driven by virulent intent during the Atlantean Root Race represents ark of a particular vintage that brings through a particularly potent lived experience. So, ark is a direct reflection of the life or series of lives that have been experienced; for example, whether the life was potent i.e. full of emotional and physical experiences lived through crises, or less potent such as in a resting life; whether that life was focused in light or dark. A dark life of virulent intent will generate more ark than a life lived subconsciously where the form was ridden by different levels of awareness.

Ark is not dissimilar to wine; each bottle of wine is built upon a particular vintage and through the growing conditions of the grapes; there are good years and poor years. So it is with ark: the vintage of ark can be potent or weak, can be strong and bitter, or occasionally sweet and sublime. For the most part, the ark that has been generated during the root races has been bitter reflecting the pattern of dark energy that it is composed of. And although there have been cycles of light and dark washing through the root races in different ways, each cycle will generate experience as ark of a specific vintage.

Ark can embody specific types of experience such as despair, pain, cruelty, fear or hatred; these different experiences can be mixed and combined to produce different lived experiences that can be absorbed by other life forms and beings on the inner planes. The type of experience, the timeline and the form that accumulated all combine to give each piece of ark its uniqueness.

Ark is a commodity. The five Perfect Masters are the primary farmers who harvest it from the shadow planes, absorbing it and then offering it to the Father as lived experience in matter. More advanced and experienced souls can also learn to generate and absorb ark in a variety of different ways. Once harvested by absorption, ark can then be used as a currency of experience on the inner planes. Souls that have not incarnated can acquire ark and through it live the experience without going into physical form. Divine beings also absorb ark and rather like a vintage wine can drink it and become drunk on the experiences. The more virulent the ark, then the better the vintage. Ultimately, however, it is the five Perfect Masters, the Avatar and the Father who will drink and absorb ark. For them, the quest is always to absorb ark that is new, potent and especially strong. So ark that holds virulent despair and other frequencies is a high value commodity on the inner planes.

Throughout the different cycles of grace that have permeated the very fabric of each root race, the forces of light and dark have played off each other in the continued quest for generating more ark. Each side has sought to build up a store of ark, rather like a series of vintage wine cellars. Through open and hidden challenges between the two sides, ark can be stolen, defended, destroyed or sold to the highest bidder. Whichever side has accumulated the greater amount of ark is usually in a better position for bargaining.

Ark, then, is one of the key commodities that have been generated through the succession of root races. Nor is it just limited to Earth. All of the lived experiences in the eighteen thousand Earths generate ark; ark from the Crab Nebula or the Pleiades will embody a particular vintage or quality, some of which is extremely ancient and potent. Ark can also be found in the other planets of the Wheel of Life. Each cycle of thought and expression that passes through each star system and planet will build ark, just as each cycle of light and dark will form ark that holds unique experiences. Ark can also be extremely ancient, dating back to the earliest pattern of lived experience in the Universe and like a rare vintage will be difficult to obtain. More recent ark may be more popular and easier to find; either way, ark is always unique and specific to the experiences held within its essence.

A major balancing of the karmic accounts is now taking place as the planet shifts from the Fifth Root Race into the Sixth Root Race. This can be seen in the speeding up of time and in the resultant speeding up of karma. Our life experiences, lived through our physical, emotional and mental patterns, are all becoming quicker. Each day can be a roller coaster of experiences that previously would take place over weeks or years. The astral levels are now completely open, and everything that has been hidden from view, especially in terms of negative energy practices, is being flushed to the surface into human conscious awareness. The rise in child abuse, child abduction, pornography, rages, genocide, bizarre diseases and more virulent infections, and other types of negativity are all part of this pattern. This pollution of many people's minds and hearts is due to the dense negativity that has to be cleared from the lower astral levels. Without the proper techniques for balancing and clearing, it is easy to become drowned in these gross, negative frequencies.

This clearing not only covers everything that has taken place in the Aryan Root Race, but also includes, as we have seen, all of the old karmic patterns from the Lemurian and Atlantean time periods. The Lemurian energies are pushed through the Atlantean, which in turn are pushed through the Aryan. All of the frequencies and energies from these root races are condensed into our individual and collective awareness, both consciously and subconsciously. The energy streams being collected and transmuted have to re-balance the root race accounts before the Sixth Root Race can truly get underway. This represents a massive amount of ark that has to be absorbed before being passed on through various intermediaries to the Perfect Masters for final processing. Everything is then offered to the Father as part of the return.

Another way of looking at this is to imagine each root race as a self-sustaining pattern in a tapestry; it is connected to the previous root race in the overall grand design yet within each root race tapestry there will be threads of light and dark, and many other frequencies. Some of the designs and schemes will appear very dark, while others will have patches of light. In essence, an energetic pattern has now been invoked which is leading to the bleaching and clearing of this old tapestry. Most of the patterns, with a few exceptions, are absorbed by the bleach until all that remains is a vast fabric of clear thread which is featureless, since all of the colours of the fabric will have been absorbed. The exceptions are those portions of the tapestry that held a creative light pattern – they have been retained and will be used for the future design. This is similar to what is now taking place; all of the old frequencies have to be absorbed and removed from the planet on all levels – mental, astral, etheric and physical in a grand clearing; cellular, individual, group and planetary. Once this has been completed and the astral levels have been cleared, then a new cycle of light and grace can begin. So, just as the pendulum has swung heavily into the dark in the past, it is now time for the pendulum to swing into the light. This time, though, it is with a difference, because the new pattern of light and dark that is being generated is profoundly different from the old.

CHAPTER 9

Devic Expression in Matter

The Devic Pulse

Devic life is like the form behind the substance or structure, although it is of itself, formless. Devic life is the superglue that holds everything together — from every atom and molecule, to complex molecule and cell; every organ, organism, living creature; every plant, animal and human; every mineral, rock, and continental plate. It is the essence within all aspects of the planet's physical form, from the gases in our atmosphere, to the presences within our volcanoes and to the elemental focus of water. The devic pattern is the living awareness that imbues absolutely everything within our physical world: it spans from the subatomic particle to the largest stellar cloud and supernova.

The devic life pattern is founded on slow moving energy and was birthed out of the initial pattern of chaos and order. As order expresses itself and comes into contact with the flow of chaotic energy, then the pulse of order creates a shape which is immediately filled by the devas. It does not matter what the shape is — whether it is a cell, a tree or a galaxy — the deva rushes in to fill the vacuum. As the deva goes into the substance of form, then this is a way in which order and chaos come together.

Chaotic energy seeks experience, and once the soul aspect finds itself in the Mineral Kingdom, it begins a slow process of experiencing the devic focus as broadly as possible. The light frequency in the Mineral Kingdom is extremely slow, comprised of approximately ninety-eight percent dark energy. It is never one hundred percent dark energy since this would mean that the form and all that inhabits it would cease to exist. The Mineral Kingdom is therefore a darker pattern of energetic expression that slowly builds an array of lighter frequencies through gross experience in matter. The devic flow of energy may feel slow and almost treacly, and within the apparatus of our interpretation may appear black, or dark brown or possibly dark green. Other frequencies are possible and as experience is gained in recognising the devic presence in different living forms, then the energetic sense may come across as something completely different.

Devic life has its own intelligence and understanding of the world around; devic life seeks to gather experience through riding the collective focus within different building blocks of physical expression. These building blocks can be like the minerals and rocks, or the plants and trees, through to the insects, fish and mammals. Devic life imbues all of these physical forms, and by gathering experience in each of these different substrates, builds up a massive amount of experience in matter. The diversity of devic expression in physical form is staggering, and yet it retains within its essence, a collective focus and an active intelligence.

Whatever we do, how we live our lives, involves at all times a negotiation and dialogue with devic life, irrespective of whether we are conscious of it or not. When we visit the woods, or move to a new place to live, devic presences are always around, and can either work sympathetically with us, or unsympathetically. If we go rock climbing, we are negotiating with the devic presence in the mountain. If that presence is unsympathetic then we may slip and fall. Whenever we eat food, we are absorbing the devic essence in that food. Humanity is generally blissfully unaware of this whole diversity of different life that exists right under our noses. The concept that there is an active consciousness and intelligence in rocks seems absurd, but once we start to open ourselves up to a different type of communication and experience, then it soon becomes apparent, that there is more than meets the eye. Devic presences in rocks can appear like faces, while in hedgerows and forests we sometimes feel that there are eyes looking out at us, although we cannot put our finger on what it is. This is all part of our connection with the devic expression. Of course, at one time, we have been through this pattern – it is just that we have completely forgotten what it was like.

The devas are also creators of physical form: they inhabit all physical form and through experience build up their own pattern of energy from the very small to the extremely large. The Earth, for example, started off as a few molecules of gas and dust, which slowly grew – the devic pattern built up from the small, until eventually after aeons of time, a whole new planet was formed. The devic pattern was then extremely large and housed one main devic presence within which existed millions and millions of smaller presences, each with their own level of awareness and consciousness. Each presence is collectively focused, yet separate within its expression.

Each soul aspect, when it arrives at the bottom of the Zero Plane, enters the devic pattern of life. Its awareness becomes magnetised to the devic pattern and it lives the devic experience in matter. Devic life therefore has active awareness and consciousness that, with experience, can build and build. Just as each soul has built up experience through its descent down the inner planes, it now begins a journey exploring the huge diversity of devic expression that is then manifested through the massive array of different physical life forms. The soul aspect will explore different streams of devic expression, starting off with the slowest and grossest, before graduating onto the quicker and more active devic streams in plants and animals. All the time, each soul aspect will use a huge range of physical uniforms, starting off with the simplest atom or molecule, before progressing onto larger and more complex vehicles of experience. Each uniform provides the means for the soul, as a devic presence, to build experience in matter. The devic pulse embodies a slow stream of light at first, and as this light pulses out, then information is gathered through the different energetic responses that come back.

Part of the experience is to allow the soul to experience the devic pulse – the pulse of devic light that is present in all matter. This pulse can be what is hosted within a small crustacean, such as a crab, or it can be held within the dance of a small flower, or it can be felt in the slow flow of energy in a rock formation. Whatever its origin, this devic pulse is the expression of devic life – it is the moment in the present when the devic expression is interacting and bridging the gulf between the soul experience and the physical experience. It is the expression in the now when all time stops and all that remains is a pulse of light – a pulse of life that hosts the essence of devic intent and devic expression. To feel this pulse is to tap into the devic flow of energy. For some people, this pulse is subconsciously felt when walking in the hills – when for a split instance, there is a timeless moment, where we feel at one with our surroundings, when our energetic system is in tune with devic life. This recognition, as it expands in our conscious awareness, can be the start of a new bridge with devic life. The devic pulse, as the manifestation of devic light, will vary according to the type of devic life form. It will feel different dependent upon the level of devic life that we tap into. It will feel very different in the mineral as compared to the plant, or the animal.

Within this pulse, there is also an expression of love, since at the source of everything and within everything there is the distant echo of divine love. Within the chaotic streams of slow frequency energy there remains a background ripple of love that originated from the Seventh Plane. It is retained, almost like a distant hologram of its original focus, within devic light. To become one with the moment of the devic pulse is to feel this distant echo.

The Mineral Kingdom

The soul aspect, as it enters the lower levels of physical form, becomes magnetised initially to the Mineral Kingdom. This stream of energy occupies the levels between 0.0 and 0.2 in the Zero Plane and the soul aspect enters a long pattern of soul expression within the mineral dance. This is a collective pattern of unconscious awareness, and the vibration of energy is extremely slow. Rock hosts ninety-eight percent dark light. Within the Mineral Kingdom there is a diverse array of devic expression that each soul aspect will sample through the slow development of gross form. Devic life is initially without structure and there is a devic presence in every living thing, including mineral and stone. It is just that usually the vibration is so slow that we may not see it or feel it, since the timescale for response is so long.

The devic pattern within the Mineral Kingdom ranges from the microscopic to the extremely large and the devic essence is the superglue that holds everything together. Every cell, atom, molecule has a presence which is based on the underlying devic pattern. Each soul aspect enters this physical realm and builds up experience, first for example, as a grain of sand on a beach. The timeline may be extremely slow, so hundreds of thousands of years in Earth time may pass before that soul aspect will progress from a sand grain to a more collective conglomerate of other grains, which ultimately will build a rock, or become part of a sedimentary rock strata. Throughout this time, the soul aspect will experience the collective devic presence, as it builds. Since time is an illusion, the experience of time as a grain of sand will be completely different from what we call time. So when we begin to feel the devic presence within a rock, it may seem extremely slow; our concept and experience of time is much more rapid than the time experienced by the grain of sand. What we would perceive in a few seconds, might take a stone ten years to absorb.

Another way of looking at it is through time-lapse photography. If we took multiple pictures of a rock over a long period of time, and then speeded up the picture frames, then we might see the intelligence within the rock form before us. From the perspective of the rock, the presence of a human nearby will register in an entirely different way: the presence may be detected but because time moves so slow, the afterglow of the presence may remain within the rock's experience for some time afterwards.

Eventually, the soul aspect may graduate into a different pattern of rock, as the forces of nature work their way through the elemental dance. Alternatively, the sand grain may reflect a mineral pattern that ultimately is absorbed into a plant and the devic presence then becomes held in matter in a different way, and that soul aspect experiences devic life from a whole new perspective.

The devic dance of life within the Mineral Kingdom can

follow many different patterns. One way of conceiving of it is like a stream of consciousness housed within slow frequency, dark light. The soul aspect enters the Mineral Kingdom at a starting point, and then through experience, and multiple physical patterns of minerals and rocks, builds up a flow of awareness within time. The devic flow underlies the physical pattern of rock formation, whether through volcanic eruptions, the crushing and grinding of rocks together through continental drift, or through the dance of erosion due to other physical forces. Whatever the pattern, the soul aspect will experience the gross world within a collective apparatus. It will experience itself as a grain of sand, it will experience the physical realms as a mountain, and with more experience, it will build up a substantial level of devic knowledge and understanding. Within it there will be other aspects of collective awareness, yet all the time the soul will gather more and more layers of devic expression.

Devic awareness and expression operate according to the dictates of Natural Law. Devic experience in matter allows the soul to gather information about the gross, physical levels. With time, that information will turn into an understanding and an appreciation of the devic pattern of life. Each soul aspect will begin to feel the essence of devic power, whether it is expressed through an earthquake, a flood, or a tidal wave. The soul may feel the raw power like a mountainous presence; a presence that looks out onto the land, imbued with the devic recognition of all that it is and has become. As the soul aspect gathers more and more experience in the Devic Realms, it will begin to gain experiences through different patterns of devic light; some will be slow, heavy and solid, like the essence of granite, while others may be lighter yet contained within the essence of mineral life. For example, crystals and gemstones resonate to a different underlying set of devic frequencies and patterns of intent.

To begin to appreciate these different types of life within the rocks and minerals requires the suspension of our normal belief systems and the emptying of our mind. Any bias or prejudice on our part will hinder our ability to connect with these different life forms. However, the devic presences can be felt in a number of different ways.

Looking at rock formations, or even patterns within stones can, with a little practice, begin to uncover hidden facial features, such as eyes, a mouth or a nose, almost like there is a presence there. Sometimes, a face can be seen in a mountain, or in an outcrop of rock. This will provide a key to the underlying devic presence. Detecting these presences can be enhanced using a camera and recording, in a frozen moment of time, a face in the rock. Usually our minds will fight this image, but once we are free of this prejudice, then it is possible to sense the qualities present in the face. There may be a timeless, granitic power that feels cold and yet extremely solid. Other feelings may also come in, such as whether the presence is sympathetic or quite grumpy. Quite often these old devic presences can reflect a sluggish and almost angry nature, as if they are locked in time. It is no accident that some mountain ranges and rocks feel more 'friendly' than others. Each devic presence will reflect a wide-ranging set of feelings that can touch us at a deeper level, depending on whether the underlying reflective pattern is more negative than positive.

With practice, it can become possible to entertain a dialogue with these different devic presences. At the core of any such interaction is respect for another life form. If we begin a conversation with the devic presence of a mountain with a lack of respect and attention to protocol, then the devic presence will not engage with us. This may sound strange at first, but it is worth considering that when we go walking in the mountains, we are in fact, entering a different realm. We are entering 'their' territory, and as such it is always worth asking for permission to enter. Through being open and centred, a response can be heard. It may be a whispered 'yes' or 'no', or 'wait.' Through an intuitive dialogue, it is possible to build up an entirely different experience of devic life.

Devic expression within the Mineral Kingdom takes on a diversity of different forms, including the basic mineral and rock patterns, through various metals which host a different vibration, to the formation of crystals and gemstones, and then into different devic life forms that are invisible to our normal, naked eye, such as the fairies. These life forms occur at the upper end of the scale of the

Mineral Kingdom and reflect a more evolved pattern of life, containing a higher percentage of light. The soul will entertain these different life forms within its experience: it may undergo many different patterns of expression as a fairy, working with these numerous devic streams of light. For some people, this may reflect an important pattern of their evolution, where a dialogue in matter as a fairy represented an important doorway of devic expression. Other people may have focused on other types of form, such as gnomes or other elemental beings that host a myriad of different expressions of light. All of these different forms build more and more experience in the developing soul.

Crystals are amplifiers and are the devic equivalent of the purer love vibration. Each crystal and gemstone will reflect a different frequency pattern and will retain inside, the prevailing energies of the place where they were originally formed. Because of their energetic pattern, some crystals such as quartz can be used as more direct amplification devices. It is important to remember, though, that each crystal or gem will house different frequencies that may or may not be harmonious to our own energetic systems. Working directly with crystals can help build up a different appreciation of devic life.

Crystals also represent a more ordered structure, and as such, can house higher energetic pulses that are anchored within the physical structure of the crystal itself. In one sense, this reflects the constant layering of different life streams that goes on all the time. While our mind would like things to be simple and direct, there are, in reality, many different levels of life that are superimposed on one another. A crystal may house the specific underlying devic presence, and yet hold within it, a higher set of frequencies from different levels of light. This overlaying of one energy pattern by another is all part of the different streams of devic life.

The Plant Kingdom

After experiencing multiple life forms within the Mineral Kingdom, through the underlying pattern of devic expression, the soul eventually progresses into the Plant Kingdom. This can only occur once all the gross sense impressions of the soul have been saturated in the Mineral Kingdom. Only then is there sufficient experience for the next stage of development of consciousness to begin. This next stage takes place in the Plant Kingdom, where the developing soul experiences a combination of inanimate and animate life. While the Mineral Kingdom hosted consciousness within what we would term inanimate life, the Plant Kingdom represents a mid point between animate and inanimate life. The Plant Kingdom covers the levels of 0.2 to 0.4 in the Zero Plane and offers the soul a different level of awareness and consciousness within a new pattern of life. The Plant Kingdom contains approximately sixty percent dark light. The physical form is held erect and the diversity of plant life amplifies the range of different experiences for the soul.

The devic pattern of expression in the Plant Kingdom is different to the Mineral Kingdom. Devic life is hosted in grasses, bushes, trees and flowers. Some plants are very much collective organisms where a whole host of devic presences can be found. Each type of plant represents an opportunity for the soul aspect to gather more experience in gross matter and to work according to a different pattern of time. Time in the Plant Kingdom moves faster than in the Mineral Kingdom and so the soul can cycle through different physical forms more rapidly. For the first time, the soul also encounters some of the more fundamental characteristics of animate life, such as reproduction. Increased consciousness is experienced through plant life, as well as an increased diversity of form.

The evolving soul will work its way through all the different plant types, including algae, ferns, flowering plants, grasses, and then through different bushes and trees. The diversity of the Plant Kingdom is huge, and for the developing soul aspect, the patterns of experience based upon a vertical physical expression, as opposed to the recumbent expression in rocks, gives a broader base to developing awareness. The devic platform within the Plant Kingdom is also freer flowing, as different streams of light have been built up through the huge reservoir of physical form. Furthermore, the Plant Kingdom plays host to a broad range of other life forms both from the Mineral Kingdom, and also from the stars and beyond. The diversity and differences of devic life form are awe-inspiring.

To build up a connection with these different devic forms requires patience, focus and an acceptance of a range of different impressions. Some communities, such as Findhorn in Scotland, have done this most effectively, through cultivating a respect and deeper understanding of devic life in plants.

The devic presences in plants provide a different focus to that of minerals, metals and crystals. In plants, the devic feel is quicker, brighter and can hold a broader diversity of energetic streams. Feeling the devic presences within flowers and other plants is very different from the presences found in rocks. Sometimes, it may feel as if flowers sing to us, or like a tree may call to us. Within flowers and petals, multiple devic presences can be found, just as trees are collective organisms which host a myriad of different life forms. Different devic faces may appear to us, sometimes singly or in chain formations. As we open ourselves up to these different patterns, we can begin to feel the flow of the underlying devic form.

Trees, in particular, can host a divergent pattern of devic life, from the very small, to the larger collective essence of the tree itself. Trees can also act as recording devices to life around and on how life locally will have developed through time. Merging our energies with a tree can provide a brand new experience and can open us to an entirely different perspective. This type of dialogue can bring through a host of different devic presences. When working with trees, it is useful to divide their physical form into three distinct areas: the root system, the main trunk, and then the branches and leaves. Each system has its own distinct energetic focus. The roots anchor the tree into the ground and also connect it with other presences in the area, while the branches can act as a receiving and transmitter dish for a range of different frequencies. Some of the older trees on the planet, such as the Giant Redwoods of California, can host stellar frequencies and are a direct bridge with the stars.

As with the Mineral Kingdom, the soul aspect eventually

becomes completely saturated by all the gross impressions that it has experienced in the Plant Kingdom. It is at this point that is ready to enter the Animal Kingdom and enter a new stream of consciousness.

The Animal Kingdom

The Animal Kingdom occupies the plane levels of 0.4 to 0.6 and provides the developing soul with a new range of gross experiences based upon physical movement, reproduction, and an increased level of awareness i.e. it is animate. In the Animal Kingdom fifty percent dark light is dominating. The diversity of experience that is generated through the Animal Kingdom is even greater than in the Plant Kingdom. The soul experiences a whole host of new physical forms through which to gain further experiences in the gross world. The invertebrate pattern, which includes insects, worms and crustaceans, focuses on crawling although it does include some winged forms. Physical sensation is experienced on land and in water. Once this pattern has been saturated, the soul then focuses on the vertebrate pattern of existence, in fish, reptilian and bird form, until ultimately becoming mammalian. The fish gives experience in water, while the bird form allows freedom of expression in flight. Eventually, the mammalian form gives experience primarily in quadrupedal locomotion. In all forms, there is a struggle for survival, and the karma generated through the progression of experience in the Animal Kingdom is carried over ultimately into the human form. The soul aspect experiences life as a predator and a prey.

Within this dance of life, the devic awareness continues to build in different ways. Devic expression focuses on survival within the physical and through the diversity of experience. The devic presence in the animal does not experience pain or emotion, but does have sensation. Sensation is experience, and the more that can be gathered then the more the devic expression of life becomes fulfilled. Today, the devic expression in animals is becoming more potent: for example, venoms and poisons are more powerful, and while humanity has learned to control the larger animal predators, the devic intent in all animals is building. It should be understood, however, that this is different from the succession of species through the planet. Some species of animals are now ready to go home, such as cattle, and will be replaced by different life forms in the fullness of time.

As the soul builds experience through the diversity of animal life form, it continues to build karma. Countless lifetimes will be spent working through all of the different animal forms, until eventually, the soul becomes saturated with the different impressions. At this point in time, the soul will then work through a particular animal species that will become its eventual doorway into the human form. Many lifetimes may be spent working through the experience as one species of animal. Incarnating as a domestic pet is also one way in which the soul can become acquainted with and used to the human frequency, although on another level, the domestication of pets does not necessarily speed up the evolution of that animal form.

There are five main doorways through which the soul may pass from the Animal Kingdom into the Kingdom of Human Beings. These are the cat, dog, elephant, hippopotamus and monkey. Each doorway gives a specific access point and each soul will have worked towards building the appropriate experience to pass through this doorway into human form. It is at this point of evolution that the soul then enters a uniquely different pattern of development that involves involution in human form. All souls, then, on the path to becoming conscious in human form have to progress through this evolutionary pattern. The evolution referred to here is different from evolutionary theory in modern biology, and refers to the progressive evolution of consciousness from the stone stage, and then through the plant and animal stages. Once the soul enters the human form, it will eventually begin the process of involution where it will slowly disengage from the physical gross world.

The soul's journey through the Mineral, Plant and Animal Kingdoms will have given it solid experience of the Devic Realms. The soul will have explored different types of devic light and a broad range of devic patterns of experience. During this process, the soul may specialise in a particular type of devic experience, such as through the mineral path or through the animal path. And although the soul will have become saturated by different devic experiences, it will not have fulfilled the full totality of all devic life form. This is only usually done by those souls that are specialising on the devic pattern alone rather than on pursuing the evolution of consciousness through the human form. The situation is somewhat similar to those souls that followed the angelic pathway, although in this instance it is to follow the full breadth of the devic path.

The Elements

Apart from the different devic forms that the evolving soul will experience, there is another grouping of devic form that is extremely important – the elements. The elements are the principal building blocks of the physical world and are known as Fire, Air, Earth and Water. Each element has its own unique expression of formlessness manifested in form, and each element works with the other elements to manifest creation and destruction within the natural expression of the planet's development.

The element Fire is present in all manifestations of fire, from the smallest flames in an open fire through to the largest volcanic eruptions. Fire is also the dominant element of the Sun and all other star systems. As with other devic forms, presences can be seen in open fires, and in the dance of magmatic eruptions. Fire interacts with the other elements to birth different combinations of expression of the elemental forms.

The Earth element expresses the physical aspect of the planet, such as the land, the soil, the deserts, the mountains. Its expression is different from Fire, and is best recognised as an earthy quality. The Earth element embodies the essence of the soil, the land and all rock formations. Like Fire, it interacts with other elements as part of the devic flow of energy. Earth can work with Air to produce erosion and a change in form, just as Fire and Air interact.

The next element Water imbues all of the oceans, streams, rivers and lakes on the planet. The element is strikingly different to the others and can be passive and quiet, and at other times destructive, as in hurricanes or tidal waves. The Water element has a very different quality from the other elements, and once felt, is never forgotten. For example, the glassy seas of the Caribbean give a sense of the purity of this element.

The final element is Air and encompasses the atmosphere, the wind patterns, the clouds and all convection streams that encircle the planet. Air dances in partnership with the other elements, and to feel the freedom of the wind as it blows across the savannas can open up an entirely different aspect of the devic dance. The annual hurricanes in the Caribbean reflect the devic pattern and again through careful observation, the different, underlying devic presences can be seen.

Each of the four elements comprises the blueprint and expression of form on the planet. Their interaction and focus provide the impetus to all planetary changes, whether they are destructive earthquakes, forest fires, floods or tornados. The elements also dictate the creative flow of form building – through the flow of magma, the slow march of continental plates, the uplifting of mountain ranges and the steady inevitability of erosion processes. In each aspect of devic expression, the underlying devic presence can be felt. Each of the elements dances to the manifestation of devic power that creates the physical world for all other life forms to then play out the life pulse. The elements also host the creative and destructive flow of devic form on the other physical planets and stars in the myriad solar systems and galaxies, although the expression or mix of elements will be uniquely different and be brought through a range of different substances.

Devic life therefore embodies everything in physical form and through the creative focus of devic light, builds a constant flow of form. Order and chaos interact in different ways and devic light then imbues all physical form, created out of the patterns of slow frequency light. Yet when these parts develop and build through the different devic manifestations of form, then different streams of devic light develop that allow life to constantly change and develop. Devic life is in everything and everywhere – the pulse of devic light imbues all matter in the physical realms and provides the fundamental building blocks for all different manifestations of physical life to take place. Without devic focus and expression, there would be no physical life. Similarly, devic light provides each soul with a vehicle of collective experience held within different degrees of unconscious and conscious awareness. More evolved devic patterns will host an active and powerful intelligence that are capable of holding multiple levels of collective awareness and different streams of consciousness. Some of these streams of devic life will be explored in more detail in Chapter 21.

CHAPTER 10

Human Involution

Through the diverse journeys in the Mineral, Plant and Animal Kingdoms, the soul retains the connections it built up with its mental and subtle forms, although these are never consciously recognised. The soul also builds up impressions through its various journeys. These impressions are diverse and, from the pattern of evolution, are gross or physical impressions. All of these impressions are carried through into the first and subsequent human lives. The start of the human form represents the conclusion of evolution and the start of involution. In human form, the soul experiences full consciousness in Illusion. It is not, however, conscious of itself as One, eternal and infinite. In the human form, the initial platform of light is twenty percent dark, slowly decreasing to around two percent in older souls on the Sixth Plane. However, this percentage of light and dark can be amplified in either direction – more into the light or more into the dark.

Each plane has millions of sub-planes and each plane holds a principle of thought held in bondage through experience, latent or active, collective or individual. Each lower plane is also like a shadow of the immediate higher plane and each plane has its own rules of engagement and has to be mastered through experience. Each plane is illusion. It is also helpful to understand that the pattern of movement down and up the different planes of consciousness is like a spiral; the soul as it comes down spirals into compression in one direction, and then as it goes back up will spiral in the opposite direction and expand.

The Zero Plane

The human existence begins at level 0.6 in the Zero Plane and passes through all of the planes up into the Seventh. The focus of energy from 0.6 to the top of the Zero Plane is very dark and slow, and reflects primarily the lower spectrums of astral light. In the first few human lives, the resonance from the previous animal lives will be strong, and the animalistic urge predominant. It will take many millions of lives to work through this pattern. Ninety percent of humanity is anchored in the Zero Plane, where the light and energy is slow and extremely dense. This also means that ninety percent of humanity does not think for itself, but rather reflects the prevailing structure of thought. The soul aspect is entirely focused on the physical realms and will go through many lives experiencing a whole diversity of different experiences. Generally, these experiences will be stacked one on top of the other through the law of opposites. In one life, a soul aspect may experience great poverty and then in the next life great wealth. In one life, a soul aspect will be a female and in the next a male. The reason for this continual dance between opposite polarities is to allow the soul aspect to begin to unburden itself of all the impressions built up during the process of evolution and for the release of sanskaras[1] built up during the human reincarnatory pattern. This process of evolution also built up a vast reservoir of subconscious experiences, which although hidden from consciousness, are nevertheless present and need ultimately, to be balanced. The soul aspect, therefore, moves between opposite polarities in an attempt to balance both the conscious and unconscious impressions. Each of these impressions will carry a karmic charge and the reincarnatory programme is specifically designed to burn off the karma of the process of evolution and the karma generated in each new lifetime in human form.

In the Zero Plane, the soul aspect in human form is exclusively focused on the outside, physical world; animalistic drives such as satiation of external desires and animal instincts predominate in every thought, emotion and action. Because the soul is focused entirely on gross consciousness, it has no awareness of any of its subtle bodies.

Such soul aspects move through the sway of different energies and are bound in Illusion. The constant cycle of birth and death provides different opportunities for processing both conscious and subconscious impressions and each soul aspect will follow a permutation of many lives where there is little conscious choice of physical form. Karma directly dictates the burden of opposite experiences.

Each life is like a uniform where more and more experiences are gathered. Each life is an interplay between the old karma that has to be burnt off through lived experience, and the new karma that is gathered by the thoughts, emotions and actions in that lifetime. Although the soul aspect is trying to unburden itself of past sanskaras, it is at the same time becoming increasingly burdened by new karmic entanglements. The impressions of the previous lives in matter push through subconsciously, while in each lived life, there will come a point when the next life will call to the soul aspect in matter. Death represents the dropping away of the old uniform, and the point where further impressions can be digested in the subtle realms before adopting another physical form through birth. Each soul is called back into physical form due to the burden of karma that has to be processed.

Each soul aspect has one permanent atom that records all of its experiences in the mental, emotional and physical permutations of life. This atom is radioactive and pulses out a series of frequencies that build throughout the soul aspect's journey. When the soul aspect drops its body, this permanent atom is left in a band of blue energy that surrounds the planet. This band of blue energy, the ring-pass-not, houses all of the permanent atoms of all the soul aspects that are not in physical matter. When a soul aspect is ready to reincarnate, it will pick up this one permanent atom on its journey back into matter and will then retain it within the heart centre for the duration of its life in human form. The permanent atom splits itself into two more aspects in the human vehicle, one atom that is feminine, and one atom that is masculine. These subsidiary atoms will then pulse more or less dominantly according to whether or not the life in matter is female or male. As more and more lives accumulate, then the different feminine and masculine life experiences are reflected in these two atoms.

The average soul aspect will undergo approximately one million life times in the Zero Plane. It will experience a diverse array of life experiences and will go through a whole range of patterns of life and death. Animal instinct is never very far from the surface and the soul aspect focuses almost exclusively on gathering information through experience. The subtler impressions of the astral levels will also flow through but will remain sub-conscious. Eventually, there will come a point where the soul will have saturated the external focus in the physical realms and will feel the call of looking inwards rather than outwards. This is usually a gradual process and the shift between the Zero and the First Planes is the demarcation point for the start of this process of involution, where the soul aspect begins to look inwards and gradually disengages from the gross world.

The First Plane

The transition from the Zero Plane to the First Plane is the most difficult. Between each Avataric Age, the transition zone between the two planes becomes thickly layered, so that souls find it extremely difficult to pass through. It is like a thick crust of dark energy forms at the top of the Zero Plane, and souls can only move through it using special boreholes. This layer can be quite thick and is like an impenetrable wall of dark energy. In an Avataric Age these boreholes are re-opened and so the flow of souls from the Zero to the First Plane increases. Outside of an Avataric Age, the holes become encrusted and become blocked so that it again becomes very difficult for souls to progress.

The First Plane represents the initial point at which the soul becomes conscious of the astral levels through the vehicle of physical form and where its focus is not just exclusively in the physical or in the gross. The soul aspect anchors its awareness in the First Plane, from which it can experience the different frequencies of astral light. The light in the First Plane is still extremely dense and slow when compared to the higher planes, but it represents a significant difference from the Zero Plane. A soul aspect entering the First Plane from the Zero Plane would notice the difference in light: it would feel lighter and brighter, and in the space, which is larger than the Zero Plane. In moving into the First Plane, the soul aspect is therefore able to begin to experience the different frequencies of astral light through its astral body, thereby building up a whole host of impressions and experiences while still in physical matter.   In successive life times there is a gradual pull to look inwards that is constantly counteracted and worked through the karmic patterns of external desire that have been built up in the Zero Plane.

Just like the Zero Plane, the First Plane can be subdivided into ten sub-planes. The soul aspect will work through each of these sub-planes sampling different levels of astral light and like the Zero Plane, will require approximately one million life times to progress through this plane. The rules and regulations that govern the First Plane are different from the Zero Plane and each subsequent plane that the soul aspect passes through has its own unique set of rules and regulations. The First Plane soul aspect experiences different things from the astral levels – different sensations such as smell, sound and sight, all of which are subtle and more refined than the physical. The First Plane soul aspect can pass back down into the Zero Plane to re-experience some of the gross experiences or to work a specific pattern of past lives. Eventually, though, the soul aspect becomes saturated with the First Plane energies, and having worked through approaching two million lives, will then prepare to move up into the Second Plane.

The shift from the First Plane to the Second plane is not as difficult as the previous transition, although the soul aspect will again have to cross the abyss of limitation between the two planes, and pass through the neutral or static zone before moving into the higher light streams of the Second Plane.

The Second Plane

In the Second Plane, the soul aspect experiences a different level of astral light that is brighter than the First Plane. The space occupied by the Second Plane is larger than the First Plane and souls can move about more freely in this more expansive light. Astral light still dominates this plane, although the mix of mental light that permeates this astral light is a higher proportion than in the First Plane. This mental light is not found in the lower parts of the Second Plane, but in the higher levels such as 2.8 and 2.9.

Second Plane soul aspects are now coming to the end of their apprenticeships as young souls, and in this plane there are often a series of choices that the soul aspect can make. It should be appreciated that these choices are not exclusive to this plane level, and can arise in the First and even Zero Planes. It is just that the soul aspect is now starting to build sufficient experience in matter to exercise choice in the future pattern of its development. Of course, this choice will reflect the initial pattern of soul development that was agreed at the start of its downward journey from the Ocean of Life, and will reflect the pattern of sponsorship that has already been established. Nevertheless, the developing soul, as it looks more inside, rather than outside, can begin to exercise choices about its future evolution.

In the journey back up the inner planes, and in the pattern of involution, or looking inwards and disengaging from the physical, astral and mental realms, a developing soul can follow one of two major paths. Meher Baba has described these paths as the Path of Intoxication and the Path of Sobriety. In the former, the soul aspect chooses to focus exclusively on the inner light of the Divine, to the exclusion of all else. These soul aspects become God-intoxicated and are known as masts. For the most part, they have existed in the East, primarily in India, where the physical platform of life's diversity can support them. These masts are special souls who are so deeply focused on God, to the exclusion of all else, that they have no concern or interest in the outer world. Often they cannot physically look after themselves since they are so wrapped up in the Divine. They have no interest in any external life, no physical desires and to some would appear almost insane. Yet such a diagnosis could not be further from the truth, for these special souls are so focused on God that they are like His gemstones of love. They are, quite literally, intoxicated by

God and His Light. They focus on the diluted essence of His Light and Love to the extent that such energy can be supported in the plane level that they operate from.

The electronic and energetic set up of masts is also very different from everyone else. Their chakra systems are focused inwards and not outwards, so that the pattern of energy that flows through them almost works in reverse. All of their chakras adopt a different polarity of energy whereby they can focus exclusively inwards. Once a soul aspect has chosen the Path of Intoxication, it will continue in this pattern all of the way up the inner planes until eventually it becomes God-realised. Masts are therefore unique souls that have chosen a path that is very different from most of humanity.

In contrast, the Path of Sobriety means following a path of communion or absorption with God. To achieve this, the soul aspect has to build inner experience and understanding of God, as reflected through the different subtle bodies that are built on the journey up through the inner planes. For example, yoga and forms of meditation would be involved in this path, since both seek to provide a greater inner awareness of self while juxtaposing this with a deeper connection with the divine. Lifetime after lifetime will be spent in developing these different skills.

The second shift that sometimes arises during the Second Plane is for the soul aspect to reach a crossroads or junction point where light and dark are entertained. This may happen in one life of choice where first the light will offer a contract of development where the principles of light are observed, and then the dark will offer a different sort of contract, where the principles of dark are offered. The soul aspect in physical matter, or at the point of death, will have to choose between these two patterns of experience, and depending upon the choices made, will then follow, over many subsequent lifetimes, a pattern of light or dark. This choice may be entertained in many different ways through many different life times and on different planes, but those soul aspects that choose the dark, will then build up experience and ark that ultimately will have to be balanced. This choice is not always offered in the Second Plane, and is often invoked in the Third Plane, once the soul has gained further experience in matter.

The Second Plane soul, as it builds more experience and understanding of the astral levels, will live these experiences in physical matter. To all intents and purposes they will live normally, yet their focus will be much more on the inner, astral levels, than on the gross, physical levels. Mental impressions will also be reflected through the astral levels so they will experience various aspects of the mind including thoughts and emotions filtered through the mind. In occasional lives, these souls may be able to perform minor miracles or will develop patterns as healers or seers of some repute. Today, many musicians that work with some of the newer energies are anchored on the Second Plane. It is also in the Second Plane that the soul aspect begins to build up power, in preparation for future experiences on the Third and Fourth Planes. As with the pattern on the First Plane, Second Plane soul aspects can move into the First and Zero Planes.

Eventually, the soul aspect will become saturated with the Second Plane and will be ready to move up into the Third Plane. By this stage, the soul aspect has usually progressed from a young soul into a middle-aged soul and is now ready to become more intensely absorbed in the astral, and eventually, the mental levels.

The Third Plane

The Third Plane hosts a higher degree of astral light than the previous planes, and also houses a higher proportion of mental light interwoven within the astral light. The astral light is more consistently higher astral and the space in this plane is larger than any of the previous planes. The soul aspect is much more fully attuned into the astral levels, and irrespective of whether operating within the focus of light or dark, will experience a much greater degree of astral power and light. The Third Plane soul aspect can move with ease between the Third and Zero Planes, and experiences a much greater degree of flexibility in terms of power: some soul aspects will demonstrate major miracles and will have specific lifetimes of power.

At the same time the process of involution is beginning to

gather pace; while the First Plane hosts both the gross and the astral, the Second and Third Planes are exclusively astral and so focus on the emotional and higher astral light. This is particularly so in the Third Plane where souls may typically have experienced between three and four million lives in matter. Their pattern of reincarnation is becoming more practised and in contrast to the first million lives or so, such soul aspects can exercise greater choice and planning in each lifetime. Their inner awareness is developing all the time, and their ability to work with either light or dark is also building. However, in both the Second and Third Planes there can be a virulence to the dark intent and some of the major tyrants have been stationed on either the Second or Third Plane. The Third Plane can also represent the point at which light and dark petition a soul for its future focus.

By the time the soul aspect reaches the Third Plane, it will also begin a pattern of meeting its soul mates, as a means of opening itself up to remembering who and what it is. This process may have started in the Second Plane and occasionally in the First Plane, but by the Third Plane, the soul aspect has undergone sufficient experience in matter to be able to cope with the potent energies set up by an interaction with a soul mate. Meeting a soul mate in physical matter initiates a stream of energy where both recognise something about the other, and often feel exceptionally strong ties of love. The pulse of recognition of the "same" inner essence opens up new streams of experience in the heart and other chakra centres. Everything is speeded up and larger amounts of karma can be processed through the energy that is manifested in such meetings. The pattern of meeting other soul mates becomes more intense as the soul aspect pushes up into the higher planes, and this is all part of a process of gathering more experience and handling higher frequency energy.

Eventually, after another million or so lifetimes, the soul aspect is ready to transition from the Third into the Fourth Plane, where a new threshold is engaged.

The Fourth Plane

The Fourth Plane is the plane of power and is the transition plane between the astral and mental spheres. It retains forty percent mental light and sixty percent astral light. Although the soul has already started turning inwards to recognise the astral levels, the Fourth Plane represents the first point at which the soul actively searches for something else inside – the mental streams of higher light and love. The frequencies of light are much brighter than on the Third Plane, and the soul aspect is able to move between the Fourth Plane and the other lower planes. Often a Fourth Plane soul aspect may be anchored on that plane and yet be working with specific contracts on the lower planes, such as the Second or First Planes. Again, the soul aspect can spend up to a million lives experiencing the Fourth Plane, so that by the time it has completed its journey through this plane, is ready to enter the higher planes and become an older soul.

On this plane the soul aspect becomes conscious of infinite energy and is equipped with full power to express it. At the same time that the soul aspect experiences this intensity of power, it also comes into contact with a profoundly different quality of light more directly – mental light. Here the soul has to absorb the intensity of mental light while not becoming obsessed with using the full power at its disposal. The intensity of the mental light can burn the thoughts and emotions of the incarnating soul aspect and often it will have to pass through a period of darkness where the polar extremes of intense desires and emotions have to be tempered against the desire to utilise the infinite power.

In the Fourth Plane, if the total power at the soul aspect's disposal is abused, such as in raising a person from the dead, then the liberation of this total power may result in a stripping away of all consciousness and experience gained up to that point. The soul aspect is, quite literally, disintegrated, and returns back to the start of the process of evolution in the Mineral Kingdom. This soul aspect then has to pass through the whole process of evolution from the Mineral Kingdom, and then back up through the planes to regain full consciousness.

The soul aspect is confronted in the Fourth Plane by the choice of utilising the power for the benefit of others, both in either material or spiritual terms. If the power is utilised for selfish and negative purposes, then the results can be devastating. For the soul aspect the challenge then is to remain in a certain degree of balance while connecting with the majesty and brilliance of mental light without the sufficient experience or understanding to temper and subjugate the mental thoughts that assault his or her experiences in the physical realms. And if the soul aspect is able to use the power for the benefit of others, this action will still incur karma and bind the soul aspect for future lifetimes.

The pattern of mental light that arises in the Fourth Plane is potent and yet the developing soul aspect will not yet have full access to his mental capacity because it is not fully activated until the Fifth Plane. So there is limitless power of the Fourth Plane that is juxtaposed against the limitation of the mental alignment. It is this polarity that presents such soul aspects with significant challenges.

A soul aspect's pattern of development through the Fourth Plane may be based on lifetimes of gradual accumulation. Life times will be spent in minor positions of power until in one lifetime, the full potential of power is presented to that soul aspect. The soul aspect may take up a position of great physical and material power in the world, or develop significant power through other means.

Souls that enter the Fourth Plane also move out of the realms of what are termed Heaven or Hell. Until the end of the Third Plane, the astral impressions created through a soul aspect's lived experience, both conscious and unconscious, can on death, lead to a direct astral experience of what may be termed Heaven or Hell. This experience is bound up in illusion, and yet may appear very real for that soul aspect. Once the soul progresses into the Fourth Plane then these illusions from the astral levels can no longer be experienced. The Fourth Plane soul aspect, if it neither uses nor misuses the power available, will gradually work its way through the sub-planes before preparing to enter the Fifth Plane.

The Fifth Plane

With the progressive involution of the soul aspect through the

Fourth Plane, its consciousness eventually identifies with the mental planes. In the Fifth Plane, the soul aspect experiences mental light in the function and application of mental thoughts – these thoughts can be experienced as good or bad, spiritual or material, high or low. Whatever their content and focus, they are always experienced as mental thoughts. The soul aspect of the Fifth Plane identifies with the thoughts of others and as such can identify with them. The pattern of light on the Fifth Plane is also extremely bright and the space in the mental planes is vast and much, much more expansive when compared to the lower planes. Souls on the Fifth Plane have truly turned inwards and are searching for God.

As with all the other planes, the Fifth Plane can be sub-divided into ten sub-planes, and the soul aspect will progressively move through them. In the human form, a Fifth Plane soul aspect will work through the gross and astral levels, but through the mental sphere. The soul aspect on the Fifth Plane is incapable of performing any miracles, and instead focuses on seeing different patterns or streams of mental light. The soul aspect can also work with the thoughts of others.

Soul aspects stationed on the Fifth Plane are generally older souls and have progressed through a large proportion of lives – often between five and seven million – and are slowly building up a pattern of working through their karma. They have worked extensively with physical and astral karma, and are now focusing more on mental karma. Soul aspects can develop to this plane level through specific spiritual practises, while certain yogic practices can allow the soul aspect to involve to this level of consciousness. However, to progress beyond the Fifth Plane always requires the guidance of a Perfect Master. In the Fifth Plane, the soul aspect is also focused more on searching for the face of God and turning ever inwards to find the true essence of self. By the time the soul aspect has reached the Fifth Plane, it will usually have worked through significant patterns of light and dark, and if it has entertained a major pattern of development with the dark, it will usually have passed beyond this set of experiences in search of the light. Typically, the shift away from darker practices may occur during the Fourth Plane, although soul aspects on the Fifth and Sixth Planes can become easily led back into older addictive patterns. Unlike the Fourth Plane, the Fifth Plane soul aspect has no power, and this pattern is carried through into the Sixth Plane.

For the involving soul aspect that has now reached the Fifth Plane the focus is very different from the Fourth Plane. There is an absence of power, and instead the mental focus is used in working through the different streams of energy. In the lower sub-planes of the Fifth Plane, there is a mix of mental and astral light that turns into pure mental light by the time the soul has progressed through the first few sub-planes. Those souls that have become God absorbed at this point usually go on to complete their journey as masts, merging their journey with the Path of Intoxication. In the Fifth Plane, it is also typical to talk of soul aspects as saints where in one life in particular beneficial actions and works are done on behalf of others.

By the time the soul aspect reaches the Fifth Plane, it will have had at least one life in matter where it has petitioned either consciously or subconsciously on the inner planes during that lifetime to return back to God. This petitioning will have set up a chain reaction of lives where the soul aspect will work progressively to balance its karma and ultimately to meet up with a Perfect Master to complete their journey. The majority of involving souls, once they reach a certain stage of maturity will also entertain a life where they will be given a glimpse of their pathway home. This might occur in a spiritual life, or arise in a vision or a dream; that one lifetime may also embody a level of light and excellence that can help provide the barometer of spiritual excellence for all the future lives; the one life where the soul aspect got everything right and where in balance and harmony the pulse of light formed a new pattern and a new understanding of what the path up through the planes entailed. This one life would then pulse at a higher octave than all the previous lives that the soul aspect had gone through.

Eventually, the soul aspect will be ready to progress from the Fifth into the Sixth Plane and by this stage will need to have met a Perfect Master in a lifetime of importance. Up to this point, the soul aspect will have built up lives like millions and millions of beads on a series of chains. If, for example, there are one hundred and forty four chains or threads and the lives that the soul aspect has experienced are divided up onto these threads, then there will be patches of light and dark all over the threads. The vast majority of lives will pulse in a fairly dull way as the soul aspect has built up experience and then worked through the ongoing karmic pattern. Within that, however, there may be two or three lives that pulse more brightly and that provide the focal point and standard for the final stages of involution.

The Sixth Plane

The progression from the Fifth Plane to the Sixth Plane has to be undertaken under the supervision of a Perfect Master, just as the final journey across the Sixth Plane can only be done with a Perfect Master. The mental light on the Sixth Plane is the brightest of all the planes, and this plane is also the largest. The energetic pattern is extremely fine and soul aspects entering it usually have been through six or seven million lives. This journey has ensured the progressive burning off of old karma and sanskaras, and by the time the soul aspect is in the Sixth Plane, the need for opposite and diverse impressions has grown fainter and fainter. In the lower planes, the soul aspect may still encounter polarised opposites in successive lifetimes but in the Sixth Plane the soul aspect is fully conscious of the mental body and is in full awareness of mental light. There are very few impressions left and in progressing through the Sixth Plane, the soul aspect begins to see God in everything. The soul aspect retains only a very small proportion of dark light and is focused inwards and balanced.

In the Sixth Plane there is ninety percent mental light and ten percent astral light; the astral light resides at the bottom end of the plane. In this plane, the soul aspect experiences the full extent of the mental, feeling everything through mental thoughts and experiences. Unlike the Fifth Plane, where the focus is in pure mental thoughts, in the Sixth Plane feelings are also worked through as part of the mental stream of higher light. As these streams are entertained, the last vestiges of duality in Illusion are worked through while the soul aspect experiences the different sub-planes.

At the same time, more encounters between the soul aspect and its other soul mates may take place, sometimes culminating in a final meeting with the twin flame. This usually takes place at the end of the soul aspect's journey through Illusion. However, it is important to recognise that not all soul aspects will journey up the inner planes in the same way. While one soul aspect may be anchored on the Sixth Plane, other aspects may be positioned in the lower planes, reflecting their own separate path of reincarnation and involution. So sometimes one aspect will be on the Sixth Plane, while another may be on the Second Plane, and others on the Third or Fourth Planes.

Compared to the First Plane, the size and light of the Sixth Plane is huge and soul aspects cannot negotiate the massive expanse of the Sixth Plane alone. Instead, a Perfect Master is needed to guide a soul aspect across the huge expanses of mental light until eventually the soul aspect is prepared for the final abyss and the eventual crossing into the Seventh Plane through the process of God-realisationship. It is only at this final point that the soul aspect wakes up to consciousness in reality and leaves behind the duality of separation that has been experienced in Illusion.

Throughout the process of involution, the soul aspect has created subtle bodies, and each of these subtle bodies has to be absorbed as part of the process of involution. The layers that were created on the downward journey into matter have to be absorbed, just as the subtle vehicles and experiences from all past lives have, ultimately, to be absorbed before a soul aspect can return back into the Seventh Plane. During the millions and millions of lives in human form and during the process of evolution, the soul aspect has to absorb all of the different forms. Lives that were out of balance and caused ripples through future levels all have to be cleared and all the outstanding karmic details have to be resolved. This balancing process is huge and at the same time, the soul aspect, in the final stages of involution, has to balance all physical, emotional and mental karma. Light and dark also have to be in perfect balance. To achieve such balancing can only be accomplished through the assistance of a Perfect Master or the Avatar Himself. There will eventually come a final life when the soul aspect will have worked through most of the karmic layers, and will be approaching saturation in the mental realms, as well as having achieved saturation in physical and emotional experience. Only then is the soul aspect ready to cross the final abyss and go through the process of letting go of all duality and in recognising itself as God. This process is like the final surrender and letting go of everything that the soul has experienced in Illusion, before Reality can be embraced.

CHAPTER 11

The Seventh Plane

Entering the Seventh Plane

It is said that the paths to God are as diverse as the number of grains of sand on a beach. And so it is that the final steps of the involutionary process are specific for each soul aspect. The patterns of experience within the Path of Intoxication and the Path of Sobriety will have been utterly unique. To return to the Seventh Plane, the Plane of Reality, means to surrender absolutely everything; all physical desires, emotional needs and mental thoughts, as well as to have balanced all karma generated through the journey down through the planes into gross matter, and then back up through the planes through the different physical forms. Before entering the Seventh Plane, the soul aspect still lives in a world of duality and separation, and it is only through moving beyond this state of Illusion, that the soul aspect can truly enter the Seventh Plane, and in the process become God-realised. Once in the Seventh Plane, the soul aspect is no longer that — it becomes at one with the Oversoul. Different soul aspects from the same soul may become God-realised at different points in outer, physical time, and yet in the Seventh Plane, they will become merged in the unity of the Oversoul in harmony together. Once all of the soul aspects have merged back into the Oversoul, then the soul is said to have completed the full involutionary cycle.

The transformation from seeing God in everything on the Sixth Plane to the realisation that "I am God" is a profound and seismic shift in awareness. All separation and duality has to disappear and be replaced by the true manifestation of the Real "I". In experiencing this transformation the soul aspect has to move from Illusion into Reality, as a lived conscious experience, and has to go through the one real and permanent death – the death of all illusion. What remains after this death is the conscious awareness of nothing, like a vacuum of nothing where the soul aspect realises that in this nothingness there is the fully conscious awareness of the true reality within it. This crossing over from Illusion into nothing is to cross the final and deepest abyss and can never be undertaken alone. It is only through the grace of a Perfect Master that a soul aspect can enter the Seventh Plane. In letting go and releasing all sanskaras, karmic ties, all subtle vehicles, the soul aspect crosses the abyss into nothing, where the essence of the soul that was originally in unconscious bliss at the initial separation from the Divine Ocean, can now enter the Seventh Plane in full consciousness of the Reality that is eternally and infinitely present. All cordings are stripped away from the soul aspect and the mind and all other aspects of the personality are annihilated in the process. Absolutely everything has to be surrendered. The soul aspect at last becomes aware of itself as being God, as being conscious of itself. It is only when this state has been attained that the soul aspect has become God-realised. The soul aspect can then function in full freedom from impressionable bindings and has no physical karma. It is like the dreamer awakens from the dream of illusion and is then in a state of wakefulness and full consciousness of the 'I am' state. Rather than identifying the 'I am' with a particular state of illusion, such as in the physical, astral or mental realms, or in particular human lives, the soul aspect knows the 'I am" to be 'I am God'.

It is this fundamental and profound recognition at the soul level within conscious awareness that enables the soul aspect to become freed of all ties to the worlds of illusion. All physical, emotional and mental ties are seen for what they are – illusion within a dream state, and inside the soul aspect wakes up to the true reality of no separation, just a unity and oneness with the divine. The full journey from unconscious bliss, through to conscious bliss in the Seventh Plane has now been achieved.

In the process of God-realisation there is a complete annihilation of all the links with the physical, astral and mental realms. All of the remaining subtle bodies are stripped away. The soul aspect has to enter an entirely different realm of consciousness, where the consciousness of the different levels of Illusion, as manifested by the physical, astral or mental spheres, are replaced by a living conscious reality of God. The advanced soul has to surrender everything, both conscious and subconscious; all last vestiges of karma are taken away and the soul aspect then stands entirely alone in a space that is best described as the one true abyss between Illusion and Reality. To cross this abyss requires absolute trust and faith, combined with an unwavering focus. In crossing this abyss, the soul aspect then enters the true realms of Reality where it becomes One with the Oversoul.

All of the chakra centres also have to be cleared of any old energies. The different patterns of cordings and energies have to be stripped out so that each chakra just becomes brilliantly white. When this is accomplished then the soul aspect is ready to move forward. There also has to be a balance in the two atoms that reflect the pattern of masculine and feminine lives: once the process of God realisation occurs, these two atoms merge and return back into the one permanent atom. This permanent atom then remains in the heart centre of the newly God-realised being.

A Perfect Master will always oversee the process of God-realisationship. He removes any remaining karma and the final stripping away of the subtle vehicles, before ensuring that the soul aspect crosses the abyss between the Sixth and the Seventh Plane. The soul aspect may feel the complete annihilation of absolutely everything and feel utterly alone in the nothingness of existence, but the Perfect Master will keep a watchful eye on the transition. And once the soul aspect has crossed the abyss, then in the unveiling of full conscious Reality, the soul aspect lets go of any separation and duality and recognises itself as being one with God, and part of the eternal essence of the Oversoul.

In any one cycle of thought, there are usually very few soul aspects that become God-realised. It can be as few as one in several hundred million, and in some cycles of thought it has been less. In the past, the process has been surrounded both by secrecy and glamour: secrecy in that the mechanics of the process have not been revealed and glamour because it is seen by all advancing souls as the ultimate key to becoming more. Furthermore, when a soul aspect usually enters his or her last life, the actual process has taken place at the point of physically dropping the body or several days afterwards. In such cases, there has not been a necessity to provide any information or understanding of the process. The move into the Seventh Plane has been accomplished using the higher, mental body of the soul aspect.

There are many, many obstacles to the successful completion of God-realisationship. In the annihilation of all desires, emotions and attachments, all conscious and subconscious impressions have to be wiped clean. Consequently, any attachment to the actual event itself is a hindrance; any attachment to the outcome becomes an obstacle. In effect, the soul aspect must have no expectations, no attachments, and no ties that bind whether it is with other people or with material objects. The focus of the will has to be utterly ruthless in paying no attention to such emotions and desires. If they become the object of attention and focus, then energy will flow into them and they will become more activated, and harder to pass through. From a state of detachment that is not of the mind, but focused through the heart, it can become possible to work through the various pitfalls of impressions and old feelings, without becoming attached to them. This stance of no importance has to be maintained all the way through the various different types of surrendering that have to be offered up. By a conscious act of surrendering absolutely everything to the Divine, only then can the soul aspect progressively free itself of all karma and sanskaras.

For the living personality, the final life may be one of great difficulty, filled with many trials and tribulations as the last vestiges of karma are burnt off. The soul aspect may meet its Perfect Master in the physical realms, or the process of stripping down and preparation may take place through an inner connection. A soul aspect may live its final life in destitution on the streets and yet the light that is building up behind them will be a reflection of what is to come. And in the final life, as all the previous, outstanding millions of lifetimes are gathered, the one life out of them all that was of greatest spiritual value will come to the surface and be a reflection of the current life of spiritual life and death. The final life, then, is the final accounting of everything that has been gathered in Illusion, and once this final accounting has been completed, all personal karma on the physical, astral and emotional, comes into full balance. With positive and negative karma perfectly balanced, the soul aspect will then be ready for the final abyss and the process of remembering its true essence and self.

One of the main challenges that any soul aspect has through all of the millions and millions of lifetimes is to remember everything that has happened. Of course, if we could remember in an instant everything that we have ever been and done, then our nervous systems would not be able to cope with the informational and energetic overload. Yet, there has to come a point in the soul aspect's involution, when in the physical form, he or she starts to wake up to what they have been. This waking up process means to allow the past to flow through, to be absorbed and to be surrendered in its entirety; yet to feel the presence of the past in Illusion flow through can help that soul aspect to recognise that it is so much more than what is presented in the physical. This waking up to the immortality of the soul aspect, through light and dark, through each successive pattern of lifetimes, can help provide a focus on the bigger picture, rather than the smaller, three-dimensional picture.

Soul aspects will entertain their last lives in a multitude of different ways – they may be entirely unconscious of what is to come and only when they drop their bodies do they become aware of their status and imminent transition into God-realisation. Other soul aspects will become more aware of who they are and where they have come from, and if working directly with a physical Perfect Master in matter, will undergo a rigorous and extremely focused pattern of teaching and stripping down. The Perfect Master will, quite literally, strip away any unwanted karma and will effectively steal all the old karma from that soul aspect. The Perfect Master is the master thief who will go on stealing from that soul aspect until he or she has nothing left. Once this is done, they will be ready to progress onto the next stage. The whole ritual of ownership is removed – all glamour, all desires, all emotions are taken away so that the soul aspect can achieve an ever-finer point of karmic balance. After such rigorous training and discipline, the soul aspect will then be ready to face the final abyss, secure in the knowledge that all attachments have been removed, and that even any attachments to attachments or outcomes have been cleared away. The soul aspect will then be ready to face the journey into nothingness with balance and no concern about the outcome. Only in this point of true balance, can the soul aspect then cross the final abyss, before being met on the other side, at the bottom of the Seventh Plane.

Every soul and soul aspect that crosses into the Seventh Plane has a unique story to tell; a story that describes the different experiences that it has been through in its journey from unconscious bliss into fully realised conscious awareness of what it is. It is this story that is then effectively passed onto God. All of the ark that has been gathered through the millions and millions of lives is then passed onto the Father for digestion. The Father always looks forward with avid interest to each soul's complete story from beginning to end, and the more virulent and bizarre the story, then the more He is entertained. So souls that have been through experiences in dark and light and have plumbed the very depths of existence and also risen to the pinnacle of spiritual achievement will always please the Father. So by the time a soul aspect reaches completion, it is never about judgement, it is about diversity of experience. For in absorbing this diversity, the Father comes to know a bit more about Himself.

One way to look at the process of completion is to imagine that the soul aspect wears a headdress composed of feathers: there is one feather for each lifetime, and on completion the soul aspect will have gathered 8,400,000 feathers which then appear like a fan above the head. The feathers will each be a different frequency and colour, and once they have formed this fan, then each soul aspect will have a unique fan of completion that is rainbow coloured. Once the soul aspect becomes God-realised, the fan will then become clear as all of the frequencies from the past lives are absorbed.

To become God-realised is to undergo the final and ultimate death. Those souls that retain a physical body therefore undergo the final death in physical form, and once God-realised vibrate on a totally different level – in the Seventh Plane. Such beings do not have any personal karma. Usually once physical karma is perfectly balanced, then there is no physical reason to remain alive – the physical form has completed its role as a vehicle and mechanism for absorbing experience while in living matter. It is for this reason that the physical body is normally dropped at the point of God-realisation. However, for those God-realised beings that remain in physical form, a new type of energetic balance and understanding is required. With no physical karma, these beings have no subtle bodies, and so have to borrow astral and mental bodies to process astral and mental streams of light. The state of God-realisationship is one of detachment – there are no desires, emotions or needs and there is a disinterest in all matters relating to the physical world. To live in the physical world, the God-realised being has to borrow karma and therefore works other people's individual karma or group karma.

The Oversoul

Once the soul aspect and the soul becomes God-realised, it then exists for eternity in the Oversoul. The Oversoul is everything – it is the unity and the reality of all souls that recognise, in conscious awareness, that there is no separation and no duality; that all exists as One in the everlasting and permanent essence of the Father. Once the soul associates with its own self, it then associates with the Oversoul since each soul realises that there is no separation at source from the Oversoul. They are one and limitless, infinite and eternal. All souls that reside in the oneness of the Oversoul are like soul mates, yet the meaning of this term is different from the pattern of soul mates in Illusion. In Illusion, each soul aspect may encounter its other soul mates from time to time, as part of the developing pattern of experience in matter. Once the soul aspect is God-realised, it then recognises itself and all other souls in the Oversoul as One. This recognition means that all souls become truly merged in the Oversoul.

One way to conceive of the Oversoul is to see It as a large mushroom without any stalk. Underneath It there are the individual soul units in a collective sense, like a family network, and then underneath them, there are the primary higher, lower and middle soul levels, and then the higher, middle and lower mental levels and astral levels. Within the Oversoul all souls are merged in unity; and then connected to the Oversoul, through the different levels are millions and millions of threads of those souls that are undergoing the outer manifestation of experience. The Oversoul has a directive of energy and the individual souls beneath it start to flux and the principle of light that is required comes down. Each soul then receives a principle of light for its own experimentation, depending on where it is in its own journey.   The Oversoul pulses and radiates Divine Light: it is a manifestation of the Source, an expression of the Father's Will and the home for all of the different expressions of higher soul light that give rise to the different soul families.

The First Divine Journey

Once the soul has passed into the Seventh Plane, it then encounters a whole new pattern of light and existence. Bound in Illusion for millions and millions of lifetimes, it now has the opportunity to begin to know itself as God through a variety of different levels of experience in the Reality of the Seventh Plane. This process of uncovering deeper and deeper layers of existence through conscious reality, of manifesting within different levels of Divine Consciousness and Divine Expression, sets out a series of Divine Journeys.

The soul, once separated from the Ocean of Life, forgets the experience of Unconscious Bliss. It sets out on a journey to rediscover this bliss, yet through a pattern of experiences that help it to wake up into full consciousness of Self; to become aware that the Self is part of God, is God. Once the soul becomes God-realised, it then comes full circle and enters a state of Conscious Bliss. In this state of bliss, the soul enters what is known as the First Divine Journey.

In this bliss state, every moment in every facet of the experience is in bliss, and for the soul in this state, it is like having a never ending chain of experiences and events which are all soaked in pure bliss, and which are not repetitious or boring. It is like entering a field filled with the most beautiful flowers and being in a state of constant rapture at each and every flower that is seen. The exquisiteness of the first flower induces a blissful feeling, and then every subsequent flower seen produces the same blissful state yet the object of attention is in a state of constant change. The soul in the First Divine Journey never becomes bored and because it is in a state of perpetual bliss, believing this to be the essence of God in Its Totality and Universality. The bliss captures the soul in a never-ending moment from which the focus is always changing but is constantly in bliss. For souls entering the First Divine Journey this is often taken to be the end point of their evolution and they become trapped and enchanted in the bliss.

To humanity bliss is anything but slow; bliss is this magnificent remembrance of the Father. If we go back to the Primary Spark and the flow of light down through the Seventh Plane, then all of these vibrations that came down gave the contemplations from the one Primary Spark, through sequence after sequence of splitting, millions of times over. So the one Primary Spark started to expand outwards in the lower Divine Journeys, like a big pyramid, and so what is present in the First Divine Journey is billions and billions of variations of what the Father probably was, what the Father probably is, and what the Father probably will become.

Over the aeons and aeons of time, millions and millions of souls have become God-realised and then entered the First Journey. The First Divine Journey can be split into ten sub-levels, just like the lower planes. So the lower part of the First Divine Journey will incorporate the first three subdivisions, the middle, the next three and then the higher part, the reminder. When a soul enters the First Divine Journey after becoming God-realised, it hits the first sub-level and then the second and third. The impulse of the soul slows down because it is an individual soul coming into a collective stream of consciousness that simply takes it out of the way. It moves sideways becoming perpetually entertained by all those sparks that call to it and present millions and millions of representations of what God was, is and will be. They become caught up in the perpetual moment of bliss. So the result is the dance and the music claims the soul because it does not have the endurance as an individual collective component coming home to endure and to move through these patterns of light. The only exceptions to this are the Perfect Masters.

Consequently, very few souls have progressed through the First Divine Journey because they have had insufficient power or focus to move on through it. They have become trapped in the bliss, seeing it as the end point, rather than as a point of limitation within the totality of all that is God. Consequently, since the beginning, the First Divine Journey has filled up with millions of souls that have chosen to remain within it. They have not moved on and this has represented a point of limitation within the unfolding of the Father's Play.

Those souls that remain in physical form once they have become God-realised enter the First Divine Journey and from that station experience everything around them through bliss. They are dead in the normal sense of experience in Illusion because they have no astral or mental bodies, and their physical shell only remains present due to the karma that is borrowed off others around them. They have no personal karma and work, instead, different patterns of group karma to remain in physical matter. Anchored in the First Divine Journey means that such souls are in a state of constant bliss, and this accounts for the belief that God-realisationship automatically leads to a state of constant bliss. The bliss is the first step, not the last step. It is the first part of the next major voyage into deeper layers of Reality and into merging with the essence of the Father.

A God-realised being who is in physical form and who is in the First Divine Journey can work directly with the bliss frequency. In the past, very few souls ever progressed through the First Divine Journey, and those that did were entitled then to enter the Second Divine Journey. On completion of the First Divine Journey such souls would have mastered the first stages of bliss, which can be viewed as a golden frequency.

The Second Divine Journey

The very few souls that do enter the Second Divine Journey either go on to become Perfect Masters or are more advanced souls such as Paramahansas. If the First Divine Journey is the conscious experience of "I am God" in infinite bliss, power and knowledge, then the Second Divine Journey builds a new platform where the soul experiences itself as God and man simultaneously in infinite, power, knowledge and bliss. The Second Divine Journey also has bliss as the predominant frequency, and the bliss experienced here is different from the First Divine Journey. One way to describe the difference is to say that the First Divine Journey embodies black bliss, while the Second Divine Journey is the essence of white bliss. Both are states of bliss, yet are different, like opposites.

The First Divine Journey is infinitely large and the Second Divine Journey is even greater than this; like the First Divine Journey it can be spilt into ten sub-levels. God-realised souls who have retained a physical body and who enter the Second Divine Journey experience a subtly different form of bliss, bridging the twin experiences of "I am God" and "I am my own physical being or creature". The gulf between the First Divine Journey and Second Divine Journey is known as the Divine Junction[1], and it is here that the soul builds up the alternate experience of "I am God" and "I am human", until at the end of the Second Divine Journey the two states can be experienced simultaneously. It is here that the soul experiences itself as abiding in God or being God, as opposed to the "I am" state.

Even fewer souls ever complete the Second Divine Journey, and those that do will have mastered a different aspect of God. If the dominant divine colour of the First Divine Journey is gold, then the dominant colour on completion of the Second Divine Journey is white. Once the Second Divine Journey is completed, the Third Divine Journey beckons.

The Third Divine Journey

The Third Divine Journey is where those souls that are to become Perfect Masters eventually live the experience of living as God. The Perfect Master becomes the Man-God on completion of the Third Divine Journey. This Divine Journey is completely different from the first two Divine Journeys and embodies grace. Grace implies the earned favour of God and it is through the Grace of God that the Perfect Master is made manifest.

It is in the Third Divine Journey that a segregation of energies or birthing of opposites is made manifest. Here the Primary Spark originally split itself up into the law of opposites — male and female, light and dark, chaos and order, and as that came down it drove the vision of the Father down into the slower, grosser levels of matter. This pattern of energy is expressed in the essence and lived experience of this Divine Journey.

In traversing the Third Divine Journey, the Perfect Master has to live through all of the emotions and the feelings in the planes of Illusion and begins a journey that is the Second Descent (as opposed to the First Descent from the Ocean of Life into the mineral form at the bottom of the Zero Plane). In this descent, the Perfect Master, who is conscious of himself as man and God simultaneously, drops down from the Seventh Plane into the Sixth Plane to live the emotions and experiences in Illusion. He then passes through all of the planes again, through the Fifth, into the Fourth, the Third, the Second, the First and then ultimately into the Zero Plane down to 0.0. From this vantage point in Illusion, the Perfect Master experiences the living emotions and feelings of all the planes and he then begins his ascent back up to the Seventh Plane as he then absorbs everything in Illusion inside him. He completes the Third Divine Journey at the point at which he returns into the Seventh Plane, goes back through the First and Second Divine Journeys and has absorbed all of the experiences in Illusion as emotions and feelings.

The Perfect Master, at the completion of the Third Divine Journey, is simultaneously in every plane all the time and actually lives the life of God in this state. Together with living the life of God, he lives the life of man, and yet he is simultaneously in all the universes, and in all the worlds and on all of the planes. He is infinitely connected with the Universe. On completion of the Third Divine Journey, the Perfect Master has absorbed the first three Divine Journeys and is living in all of them, as well as in Illusion. The divine frequency of the Third Divine Journey is blue and the Perfect Master is then able to host the gold, white and blue frequencies in his living essence.

The Fourth Divine Journey and Beyond

The Perfect Master, while retaining his physical body, does not progress beyond the Third Divine Journey. It is only after dropping his physical form that he begins the Fourth Divine Journey, which is also called the annihilation. After dropping his body, the Perfect Master remains consciously and individually as God the Infinite. The experience of infinite consciousness, which is indivisible, is retained eternally as "I am God". In the Fourth Divine Journey the Perfect Master enters the Ocean of Annihilation where he undergoes a further transformation and absorption into God. This Journey represents another aspect of unveiling of a different part of God in terms of becoming absorbed into the living essence of God As the Perfect Master becomes absorbed in the Ocean, then all of the ark that he has gathered throughout creation is also absorbed into the essence of the Divine.

The Fourth Divine Journey can be split into two major patterns – the first, as mentioned, is the Ocean of Annihilation where each soul has to endure seven principle waves of Light and Dark, although the formation of this Light and Dark is completely different from what we would understand it to mean. Crossing the Ocean takes each soul to an island of light, where the Father is present. From this vantage point, the soul then moves up into a higher pattern of light, known as Air of the Fourth Divine Journey. This expanse of Air is limitless and again to cross this pattern of light requires a focus of will and endurance to withstand the hugely powerful light streams. Once the crossing of Air has been completed, the soul has then completed the Fourth

Divine Journey. The dominant frequency note for the completion of the Fourth Divine Journey is green.

Up to now the Fourth Divine Journey has represented the cut off point in terms of the description of the different states of existence within the living essence of God. Yet there is always more and the new pattern of energies being birthed through the Sixth Root Race are opening up a new description of the different Divine Journeys, and in characterising those Journeys in more detail. In the context of attempting to describe that which is infinite, eternal and indescribable, Meher Baba himself distinguished between two principal states. His description follows below:

> "*Because God is Infinite, Eternal, all pervading existence, and is eternally infinite existence, it follows that there are also an infinite number of states of God, which are infinite and eternally existing. Within this there are two fundamental states of God: the original state and the final state. The original state of God is the Beyond the Beyond State of God where eternally God "Is" and consciousness "Is Not". The final state is the Beyond state of God where consciousness "Is" eternally of the "God-Is" state of the Beyond the Beyond state of God.*" (From *God Speaks* pps. 152-153.)

For the soul that seeks to become more, there is always the possibility of pushing up beyond the initial Divine Journeys. In this progression, the soul will come into contact with more and more condensed light, and each aspect of the different Divine Journeys gives a fundamental detailed analysis of what the Father probably is, but as the soul goes up to another level, then it absorbs yet another, more detailed expression of the Father. So the First, Second, Third and Fourth Divine Journeys all give an increasingly refined expression of what the Father was, is and will probably become.

CHAPTER 12

The Avatar & The Perfect Masters

The Avatar

The Avatar is the first soul to complete the journey through all of the planes, and since that first journey the Avatar has returned at periodic times, to go back into the Creation of the Father to unfold more. So in the grand scheme of the everything and nothing there was the original "I" which was and is the Father, which then sought expression in "I am" which then became manifested as the Son. The Father is fathomless and beyond expression, and yet out of the Father was birthed the Primeval Spark, the Son, that became the Avatar.

In the first original cycle of manifestation, the Primary Spark dropped down through the Seventh Plane and then down through the shadow planes, before returning back up. In birthing this sequence of journeys, the Primary Spark also locked everything into a sort of sequence. In so doing, the Avatar started to activate within the placement of vibration or energy – call it the imagination of the Father – a discourse of Reality and Illusion. The Father sent down a spark of His imagination that created what we know as creation, and as He came down everything was there but in a layered pattern. As the Primary Spark came down, it set off a transference of energy that started to activate other sparks that then grew according to the discourse of the Father or life that was actually put into them. While this took place the life pattern, as we know it, started to manifest, and creation from the Primary Spark started to manifest as well.

This principal journey is loosely reprised during each cycle of Avataric expression and form. The Avatar comes back down from the essence of the higher aspects of the Seventh Plane, dropping down through the Seventh Plane and into the lower planes, ultimately to the bottom of the Zero Plane, and then back up through the planes to return into the Seventh Plane. The Avatar comes in to take the pulse beat of Creation, and to make any necessary adjustments to the pattern and flow of energy. The Avatar comes down for all life – not just humanity, but all the different life forms in the Mineral, Plant and Animal Kingdoms, and for all life that is expressed in the Wheel of Life. In each cycle of thought, the Avatar will incarnate in the current expression of physical form that is dominant. So in our current age, the Avatar presents Himself in human form and walks the Earth as the living manifestation of the Will of the Father.

We currently live in an Avataric Age and this represents the time during which the Avatar is in incarnation and for the one hundred year period afterwards. This one hundred year period represents the period of outer time in which the Avatar returns back "home" through the millions and millions of levels of the Seventh Plane. Each Avataric Cycle lasts either 700 or 1400 years in Earth time, although there are sometimes intermediate periods during which an aspect of the Avatar may come down into incarnation within a variation of His Full Manifestation. The timing of each cycle is set by the five Perfect Masters in matter at that time, and it is the five Perfect Masters who call the Avatar back down depending upon the prevailing conditions. So, if in between an Avataric Age, the balance between chaos and order is shifting away from what had been established during the last Avataric Age then there is a pressure on the Perfect Five to call the Avatar back in earlier – i.e. after 700 years rather than waiting the full 1400 years.

The Avatar, when He first sets off on each journey into physical incarnation in each cycle, will begin His descent from the highest levels of the Seventh Plane. It is like He begins His Journey in the God in the Beyond-Beyond State, although this cannot be defined, and then comes down through the God in the Beyond State to the lower levels of the Seventh Plane. In the Fourth Divine Journey a different pattern, like a time lock was established, so that each time the Avatar comes down the pattern of energy opens up a series of aperture points. These openings in the Fourth Divine Journey remain open, and do not close very quickly. It takes approximately one hundred years in Earth time for these openings to close, and it is this pattern of energy that helps to maintain the irradiation of the Avatar during an Avataric Age.

As He comes down, He draws to Himself, those souls that will be part of the Avataric Programme of Work. This relates not only to those souls on the Seventh Plane, but to all those on the lower planes. As the first soul, the Avatar does not go through the same process of evolution and involution like all the other souls in matter. He is already God and it is a case of His remembering and experiencing this essential fact. In remembering who He is, He becomes the living embodiment of God in the physical realms. He is the God-Man.

Just like any other incarnating soul, He is born without any memory or recall of what He is, and it is only through meeting with the different Perfect Masters that the different veils of illusion are stripped away from Him, and He comes to recognise and live what and who He is. In becoming the Avatar, he goes through all of the planes while growing up, and then returns to the lower levels of the Seventh Plane, as the veil of illusion is lifted and he becomes God-realised again. This process is like a memory, since He is God all the time, but there is a requirement for Him to become the Avatar through the stripping away of all the different illusions.

The Avatar then passes through the bottom three Divine Journeys, first experiencing the bliss of the lower levels of the Seventh Plane, and then into the Third Divine Journey where He absorbs everything from all of the planes below into Him. He does this physically as well as emotionally. So, with Meher Baba, the experience of being God meant that He had to absorb all of the pain and suffering of all creation into His awareness and experience in physical matter. At the same time, the intensity of light was such that He also found physical pain the principle mechanism to ground Himself in matter. Once awakened, Meher Baba then set out to rewire and restructure the creation as part of the Nine-Pointed Plan.

Each Avataric Age represents a focal point of Avataric Energy and in this latest cycle, the level of energy is one hundred percent. This means that the Avatar is irradiating all of His Attributes. This has not always been the case, and during the time of the Christ, the manifested level of energy was seventy–five percent. Previously with the Buddha it had been sixty percent. And if we look back through history at the different Avatars that have graced the planet, then we can see a range of different types of expression and energetic focus. The Avataric Programme is the ongoing pattern of manifestation through the ages, of the Avatar in His different forms. So, earlier Avatars like Ganesha have made way for Krishna, Zoroaster, Mohammed and others. During each Avataric Age there has been change which has been played out in the different cycles of thought and experience in matter. Each root race has been initiated and finished by the presence and authority of the Avatar.

Each Avataric Cycle will irradiate a pattern of energy that can be supported by the living form present at that time. So today, the physical manifestation of life is now able to absorb the full irradiation of the Avatar – one hundred percent. And what we are seeing in the unfolding of the Nine-Pointed Plan is the expression throughout all of creation of the new birth of the Sixth Root Race. The bulk of humanity has tended to accept the Avataric Energy of each Age with some difficulty, and rather than experiencing the living Will of the Father as a dynamic, constantly changing expression of life, has sought to 'freeze' the particular series of teachings and energetic patterns into a series of different religions, each of which is but a shadow of the essence of the true spiritual message and divine pattern of orchestration. This 'freezing' process represents limitation, and in some cases the pattern of energy that Meher Baba has orchestrated is seen no differently. Rather than experiencing the constant flux of dynamic love and becoming within the pattern of awakening that Meher Baba has orchestrated, there is sometimes a tendency to hold onto the more superficial patterns that do not full justice to the true and undiluted rhythm of His Energy. Consequently, humanity can never claim to know the Will of the Avatar, and can never claim to be the source of balanced interpretation, because with the exception of those who have ascended into the Seventh Plane, those in the Sixth Plane and below, are all bound by Illusion and karma, and have to work through the ongoing interplay of light and dark, and chaos and order. This is not a judgement, but a statement of how the energy operates and how our different personalities may seek to limit something that is utterly limitless. Thus the Nine-Pointed Plan of Meher Baba represents the unfolding flow of different aspects of His Will in a host of different ways and what may appear to be strictly true and unchanging at one point in time, may at a later date, no longer be true. Thus the truth of today becomes superseded by the higher truth of tomorrow.

The Avatar has two hundred and twelve main agents in matter, and these agents are positioned on different levels on the inner planes. So some will be in the Zero Plane, others on the First Plane, while others stationed between the planes, and so on. Some of the agents will be consciously aware that they are working with the Avatar, while others will not be. Either way, they will be under the energetic umbrella of the Avatar and will work according to the dictates of His Will. In this Avataric Period, there has been a lot of recorded information on the actual life of Meher Baba[1] and the Avatar also has left a series of writings to focus the spiritual development of humanity. Meher Baba always said that He had come to awaken, and the central key, for every sentient being on the planet and beyond, is ultimately to align him or herself with the living Will of the Avatar. To offer everything in our lives to the Avatar is to begin this process; to surrender everything on the principles of trust and faith is to open up a dialogue with the Avatar. Yet, at the same time, it is to recognise that the Avatar never does anything the same twice over. So if He first appears to us in our dreams, then the next time, He will present Himself differently in our awareness. We, therefore, have to be flexible and avoid being dogmatic in building up a dialogue with the Avatar.

The Avatar represents everything in creation, is everything and nothing, is in and part of absolutely everything; He is all of the planes and beyond and so to connect with His Presence, in whatever way, always involves change. The Avatar will always change absolutely everything in our lives. Ultimately, as evolving souls, it is our aim and destiny to absorb the Stare of the Avatar. The Stare represents the manifested expression of the Avatar's Will, His Energetic Essence and His Unconditional Love. To be able to absorb the Stare of the Avatar means that first, every soul has to be able to absorb the Stare of a Perfect Master. So the journey of discovery and self-realisation, which ultimately leads to the Avatar, always has to come through the auspices of one of the Five Perfect Masters.

The Avatar, then, incarnates for all life, and will work with every life form present. During His Life, Meher Baba worked for 40 years in silence – true spiritual work is always done is silence. So in finding our own inner silence, we can begin to connect with this pattern. He also released the Unspoken Word, which represents so many different things on so many divine levels. In one sense it is the essence of change and the transformation of every living being into the new root race alignment. On releasing the Unspoken Word during His Life, Meher Baba sent out an energetic charge that is now coming back into the Planet – and this energetic charge represents total change on all levels.

For all of us, our minds can never comprehend the Avatar. Instead, our focus should be to embrace with our hearts, and not our minds, the essence of his living Will and Love. The Avatar knows every thought, every action and every emotion that we live and breathe; He knows everything that has ever been, is, and will be. So if our lives have been graced by the blessing and love of the Avatar, then all that we need to do is to invoke His Authority and Love, and trust in the outcome of everything that is. Through unconditional love our lives will be forged into a new type of expression and in aligning ourselves with the living Will of the Avatar, then we will be and become that which our souls have ordained on the higher planes.

The Father, Son and Holy Ghost

The new pattern of energy that is building also requires that we work and assimilate the essence of more. And the principal focus, the primary triangle of expression is the Father, Son and Holy Ghost. The

Father on any day is beyond our comprehension and understanding. He is the embodiment of absolutely everything that is present in both the everything and the nothing. The Father is immense and beyond any form of description. The Father then gave birth to the Son, which became the Avatar in physical form on Earth. The Son was the Primary Spark, the first light to lighten up the planes, and then the multiple manifestations of the Avatar through all the different cycles of thought and the ages that have ever been. The Son always embodies the manifested Will of the Father, and while the Son is all things in everything and nothing, and is unfathomable, He is separate and distinct from the Father and by coming into matter provides a path for all souls to follow.

The Holy Ghost completes the third aspect of this principal triangle and is the essence of the One, the essence of the Father and the Son. The Father and Son combined are the One, so the Holy Ghost is the essence of the One. Another way to express this is to see the Holy Ghost as the afterglow of the initial spark, the two original sparks that sparked creation – the Father and the Son. Yet in becoming the afterglow, the presence of the Avatar constantly sparks this afterglow into a spark and this is the manifested essence of the Holy Ghost. The Holy Ghost is the creative and destructive song of the Father, embodying power and love. The presence of the Holy Ghost always invokes change on every level, from the individual through to the root race. Together, the Father, Son and Holy Ghost represent the Trinity.

The Five Perfect Masters

At any one time, there are always five Perfect Masters. The Five each host twenty percent of God and each one can be defined as Man-God. The five Perfect Masters always oversee the whole focus of creation in between Avataric Ages, and during an Avataric Age the responsibility of everything is passed to the Avatar. Unlike the Avatar, Perfect Masters have been through the whole pattern of evolution and involution and are souls that have also become God-realised in their final life, and then gone onto complete the three Divine Journeys. They hold all of creation within their essence and are beyond light and dark, chaos and order, and the masculine and feminine. The Perfect Master is manifest on all planes simultaneously and yet can appear as a perfectly ordinary human being. Unlike the Avatar who is God becoming man, the Perfect Master is man becoming God.

The five Perfect Masters embody different attributes: power, knowledge, wisdom, truth and bliss. Each one also represents a series of frequencies, like a dominant colour: white, black, orange, gold and pink. During any particular period, some of these attributes will dominate over others, although power is usually a prerequisite to any pattern of change. The Perfect Master will live their specific attribute, so knowledge will manifest all aspects of knowledge, both light and dark, while truth will also reflect the prevailing patterns. Sometimes Perfect Masters will work these attributes through light and at other times through dark, depending upon the specific cycle. While power provides the 'juice' for everything, bliss is like the fixative that makes sure that everything is 'glued' into place. For any change to take place, there always has to be agreement between the five, and all of them ultimately have to live the love, service, devotion and obedience to the Father. They become and live the living will of the Father.

Three of the Perfect Masters work with humanity, while two do not, and in any one cycle of thought the Perfect Masters will embody a specific balance of male and female members. During Meher Baba's life there were four men and one woman. There are many different examples of Perfect Masters from the past and perhaps best known today are the five that were in office during the advent of the Avatar: Sai Baba of Shirdi (Power), Upasni Maharaj (Knowledge), Hasrat Babajan (Bliss), Taddujin Baba (Wisdom) and Narayan Maharaj (Truth). A living example of a Perfect Master is Amma who embodies bliss and works with humanity. For the most part, the spiritual climate in the East has been more supportive of the workings of Perfect Masters, although Meher Baba predicted that Perfect Masters would also be born and work in the West.

The Perfect Masters represent the spiritual guides and dynamic generators through which the essence of the Father flows.

Each Perfect Master hosts twenty percent of the essence of God and during his or her lifetime will work according to the specific dictates of the Will of the Father. The Perfect Master has one day in which to achieve and fulfil his or her contract. The work of all Perfect Masters is continual and carried on day and night, irrespective of the physical needs of their bodies – hence each Perfect Master lives for one day only. In Earth time, that day may last a few weeks, a few years, or decades depending upon the focus of work that needs to be carried out. Yet each Perfect Master is only in existence due to the Grace of the Father. So a day in the life of a Perfect Master is the time down here where service is and service will be the definition of life for the Master of that time.

Each Perfect Master has one hundred and forty four main agents. For those working with humanity, they will always be human, while for the two Perfect Masters that work with other life forms then the circle is composed of devic and other life forms. Each Perfect Master has a principal circle of twelve, and then arranged below this the other circles of twelve that go onto make up the one hundred and forty four.

A new Perfect Master is only made up once another one has dropped his or her body, and so the principle of "dead man's shoes" always operates. Once initiated, each Perfect Master then has to undergo a rigorous training and to follow a pre-established pattern of young, middle-aged and old Perfect Masters. A new Perfect Master can only be initiated by an existing Perfect Master, and through this pattern of initiation, then a lineage of Perfect Masters can be established. New Perfect Masters are usually initiated out of the existing membership of the fifty-one God realised beings on the planet at any one time (see below – The Fifty-Six God-realised Ones).

Once made up, the new Perfect Master has to go up through the first three Divine Journeys and then bring his awareness down from the Third Divine Journey into the Second Divine Journey and then into the First Divine Journey; from there he has to enter the Sixth Plane, and then take the three Divine Journeys into the Sixth Plane, and then on going into the Fifth Plane, bring the three Divine Journeys and the Sixth Plane into the Fifth. This process goes on down through each plane, where all that has gone before has to be brought into the next plane level; so at the Fourth Plane, for example, the Fifth, Sixth and the three Divine Journeys are condensed into it. This goes on all of the way down into the Zero Plane and then the Perfect Master comes all of the way back up. In this way the Perfect Master experiences the living essence of everything through a pattern of condensing and expanding.

Each Perfect Master has the capacity to ride the awareness of living form, either in light or dark, according to the specific directions of the Father. Perfect Masters, depending on the time period and type of work that needs to be done, will either be more or less in the public eye. Humanity is not necessary for them to do their work and those that work with other life forms will usually retain the presence of many different life forms within their agency. Behind each Perfect Master is the essence of the collective Perfect Masters, which represents all of the Perfect Masters that have ever been. The collective Perfect Masters are the combined essences of all the Perfect Masters and, as such, host all of the frequencies that they have ever been throughout the different root races. As part of the initiation programme, all young Perfect Masters have to receive the stare of the collective Perfect Masters and in so doing, absorb the collective essence of all that the Perfect Master is and has ever been.

During a soul aspect's journey into matter and over the course of that soul aspect's allotted lives, meetings either in the physical or on the inner planes will be orchestrated as part of the evolving pattern of development. If a soul aspect meets a Perfect Master in physical matter, then a contract is entered into between the Perfect Master and that soul. Sometimes such encounters can be pre-ordained, while at other times, they are opportunistic. When the Perfect Master then drops his body, the contract with that soul aspect is then passed onto the collective Perfect Masters where it is retained until in a future life it is reactivated through a further set of physical meetings with a series of different living Perfect Masters. So each soul aspect, during its 8,400,000 lives will physically meet a Perfect Master at least once.

The Perfect Masters represent the esoteric thieves of karma, for in every encounter, physical or otherwise, the Perfect Master will strip away the karma from any given individual or group. Perfect Masters need to borrow karma to stay in physical matter, while at the same time, one of their primary roles is to absorb the ark and karma of living beings and transform this dark energy into overspill. Overspill is like the pure essence of higher light that is generated as a result of his or her work, and the overspill can then be used to infuse and transform any physical or subtle event, person or object to a higher vibration. So if an evolving soul aspect receives a large dose of overspill, then in all likelihood, that will reduce the number of lives that the evolving soul requires before completion. Those souls, when they have built up enough experience in matter, will then be offered a glance from a Perfect Master, and if this is sufficiently absorbed, then a look and ultimately a stare. The stare of the Perfect Master is the embodiment of his or her essence, and through close association, the disciples of a Perfect Master will build up experience through receiving more and more virulent stares as a progressive sequence of light that will ultimately be the preparation for receiving the Stare of the Father.

Perfect Masters are generally dynamic-dynamic which means that they initiate, push through and direct the focus of energy wherever it is needed in the Universe. They are the axis or the pivot around which creation flows. They are the embodiment of the everything and nothing. They focus their will and intent and direct the energy to where it is needed and then will use that energy to ride the awareness of different living beings, including the planets and solar systems and stars. They are the initiators and also the overseers of all events that take place in the Universe. For example, Sai Baba of Shirdi was responsible for the 1st World War, and the pattern of energy that flowed through him, as a consequence of the loss of limb and life in the trenches, led to a reflective pattern within his own physical vehicle where his legs and arms would become detached from his torso. He was a 'ghouse' type of Perfect Master.

During the twenty-four hour day, the five Perfect Masters irradiate a series of pulses that can be picked up by all living form and there are eighteen pulses each day. Every pulse represents a point of silence; a point of stillness where the true essence within can be accessed and this pulse can be felt within the heart.

The Fifty Six God-Realised Ones

During any age there are normally fifty-six God-realised beings on the planet. Of these, five are Perfect Masters, while the remaining fifty-one act as the spiritual generators. The fifty-one God realised beings are normally passive-dynamic and not necessarily aware that they are one of the Fifty-Six — they are not necessarily consciously aware of their true role. Nevertheless they walk the Earth and irradiate unconditional love as spiritual generators. If we were to give a dominant frequency focus or colour to each one of these fifty-one, then it would be purple.

Unlike the Perfect Master the spiritual generators do not pass through the Third Divine Journey but normally reside in the bliss state of the First Divine Journey. Their energetic systems are like open doors in that they can host a whole diversity of different divine energies according to the strength and underlying genetics of their supporting mechanism. Principally, however, the passive state of the fifty-one God-realised beings is ridden by the dynamic focus of the five Perfect Masters. So at any one time, a number of the Fifty-One may feel the presence of one of the Perfect Masters pulsing through them. As the energy flows through, then the passive state can become a more dynamic energetic flow, hence the passive-dynamic state. The spiritual generators are also collective and represent a platform through which the five Perfect Masters can direct and control the flow of energy through all of Creation.

As spiritual generators the role of the Fifty-One is to open up to the energies coming in, to allow their systems to be used as amplification devices and to feel the energy being directed to wherever it needs to go. This will usually be an unconscious process, although each individual may feel the pulses of energy manifesting in his or her physical vehicle. In remaining usually in a passive state, they are then in a state of readiness to receive whatever divine instruction and energy flows through them.

In exceptional and special circumstances there may be more than fifty-six God-realised beings and currently there are fifty-seven. The special addition to the Fifty-Six in this instance is Mother Meera who has a specific role of bringing through the Paramatman into humanity. Her speciality role makes her a key addition to the Fifty-Six.

The Fifty-Six God-realised beings also act as the assembly or parliament for all matters and decisions of import to affect the planet and beyond. All spiritual promotions within the different planes, in the progression of a soul aspect's journey through involution will be discussed and argued by the Fifty-Six. For example, if a soul aspect is seeking a spiritual promotion, then he will need a sponsor to put his case before the Fifty-Six. Generally speaking there are always those who will support a promotion, and others who will oppose it. After discussion, a decision will then be made usually along the lines of either "Yes", "No" or "Wait". Of course "wait" can be interpreted in many different ways and can cover many lifetimes. In a rare life of spiritual importance, a soul aspect may petition to become God-realised, and this petition may also go through the five Perfect Masters or the Fifty-Six.

The Fifty-Six also reflect the pattern of fifty-six mental illnesses that afflict humanity. All of these different energetic patterns will run through the Fifty-Six at any one point in time, but generally, many of the Fifty-Six will specialise in one of these illnesses. So, for example, despair, rejection, anger, cruelty, greed, fear etc. will all be pushed through the Fifty-Six as a series of frequencies, yet each member will work one specific illness more than the others. On becoming inducted into the fifty-one, each being has to experience the full complement of fifty-six mental illnesses in the lived experience of the moment, while retaining a specific focus on one of the illnesses. The fifty-one generators do not work this through as their own karma, but as the pattern of work that each one has undertaken for humanity and other life forms.

The Spiritual Hierarchy

In addition to the Fifty-Six there is another level of spiritual recognition known as the Spiritual Hierarchy. It normally contains seven thousand members, although in an Avataric Age, numbers seven thousand and one, with the Avatar as the automatic Head. Members of the Spiritual Hierarchy are strategically placed in the different planes, from the First Plane through to the Seventh Plane. The bulk of members are either in the First Plane, or distributed between the different planes, from the First and Second through to the Sixth and Seventh. Their role, amongst others, is to oversee the movement of different souls through the planes. The remaining members are found in the Second through to the Seventh Plane in decreasing numbers[2]. For example, there are only fifty-six members in the Fifth and Sixth Planes, and eight in the Seventh Plane. The latter include the five Perfect Masters and three other members of the Fifty-Six. The other remaining forty-eight members of the Fifty-Six remain independent of the Spiritual Hierarchy. Consequently, the Spiritual Hierarchy is structured like a pyramid, with the five Perfect Masters at the top.

The role of the Spiritual Hierarchy is to undertake assigned spiritual duties across or between all of the planes according to each member's experience and level of spiritual advancement. They are the managers of the planes. Every member of the Spiritual Hierarchy is currently in physical incarnation at this time.

CHAPTER 13

The New Sixth Root Race
Programme I

Raising the Planetary Vibration

The planet is the living essence of Gaia and as a living entity in its own right has endured and survived the succession of cycles of light and dark that have flowed through the various root races. All the different life forms that have ever stood, crawled, walked, climbed, flown or swum on the planet's surface have left an energetic charge. This charge is like a memory of what the particular life form did and is recorded in the rocks, the earth, the water, and the various life forms that have remained on the planet's surface for longer periods of time, such as the trees. Like us, the planet has etheric, astral and mental body forms; the same is true of the galaxy.

Each root race has left an enduring pulse of energy that is like a recorded memory of what took place. Initially, that energetic pulse is quite strong, but with time it diminishes and fades. In each succession of change, the planet plays host to a procession of different life forms; the physical fossil record gives an indication, albeit an incomplete one, of what different life forms have passed through the planet. However, the fossil record represents less, not more of what has ever been. And the patterns of change that sweep over the planet through continental drift, sea level changes, climatic change and ice ages are all part of the ongoing process of change: the planet is never static. The planet also interacts with the Moon, the feminine shadow, and also the Sun, and the other planets in the solar system. It is also part of a connected pattern of communication with other stars and galaxies out there in space, and part of much larger cosmic cycles.

Just as physical form has evolved through the pantheon of different root races, so the planet has also changed. Following its initial formation and birthing, the vibration of the planet has constantly changed as a result of the different life forms that were hosted both on its surface and inside it. This process has been dynamic: for its part, the planetary vibration, or the sum total energetic expression of light and dark, has had to change during each successive root race. This has been brought about by the essence of Gaia and her dance with Macheldavek as she has absorbed different light frequencies and has orchestrated a majestic flow of different light streams, through the pattern of the elements, Fire, Air, Earth and Water.

The Earth inherited an older pattern of solar system energy that can best summed up as the old devic patterns. This old pattern was quite dark and was represented as a square pattern of energy. The energetic foundations of the planet were built upon this old devic pattern. This old devic presence is very strong and has required disciplining, a pattern that humanity has to exercise today. Hand-in-hand with this flow of energy, each succession of life that has graced the planet has earthed a certain series of frequencies that were imbued into their essence. So through the different root races, as the mix of light and dark was changed, and as the different subtle and physical vehicles were birthed onto the planet, then such vehicles were used to ground a multiplicity of light frequencies into the planet. So in the Lemurian times, the creative and intuitive flow of energy was pushed through, while in the Atlantean age, the scientific and intellectual flow of energy was initiated. Within each root race, multiple streams of energy, as maintained through the interplay of light and dark, were held in bondage by the physical vehicles at that time. So the Mineral, Plant, Animal and Human Kingdoms all maintained different patterns of energy that were supported by the devic focus of intent. The devas acted as the superglue and supporting structure for all physical form on the planet, as well as the planet herself.

Within this creative mix of different energetic streams and life forms, aspects of the Divine then graced the planet. The succession of Avatars and Perfect Masters and other God-realised beings all contributed to the constant flux of the planet's vibration. And throughout these cycles, the focus has always been to raise the vibration of the planet. Yet in each successive cycle, the principles of karma and natural law have had to be adhered to. So with each shift in vibration, the older, slower frequencies have needed to be cleared to create the space for the newer energies to come in. This situation is no different today where the old timeline supports old astral intent, which is unfinished purpose in matter. The old needs to be cleared to make way for the new.

This process of clearing is a vital prelude to the shift in energies that the planet needs to invoke to fully enter the Sixth Root Race timeline. And within this process of clearing, it is necessary to go right back to the birth of the planet and the inherited matrix of energies that were donated from the different solar systems. Consequently, one of the first aspects of change that needs to be invoked is a shift in the inherited devic patterns from the old solar system. The square formation of devic energy has to be replaced by the new triangle of devic light and one that can support a higher flow of mental light. The old pattern can be seen as a cloud of dark energy that surrounds the planet, and which is also held within the planet itself. The vibratory pattern of this energy is very slow and over the next few years a programme of clearing and transmuting this slow frequency energy needs to take place. The old devic pattern has to go (see also Chapter 14 – New Patterns of Soul Light).

When we go back and focus on the old root races, each one has a different pulse or virulence. The pulse of the old Adamic and Hyperborean Root Races is very weak, which means that most of the older energies and frequencies associated with them have already been cleared. The same is true of us – if we look into our past Akashic Records, then there is barely a pulse beat from those times, and the vast majority of souls now on the planet first came in either during the Lemurian or the Atlantean times.

If we go into the energies retained from the Lemurian and Atlantean times, then the story is very different. Both root races maintain a strong pulse, and many of the difficulties that humanity has encountered in more recent times are due to the echo of these old energies calling to them – especially from the Atlantean. All physical form acts as a recording device; this refers to the gross, physical measurement of different characteristics and properties, such as the magnetic patterns in rock, the climatic rings in trees, the patterns of salinity in the sea, and the gaseous content in the atmosphere we breathe. This recorded history also encompasses the astral levels where emotions and thought forms are retained. The whole planet is full of the memories of the energetic charges of what has happened at a particular place in specific times. Positive and negative Ley Lines acts as amplifiers and distributors of this energy throughout the planetary surface while water and the ground retain clear records of what has transpired. It is not especially easy to find virgin territory on the planet, where there has been little or no imprinting, although Iceland would be a fair example of this. In some parts of the world, the negative imprinting has been almost constant, with one wave of negative energy overlaying another. Cities are good examples of this, where large amounts of slow frequency dark light are retained.

It is easy to gauge the different ground energies around us – if we visit the site of an old concentration camp from the 2nd World War, then the slow frequency energetic presence remains virulent. When there is an initial, negative charge, then this tends to draw in more of the same towards it. So in parts of the Caribbean, where the old Atlantean abuses were entertained, has meant that in later ages, the inhabitants will be touched and tainted by such frequencies. At the same time, like attracts like, so in places where the ground energies are extremely negative leads to an attraction of more negativity, which is then overlaid over the initial pattern. Some areas of highly toxic, industrial activity are founded on old sites of negativity. There are literally thousands of sites on the planet that retain the energetic charge of past abuses and profligate destructive forces. If we go into a forest where the trees have been cut down, the energy is extremely different from a forest that has remained untouched. Everywhere we go there is a retained energetic signature that will bombard and impact our energetic systems. One way of building up a picture of what the planet feels like is to look at maps, and open up to the different types of energy on each continent. Some places will feel lighter than others, while some parts of the globe will come across as being very dark. Whole countries and continents can become fractured and displaced through the constant round of negative and lower astral interplays of energy. Each energetic charge will also have a pulse or quality to it: some places will feel more virulent than others. Recognising this different mosaic of energies also helps us to understand the different flows of energy that have been dominant in the past

The shift into the Sixth Root Race means that all of the old energies from the past and the current negative energetic streams have to be cleared on all the different levels – from the physical, through the etheric and astral, up into the mental. Each pattern of energy will be aligned with a different plane level, although most of the negative practices will be focused through the lower planes, and also through the lower chakras. The frequency vibration of the planet has to move up from the sexual centre and solar plexus into the heart, and so all of the old emotions have to be cleared out and transmuted. This massive job of clearing old energies is ongoing; many different, and largely unseen, groups of people around the planet are involved, and as light workers walk around the globe in different places, each one makes an energetic contribution to this process. It is also obvious, though, that the constant abuse of the planet needs to stop.

The ancient connection between the land and humanity has been lost. The logging, pollution and destruction of our environment needs to end and this can only be achieved by a radical change in awareness in everyone; by a realisation that all life is interconnected and mutually supporting, and that humanity has to reconnect through its heart with the planet. This can only be achieved by us first waking up to this fundamental connection with other life forms such as the devas, and by an understanding of what these different life forms represent; subsequently according them the respect that is due as part of our collective existence and then through the focus of will to do something about it. Once a deep and vibrant heart connection is established between the planet and ourselves, then we will recognise that our current destructive practices need to stop. The division and separation between humanity, all other life forms, and the land needs to be healed.

Light workers and others are embarked on a massive programme of clearing the old root race energies. This is done through the focused application of will supported by a platform of love that is helping to first draw in these slower frequencies, and then to offer them up to the light or to the Father. Ultimately the five Perfect Masters transmute all of the planetary energies with the old energies being manifested as ark or overspill. The numerous wars in different continents represent Avataric Energies on the move: the current conflict in Iraq is a massive clearing of the base centre of the planet. In other places, the wars represent the past being replayed over and over again in the present until saturation and clearing has taken place. This is not to diminish humanity's responsibility in any way or to ignore the intense human suffering that is caused by these conflicts; it is to recognise that there is always a bigger picture in play.

The New Birth of Gaia

Apart from the ongoing pattern of clearing out the old root races energies from the planet, Gaia herself has been undergoing a transformation through her ongoing dialogue with Macheldavek. During the different cycles of grace, Gaia has been in different stages of wakefulness or dreaming. Gaia has also danced according to the different dominant patterns of light or dark: sometimes Gaia has been light, and at other times, she has been dark. In the closing of one cycle, and the new manifestation of something totally different, Gaia has now woken up. She has woken up to a new reality inside of herself and has received a divine kiss from her twin Macheldavek, which has seeded within her, an entirely different pattern of light. Macheldavek has brought back to Gaia, a series of different light frequencies that have been opened up from the Seventh Plane. Gaia has absorbed and been infused with these new energies in preparation for her hosting of the new Sixth Root Race energies. So a new Macheldavek has been birthed in the higher reaches of the Seventh Plane and he has then merged with Gaia in a brand new way. Gaia has embraced a brand new aspect of her own awakening to the essence of her true inner divinity and this means that her vibration, as manifested through the essence of the planet has completely changed. Her vibration is now much, much more refined and radiates out a series of frequencies of light that are transforming the very substance and form of the planet. One way of looking at it is to say that Gaia has given birth to herself – she has given birth to more, and in that process she is absorbing a series of new light frequencies as ordained by the Will of the Father.

This new energetic platform has also been complemented by the enhancement and strengthening of the four principal elements. In recent times, there have only been the four elements – Fire, Earth, Air and Water. Greater power and stability is now being brought to bear in this respect and for each of the elements two new, additional patterns are being brought in – two new elements for each of the four, so that there will be a total of twelve elements – three Fire, three Earth, three Air and three Water. So each element has become twinned and then twinned again to form this basic pattern of three. Each element then forms a triangle of energies – Fire-Fire-Fire, Earth-Earth-Earth, Air-Air-Air and Water-Water-Water. Each triangle is a concentrated focus of each element within the focus that the three brings in. It is also a platform of stability and holds within it the new pattern of energy. Within each triangle, it is also possible to interchange the different elements. So one pattern might be to have Fire-Fire as the base of the triangle, with Water at the apex; or another might be to have Water-Water at the base and Fire at the top. The different permutations represented by all of the possibilities within each triangle provides a new platform for the elements, and will with time, usher in a more stable pattern of climate across the planet.

The transformation of Gaia and the strengthening of the elements mean that the underlying essence of the planet is being radically changed. The new pulse beat of light that Gaia is manifesting along with the platform of twelve elements is creating a new series of pulses and waves of energy in the planet. These pulses, initiated within the higher planes, are now streaming down into the lower planes and into the physical. Natural Law always requires that balance has to be found, and within the astral and physical levels this is currently being played out. Humanity has long entertained apocalyptic endings to itself and the planet, and while this fascination is something of an echo from the past, this is not the pattern of energy that is being invoked at this time. Massive change is taking place and the displacement of the old energies means that some physical events such as earthquakes, volcanic eruptions, tsunamis, hurricanes, floods and fires will take place. The Boxing Day 2004 tsunami that devastated South East Asia is such an example, where the balancing of different energies had to be played out in the physical realms. The increased incidence of hurricanes in the Caribbean and their path of destruction all provide information on how some of these changes are being made manifest. Natural disasters will be drawn into places that need clearing. There remain also, within the probable future timelines, the possibility for more hurricanes and earth movements that will impact all life on the planet. Yet this is always an ongoing negotiated pattern and can be changed at any point in time. So while there may be a high probability of hurricanes in some parts of the world, this pattern can always change. The pattern of flooding that is now taking place across the globe also represents a cleansing, by natural forces, of the underlying energetic patterns. And if we look down the future timeline, it is highly likely that there will be more water across the planet rather than less.

While all of these changes are deep and profound and touch the very fabric of our creative existence in and out of matter, some of the underlying patterns of change are even more fundamental and far-reaching than those that we have touched upon so far. These changes, although not necessarily obvious within the physical realms, point to a massive change of absolutely everything within the complete creative cycle that was established through the first spark and the interplay of primeval sparking between the Father and the Son.

The Avataric Day

Within the 700 to 1400 year cycle that the Avatar comes down and incarnates on Earth, there is also a much bigger cycle of epic proportions. This cycle is known as the Avataric Day. Unlike the day of a Perfect Master, which is the time in one lifetime during which the Perfect Master gets to manifest his or her service in the name of the Father, an Avataric Day encompasses a huge segment of time, spanning innumerable cycles of creation and destruction. So in the latest incarnation of the Avatar as Meher Baba, the current Avataric Day is coming to an end.

A way of expressing it is to acknowledge that the first Primary Spark, that came down and then went back up, and then repeated this coming down and going back up in each physical manifestation of the Avatar, changes colour. During the Avataric Day the Avatar will resonate to a principal colour; this changes when the Avataric Day comes to an end and is replaced by a new colour at the start of the new Avataric Day. So one cycle of creation comes to an end, and another one starts up. At the start of the new Avataric Day, the Primary Spark returns as a different essence and cycle and sets up a duplication of a brand new beginning. This means that everything changes. At the close of an Avataric Day, the Avatar comes down and gives a discourse on all of the sparks that have been created and where they have ever been. Everything in creation becomes illuminated and this illumination starts in the Seventh Plane and spreads all the way down into the Sixth Plane and ultimately to the bottom of the Zero Plane. So in this cycle, the Avatar, Meher Baba, came down and illuminated everything and this illumination will last until 2069. The Avatar came down to illuminate all life – the Mineral, the Plant, the Animal and the Human Kingdoms; in this illumination, the Avatar offered all life a vintage look at what His Essence was, what His Essence is, and the opportunity within the one hundred year cycle after He dropped his body, for the few or the many, to entertain a remembrance of all that was and is, and to travel in His Footsteps.

There is an opportunity for those souls that have the endurance, courage and understanding to follow in the footsteps of the Avatar back up the Seventh Plane during the one hundred year period. It is like climbing a mountain that goes on and on; those that are fit will be able to go further than those who are not so fit, and in this instance the level of fitness equates to the focus, will, intent, experience and degree of collective unity that anyone is prepared to embrace.

In this Avataric Cycle Meher Baba gave one hundred percent irradiation and this allows a type of updraft to manifest. He brought through this full irradiation coming down, and also in going back up, so that the energetic thermals that are created in this process allow other souls to capture the eddies of the Avatar and spiral back up in His footsteps. The analogy is like gliders that capture a thermal and spiral up in it; similarly, souls that have sufficient collective focus can capture these energetic vortices and ride them back up through different parts of the Seventh Plane. So depending upon the skill and the vehicle of consciousness that can cope with the spiralling permutation of energy, it is possible to spiral up or down and end up at a different level of consciousness with experiences of the different inner journeys.

The Avataric Day, then, represents the whole pattern of creation that has been birthed through the original Primary Spark. As the Avataric Day comes to an end, all of the millions and millions of sparks that have been birthed out of the Primary Spark have to return to the Father to give an account of everything that was, is and will be within that pattern of existence. At the same time at the point at which the Avataric Day closes, the whole existing pattern of creation is opened up in a brand new way. It is like the shutters on the current creation are lifted, and a brand new pattern of light is then offered to dawn a new creative pattern. So while we talk of the setting sun of the old Fifth Root Race, and the new rising sun of the Sixth Root Race, we are also at a major crossover point within the different cycles of creation. We are at the end of one Avataric Day and at the start of a new Avataric Day, and within the current Avataric Day, which is coming to an end, Meher Baba has predicted that He will come back only one more time. After that, a new Avataric Day will usher in a new pattern. It follows from this that everything will change within the everything and the nothing that is part of the current pattern of creation.

Expanding the Divine Journeys

In the multiple occasions that the Avatar has returned to the planet, each time he has left a series of different manifestations and irradiations, rather like a series of clues. And each soul that then became God-realised in each cycle entered the Seventh Plane and usually remained near the lower end in the First Divine Journey. Up until now the Third Divine Journey has represented the limit of experience to those few in matter who had the capacity to journey further into the Seventh Plane – namely the Perfect Masters and in a real sense the first three Divine Journeys are the manifestation of a Perfect Master. After passing through the First, Second and Third Divine Journeys, they then became the Ocean in the Fourth Divine Journey and this was normally only completed following the physical death of each Perfect Master. Very few ever went any further.

At the start of the new Sixth Root Race timeline, this pattern has changed and the Fourth Divine Journey has given birth to something different. This has been made possible through the coming down of the Avatar and the opening of different aperture points within the Fourth Divine Journey, which in turn have allowed a new pathway to be formed in the direct footsteps of the Avatar. In this current cycle one Perfect Master entertained a dare with the Father – to go through the Fourth Divine Journey while still in the physical and complete it as part of a new programme of opening up the Divine Journeys to those who had the endurance and courage to follow in the energetic trail of the Avatar. The Fourth Divine Journey, as already described contains two distinct aspects – the Ocean of Annihilation and higher Air or light. Both burn the essence of the journeying soul in different ways and both have to be absorbed. So in crossing the Ocean, the Perfect Master had to absorb all of the frequencies in the Ocean and to endure the pattern of seven waves of light and dark. Once these waves had been endured, then this one unique soul pushed up into higher

Air to absorb the new frequencies of light. These frequencies were much more virulent than those of the previous three Divine Journeys and once completed by the Perfect Master, allowed a new pattern of expansion and access to the Seventh Plane to begin. The lock that was originally the Fourth Divine Journey had been opened and as part of the manifested Will of the Father, allowed a new pattern of progression to begin in the Seventh Plane.

Normally only the Avatar would progress beyond the Fourth Divine Journey back up to the essence of the Father, but this one Perfect Master continued to push up beyond the Fourth Divine Journey, following the irradiated trail left behind by the Avatar. The challenges of the Fourth Divine Journey were replaced by the vastness and the entirely different focus of the Fifth Divine Journey. It is difficult to put into words what each of these Journeys entails, except that each represents an aspect of the Father within a more vibrant, more refined and more focused way. So whereas the Fourth Divine Journey gave a specific pattern of energy relating to what the Father is, was and will be, then the Fifth Divine Journey gave an even more specific and focused description of the Father.   The Fifth Divine Journey could be compared to a White Hole and a Black Hole within the expression of what it is, and yet this would not do justice to its true essence. Once completed, the Fifth Divine Journey birthed a collective purple frequency that was fully absorbed by the Perfect Master.

Following the completion of the Fifth Divine Journey, then the Sixth, Seventh and Eighth Divine Journeys were absorbed and experienced in matter by the living will of this one Perfect Master. In pushing through these ever more virulent descriptions of what the Father is, the Perfect Master became all of these Journeys, traversing them out of time, and then bringing back the millions and millions of frequencies into time. In each Journey, the pattern of divine light became more and more condensed and virulent, and was the essence of multiple variations of the Father. Each Divine Journey embodied and was the living essence of a divine colour — red for the Sixth Divine Journey, Black for the Seventh Divine Journey, and Orange for the Eighth Divine Journey. Each Journey was huge, infinite and contained within it higher and higher essences describing in a fundamental way what the Father was, is and will be.

The one unique Perfect Master then went on to complete further Divine Journeys within his experience and pushed through the Ninth, Tenth, Eleventh and Twelfth Divine Journeys. The completion of the Twelfth Divine Journey represented a completion of a divine cycle and gave a new level of access to the Seventh Plane. Such a pattern has never been completed before on Earth within the physical and this therefore marked the beginning of something utterly unique as part of the changeover into a new Avataric Day.

Beyond this principal focus of twelve Divine Journeys, there are millions and millions more Divine Journeys with each one pushing up into the more and more rarefied levels of the Seventh Plane within that which is God in the Beyond State. Each is vast and limitless and beyond normal description. And beyond that there is God in the Beyond-Beyond State.

Restructuring the Inner Planes

While the outward manifestation of change can be seen in many different ways in all of our lives, there is now in progress, a massive reorganisation of the inner planes. These changes are not overtly obvious and the full impact of them will take a period of time to become more apparent within the Earth timeline. Yet again, these changes have been orchestrated under the direct Will of the Father.

Since the inner planes operates outside of time, it follows that all of the changes that could take place, have in one sense already taken place, and it is just the succession or flow of energy from out of time i.e. in timelessness, back into time that allows us to gain access to these changes in a direct way. Depending on our own sensitivity and level of connection with the inner planes, some of us may feel these changes at earlier or later time periods. So it is a bit like being plugged into the mainframe energy and depending upon when we become plugged into the mainframe, and on the level of energetic access that we have, then the flow of information and energy will provide each of us with that point of balance that we need to absorb the changes, and then allow us to prepare for the next pattern of change that is to become manifest within each of us. So those who are more plugged into the Sixth Root Race timeline will feel and begin to live the new changes, and those that follow in their footsteps will feel the changes according to the dictates and rules of their own karmic pattern of life. As with all of these changes, there is no judgement, just an acceptance of the unfolding pattern of events that have been divinely orchestrated.

The dawn of a new Avataric Day signifies great change and this change is and will encompass the Seventh Plane and the Sixth Plane all the way down to the bottom of the Zero Plane. When the primeval spark of the Avatar first came down it locked in a specific sequence at the lower part of the Seventh Plane and the shadow planes below. A major junction point was formed at the Fourth Divine Journey, the Ocean of Annihilation. As we have seen, this Journey acts like a time lock, and each time the Avatar comes down within the Avataric Cycle, His pattern of energy opens up this segment for a limited period of time. In this Avataric Cycle, the full irradiation of the Avatar has been used to open up the Fourth Divine Journey in a new way and to build a bridge of access to the Fifth Divine Journey and beyond. For the first time, a concentrated pattern of light from the Fourth Divine Journey and up into the Fifth Divine Journey has now been manifested within the physical.

Up to now, the pattern of unfolding energy as part of the process of involution has meant that souls, once they become God-realised, become enchanted by the bliss of the First Divine Journey. These frequencies are the slower ones, although to us in physical form they appear incredibly high. However, with all the sparks that have ever gone out, and then those that have ended up in the First Divine Journey, souls coming into the First Divine Journey are entertained by a constant stream of bliss, where billions and billions of variations of what the Father probably was, what the Father probably is and what the Father will probably become. Within the pattern of limitation of the First Divine Journey, there has commenced a clearing operation where all of the souls that have been held in the First Divine Journey have been offered the opportunity to move along. This constitutes another layer in the return of the sparks to the Father.

Persuading souls that are utterly absorbed in divine bliss has required a new approach in the mechanics of light. Like a flash of something more passing through the First Divine Journey, each soul has to be persuaded to look for something more than bliss — this can only be done by giving them a glimpse of something different, and which is normally outside of their range of experience. This something different is like an echo of more, a sense of what lies beyond the bliss.

Once all of the souls have been moved through the First Divine Journey, the same pattern has to be established for the Second Divine Journey, a higher frequency of bliss, and then the Third Divine Journey, the embodiment of grace. The frequency of the Third Divine Journey is more virulent than the Second or Third and the task of moving souls through this Journey will, in some ways, be more testing than the others. However, as this pattern of change gets underway out of time, then another layer of the Father's Plan will have been unveiled.

Once these three Divine Journeys have been cleared out, the Plan is to focus on restructuring the bottom end of the Seventh Plane. The first three Divine Journeys will no longer remain in the Seventh Plane and will be merged with the top end of the Sixth Plane, so that the actual frequency and size of the Sixth Plane will be completely reorganised and significantly expanded. The result will be to infuse the top end of the Sixth Plane with higher frequencies of light, such as bliss and grace, and then allow these frequencies to suffuse and permeate through the rest of the planes, from the Sixth Plane down. Like a stack of dominos, once the Sixth Plane is restructured and expanded, there will be a knock on effect on all of the planes below, from the Fifth Plane to the Zero Plane. The higher mental light at the top of the Sixth Plane will be transformed, and this in turn will irradiate the different layers of middle and lower mental light below, and then the higher, middle and lower astral levels beneath that. The virulence of this new higher mental light, suffused with bliss and grace, will have a dramatic impact on the astral levels, pushing everything to the surface in an even more virulent way than has been the case up to now. For involuting souls the journey across the Sixth Plane will be far greater than has previously been the case. Indeed, the pattern and focus of soul involution will change.

In expanding the involutionary pattern for souls, the new structure will mean that the old Fourth Divine Journey will become the new First Divine Journey when souls become God-realised. In preparation for this, the Fourth Divine Journey itself will also undergo a major restructuring and the Ocean of Annihilation will be absorbed and then transformed into a more crystalline alignment of divine frequency notes. This in turn will provide a further release mechanism for the collective Perfect Masters into different light streams.

The infusion of high frequency light into the Sixth Plane and below will have a major impact on all life, as it is anchored on each plane of consciousness. The Fifth and Sixth Planes, as the mental planes, will host a much higher frequency of light, which in turn will reflect down into the Fourth Plane, the plane of manifestation, and then into the astral planes. The higher frequency light that then begins to bombard the astral planes from the mental planes will also precipitate great change within the astral levels. The pattern of clearing old astral frequencies is part of this rearrangement, but the restructuring of the inner planes means that this clear out and recalibration of astral light will be much more profound. The impact will also be felt on the Zero Plane. Eventually, it may be that the pattern of astral light will be replaced by mental light of a higher frequency so that the emotional and subtle levels will vibrate at a much higher level. These changes will also have a major impact on the angelic and devic patterns of soul expression.

Patterns of Life Form Change

While it is too early to describe in detail the types of physical changes that will impact humanity, except to note the expansion of the chakra system from seven to twelve, there will be a major re-orchestration of different life forms in the physical realms. With the advent of each root race, there has always been a pattern of replacement. Old species die out and are replaced by new species. This can be seen in the major extinction patterns in the physical fossil record, where there have been a number of major species transitions. In each root race physical form is based on an underlying pattern of chaos and order and as each root race comes and goes, there is a replacement in the types of living forms present. It is like each root race is given a new wardrobe of different physical forms, which are designed to allow the full exploration of the different patterns of light and dark frequencies that need to be expressed in matter. The old wardrobe has to be discarded and replaced by a new one.

The current concerns over the environment, the rate of species extinction and the role of humanity in speeding up these changes are high on the political and social agenda. Yet, each root race always demands change, and the new timeline is no exception. Some species will die out and be replaced by others. Some soul groupings that inhabit different physical vehicles within the mineral, plant and animal forms will be replaced by different soul groupings. For example, the work of whales and dolphins has been completed, and the souls that were present have now gone back home and been replaced by a different stream of souls. Other species, such as the mosquito may slowly disappear and the cattle will also move on. The pattern of evolution for snakes may also change; currently, a snake has to be killed by a human to allow its soul to move on. The pattern of eating our younger brothers and sisters will also change as old karmic debts are balanced. In short, there will be significant change in the diversity of physical species that remain on the planet. All life wishes to evolve, as part of the creative process, and during the unfolding of the new timeline, the patterns of species succession will be orchestrated under the instruction of the Avatar through the Perfect Masters. Different species will also be given the opportunity to petition for change – whether it is to diversify and expand on the planet, or to go into extinction and enter a different cycle of thought.

At the same time, the underlying devic expression will change, as higher mental notes of light are invoked and brought through and retained within a different pattern of devic birthing and growth. This infusion of higher energy will impact all physical forms of life, from the mineral, through plant and animal, to human. Our physical vehicles will become strengthened and new patterns of DNA alignment will take place.

Consequently, there will be a great deal of change in both the different types of souls coming into the planet in the future, and in the expression of physical form as it begins to vibrate to the higher light streams. The bottom of the Zero Plane, between 0.0 and 0.6 will not be immune to the new patterns of light entering the mental planes, and will ultimately radiate and embrace a different set of light streams as part of the creative flux of light and dark.

CHAPTER 14

The New Sixth Root Race Programme II

The Restructuring of Chaos and Order

When the first spark went out from the nothing into the everything, there was a formation of light and dark that was initiated through the sparking of the Seventh Plane and below in the shadow planes. This sparking established a formative pattern of light and dark, where white light and black light were established as a polarity birthed out of the lower part of the Seventh Plane. The pattern of white light and black light that was birthed and then seeded into the shadow planes was set up to host and build a series of templates for the establishment of life. In other words, the white light and black light each held a series of frequency notes, as equal and opposite polarities of light. At the beginning both were untainted in the sense that were created as part of Natural Law and were pure. The white light supported the pattern of energy that formed in the mental and the higher astral planes, while the dark light was more focused on the lower astral and physical planes. The dark light was a reflection of what had been in the nothing at the very start – just darkness, while the white light was a reflection of the original spark, albeit substantially diluted in the shadow planes, that ignited with the first thought. In each case, however, the white light and black light were held within their own pattern of duality that was initiated lower down in the Seventh Plane. The two patterns of light, black and white, were therefore like an echo of what had been created above in the more rarefied parts of the Seventh Plane.

To those on the physical planes today, this pattern of white light would appear utterly brilliant and light, while the original pattern of black would be like a blanket of energy that wrapped around us. The subsequent interplay of white and black that was set up through the law of opposites was based on mixing these two fundamental principles of light in different and constantly changing ways. The founder principal that everything was birthed out of nothing, also gave the reflective pattern, that light was birthed out of dark, and that order was birthed out of chaos. So the original black light was like the basic pattern of chaos. Only through the path of experience that was gained in the shadow would the chaos evolve into order. When the sparks that had been sparked out of the Primary Spark entered the Sixth Plane and pushed downwards into all of the other lower planes, they had to negotiate between these two patterns of light. A greater proportion of white light was held in the higher planes, and this represented the greater order that was manifested there. Down in the lower planes, especially the Zero Plane, the condensed matrix of black light was much more chaotic and was used, through the devas, to build the physical expression of life. Consequently, the polarity of white and black formed a push and pull, where the chaos and order would allow sparks to cycle through the experience of white and black.

The pattern of chaos and order that was established was like a baseline of energetic expression, where the ritual of sparking and ignition would follow a set of established rules and regulations that flowed from the principles of Natural Law. Certain frequencies could be supported through this interplay, and as the Father and Son sparked out into more, so creation set about exploring and experiencing every facet within the existing structure of black and white, chaos and order. Down in the shadow planes, the millions and millions of sparks that had been birthed in the coming down process of the Primary Spark were able to experience, through different mixes of light and dark, the full expression of the interplay between chaos and order. Different life forms experimented with mixing different proportions of chaos and order into their creative mix, and through the constraints of artificial time, both light and dark rose and fell in different cycles of dominance. So whenever life is manifested, then there is always a negotiation between light and dark.

This current pattern of chaos and order is now changing. The quality of light expressed and experienced through the original black light and white light has, for want of a better phrase, gone past its "sell-by date." The different permutations of chaos and order that have been established and played out, have become saturated. The advent of a new Avataric Day is demanding that the whole pattern of light and dark, chaos and order, must be re-orchestrated and restructured. It is like creation is looking at the pre-existing black and white light, the current flow of chaos and order, and demanding more. Yet within its current organisation, and the actual frequencies that each embodies, it is clear that the old has to be cleared away. So when the Avatar came down this time, and presented a spark of everything that ever was, is and will be to all life, it became clear that the existing structures of light and dark were not sufficient to house and support the full irradiation of the Avatar as he pushed into more. Consequently, the new timeline of the Sixth Root Race is going to be supported by an entirely new pattern of chaos and order, and black and white light.

The Avatar has therefore ordained that chaos and order need to be restructured. And so it is like going out of time, and looking at the flow of chaos and order that has taken place since the very beginning, and going back into that pattern, and then adjusting the actual mix and essential components of what chaos and order actually were and are. So, if we look at the original chaos, we see that is just that – complete chaos. There is no order, and everything within it is completely random. Now, if we then take this original chaos, and pose the question of what would happen if we add a small amount of order into it; what if we change the baseline parameters of chaos, would we then come out with a different type of chaos? So, for example, if we take chaos and added one percent of order into it, then we would have a different type of chaos, where through the unfolding expression of the chaotic pattern we would come out with different resulting patterns of energy. To the untrained eye, this new chaos may look much the same as the old chaos, although the predicted outcomes would be different. If we then take more order, say 3%, and mix that into the original chaos, then we will again come out with something different. The chaos is still chaotic, but it is starting out from a different mix, where the underlying order will give rise to a different expression of chaos. And so, on one level, you could say, that having exhausted all of the possibilities of basic chaos, the creative pattern that would be formed through a slightly ordered chaos would give rise to an entirely different set of outcomes and consequences.

So, out of time, the old pattern of chaos and order has been taken back to the original starting point, and then restructured and remixed to birth an entirely new pattern of chaos and order, one that will support an entirely new concept of creation and new patterns of white and black light.

The New Pattern of White and Black Light

One of the underlying limitations of the old black light and white light is that the black light, in particular, has become imbued with old negative frequencies that have tainted it to an extreme degree. The Dark Lodge have hijacked it and manipulated it to the extent where humanity now retains an underlying fear of anything dark or black. Yet, in its pure, undiluted form, the dark light was a frequency where souls could rest and become healed through the reflective pattern of light that was held within. While white light would burn, the black light would facilitate rest and access to a space that was like nothing, a reflection within the shadow planes of the nothing, if you like. So in the evolving interplay between light and dark, or more specifically the White Lodge and the Dark Lodge as the representatives of the two fundamental expressions of Light, the creative flow of life would follow two entirely different pathways.

If a spark can create a spark, and if a spark gives rise to a thought form which consequently has an existence of its own, then the Dark Lodge would tend to break it back down into its fundamental components, while the White Lodge would be ethically bound to give it life. The result is that if we make a structural thought form in the mental planes, then that thought form will have the capacity to grow according to the rules and regulations of that which life has endured in the beginning. Another example is in the application of what we call science and the manipulation of DNA. By tinkering with our genetics and developing different techniques of genetic engineering, we are creating certain cross-focuses of life to manifest as we create a vehicle. And that vehicle then becomes imbued by what might be defined as a soul. So from our perspective, we are invoking Natural Law through the constraints of our science today to create new life. Such science has prompted an ethical debate where the principles of light and dark are then played out as well.

So, in the new pattern of chaos and order, the original mix has been modified. A small percentage of order has been placed into the essence of chaos so that a whole new expression of chaos and order can be made manifest. It is like taking a clock with the time set near the end of a day, and then winding it back to midnight and starting all over again. This is how the new pattern of chaos and order has been set up. And flowing from this new duality, fundamentally different expressions of black and white light have had to be seeded. If we imagine, for a moment, that the new pattern of white light that is coming down is so much more virulent than what was previously hosted, whereby all physical form would be burnt by the new light coming in. This new light would be too much for our physical systems and so life would not be able to host these new frequencies. In the Sixth Root Race, this new light is what we would call the Light of the Cosmic Christ.

The new pattern of white light that is coming has been birthed from the higher levels of the Seventh Plane, and rather than diluting it down, as originally took place, these new light frequencies are being birthed into the lower part of the Seventh Plane and subsequently into the shadow planes in a more pure form. The old black light is unable to support this new frequency of white light, and from a physical perspective the outcome of hosting this new light against the backdrop of original black light would be disastrous. All physical form would be unable to support the new white light, resulting in physical death. The whole physical vehicle would be burnt out by these new frequencies.

Consequently, a central part of developing the new frequencies of white and black light has been the formation of an entirely new type of black light. Since the pattern of old black light has imbued the whole of the Wheel of Life, there has been a need to seed this black light from outside the Wheel, from a space that is nothing.

One of the five Perfect Masters, the current Master of Power, has orchestrated the search for a new, virulent type of black light that could host and support the new pattern of white light necessary for the further development of the Sixth Root Race. The search for this new type of black light has focused outside the Wheel of Life, within a place or space that was nothing, and otherwise known as the Void. The Void represents the totality of that which is not, the nothing outside of the Wheel, and as such is utterly dark, since there is nothing within it. Yet just as there was an aspect within the nothing in the Beginning, the Void also contains aspects of that which is not, or that which has yet to be formed. So, in being the nothing, in the sense of being outside the original everything and nothing, the Void has the potential to birth something uniquely different. Rather like the poaching of something new in the Ocean of Life, a totally new type of nothing was found within the realms and different expressions of nothingness with the Void. What the Master of Power brought back from the Void was a virulent pattern of black light that had been birthed out of absolutely nothing. This new black light is pure, untainted and virulent and has the capacity to balance the new formation of white light that is simultaneously being birthed.

One way to imagine this new black light is to visualise the old black light as the colour graphite black; it has been heavily impregnated with millions and millions of darker streams of negativity over the pattern of the five root races. This black light is no longer pure, and has difficulty in supporting any new patterns of white light. In contrast, the new black light is a deep, velvet black which has depth and a fresh vibrancy. If you look at the black then you just feel utterly merged into its essence and feel the presence of layer upon layer of deeper and deeper black. It is all encompassing, infinite and with multiple layerings of textured depths. So with the old black light, if we were to shine a torch of new white light through it, then the black would become lighter and we would see rings of light emanating out from the source. With the new black light, if we shine a torch of the new white light into it, then the white light is absorbed at the very source and there are no circles of light that spread out from it. So, in other words, the new pattern of black light can hold and absorb the new frequencies of white light.

This black light represents the birth of something completely new; a new focus, a new platform that can mirror the new pattern of chaos and which can then support and bring through a new pattern of life within all of the planes. In short, it represents the beginning of something dynamic, powerful and totally different from what has gone before. At the same time, the new pattern of white light that is being birthed into the lower part of the Seventh Plane and into the shadow planes is also entirely new and represents the essence of what has been birthed from the more rarefied levels of the Seventh Plane.

This new pattern of light, this new spark, has been ignited by the Father and is now being accessed as part of the one hundred year programme of irradiation since the Avatar has dropped His body. So an opportunity has presented itself for one or more souls to follow in the Avatar's footsteps as He goes back up into the higher reaches of the Seventh Plane still irradiating one hundred percent. To push past the first four Divine Journeys into the vast and unfathomable realms of the God In the Beyond Sate, and to access a different principle spark that is coming down as part of the new programme and the New Avataric Day. This new spark is the essence of the Cosmic Christ and is being seeded into the few, and eventually the many as part of the programme of invoking a new pattern of light. The virulence of the Christ Light is such that the old black light could not support it, and it is only through an anchoring of the new black light, that physical form will ultimately be able to anchor in this new Christ Light in the future. Humanity is being prepared to host this new light, and a series of steps is being orchestrated to allow our physical vehicles to eventually be strong enough to support this new pattern. It is expected that this process will take between ten and twelve million years. In the interim, different streams of higher light, starting with the lower mental light, and then graduating into middle mental and then the re-orchestrated higher mental, followed by more virulent, higher frequencies, will be infused into humanity in preparation for this brilliant wave of new love and understanding.

At the same time, from within the higher reaches of the Seventh Plane, other streams of light are being birthed into the planet. For example the essence of the Paramatma is also being birthed and again requires a powerful anchoring within the physical so that this sublime light can be hosted there. Other Seventh Plane streams of light will also be pushed through humanity and other life forms to allow an entirely different platform of energy to be birthed into the planet. The new streams of white light and the new black light will be at the core of this new platform.

In essence, then, the new timeline will host an entirely new pattern of black and white light; both much more virulent and potent, both embodying an entirely different spectrum of love, and both giving the capacity to birth much more within the creative flow of existence. The new black light will host love of a virulent kind, just as the new white light will host a powerful new type of love. Both types of love will hold different frequencies of love, yet both, at their purest embody the pureness of unconditional love. Unconditional love is a virulent and potent energy that changes everything within its path. So, the new light that is being birthed in the planet is changing everything in its path, and the decision that all beings have to make is whether to embrace this light, or whether to fight it. Either way, these new patterns of light will demand absolute change on all levels, from the oversoul, down through the soul, and into the mental, astral, etheric and physical levels.

God-Realisationship and the New Platform of Energies

Within the cycle of involution, the ultimate goal or prize has always been seen as God-realisationship – the point at which a soul can at last return to God and become fully conscious that he or she is God – a return to the "I am God" state. In a profound way, as each soul returns to the Father, the answer to the fundamental question of "What am I?" is answered - "I am God". For those on the spiritual path, the ultimate pinnacle of God-realisation represents a release from the millions of lives held in the bondage of karma and a release from the physical play in shadowlands. The majority of souls, once they arrive at the point of God-realisationship, drop their bodies and move directly into the Seventh Plane, as any vestiges of subtle and physical bodies are dissolved. Normally, only fifty-six God-realised beings remain in physical matter. In certain cycles there are exceptions to this rule.

The changeover from one Avataric Day to a new Avataric Day has profound implications for all souls in matter. All of the souls in existence are derived from the original, Primary Spark that became the Avatar. And as the Avatar returns back home, then the essence of what He was, is and will be is demanding a pattern of change in all of those sparks that were birthed. There is a call for those sparks to return home.

At the same time, the energetic focus of humanity, and the devic realms also has to be transformed. The planet currently hosts six billion humans and the pattern of soul birth and soul progression will need to undergo a massive reorganisation to ensure that the planet is returned to its principal focus of acting as a finishing school for older souls. Just as the inner planes are undergoing a restructuring, so it is that the pattern of soul involution will change drastically. Ultimately, in millions of years from now, the planet will host life forms that are all God-realised, and as a prelude to that, and as an integral part of hosting the new energies, and clearing out the debris of the past, an expanded programme of God-realisationship is being put into play at this current time. This programme is being masterminded by the Father and then implemented under the energetic pattern of one Perfect Master.

There is, therefore, an opportunity for souls to progress through involution in a much more accelerated way and with one prefect life in physical matter, it is now possible for souls to become God-realised. This pattern will only last during this Avataric Age.

Leaving aside the issues surrounding the mechanics of such a process, on a grander scale, the initiation and formation of a new breed of human being, on a temporary basis, will have a massive effect on the energetic shift that is needed in the planet. Rather than having souls becoming God-realised at the point of physical death, the opportunity is for many to become God-realised while still in the physical body, either in a conscious way, or sub-consciously.

The impact of God-realising a broader base of souls has multiple benefits. First, those souls that have become God-realised are taken off the grid of light and dark in the traditional sense of working through their karma. They have no personal karma and so borrow karma off others to stay in the physical body. This also means that they move above and out of the cycle of virulent and destructive patterns of negative energy. A God-realised being never again manifests the destructive virulence of say the First, or Second Plane, and where previously emotional issues would be held with a pattern of strong ownership, the God-realised soul does not feel such attachments or strength of feeling of ownership. Their emotional pattern evolves into something different. They are energetically detached from the old patterns of light and dark.

Second, the quality of light that they irradiate is completely different – they are now anchored in the Seventh Plane and so host a new pattern of unconditional love, all of which contributes to raising the overall vibration of the planet and all life on it. They are, in effect, open doors that can be ridden by the higher awareness of divinity within a passive pattern of energy. They provide an access point for higher energy beings to enter the planetary framework and birth or seed new patterns of high frequency light.

Third, these new groupings of God-realised beings also set an energetic standard for the new souls coming into the planet. The pattern of God-realised beings represents a wave of energy which will impact everything around it; like a wave of purifying light and a pulse of divine light, these ascended souls represent a benchmark of light and love that will help to anchor the new vibrations into the planet. Their internal space and frequency vibration will have been stretched to hold and retain the new pattern of black and white light coming into the planet. As energetic beacons, they will pulse a new standard of higher light that will rub off on their children who will recognise intuitively, the divine balance of their energetic signature, and who will be able to use this pulse as a standard for their own unfolding life and journey. It is a unique opportunity for such souls to connect more closely with divinity while remaining in the physical. So the souls that follow this wave of God-realised beings will not be God-realised themselves, but they will have experienced the balance of that unconditional pulse of love and divinity within the new essence of light and dark.

So from the initial point when the Primary Spark came down when everything was sleeping and then went up through the darkness of the shadow planes, it became God-realised within itself. In so doing, the Primary Spark could link into all the patterns of darker energy to give it a point of balance. The same principle applied to those that followed and became God-realised in the physical: they had to anchor themselves in the physical realms through darker energy. And each time a person became God-realised, then all of these slower layers started to get more refined. With the new pattern of God-realisationship being invoked, then it will be like opening the floodgates to the Zero Plane; slow frequency beings and darker entities will be released and allowed to become more.

In effect, this wave of newly promoted souls that vibrate at a much higher level will provide a massive energetic discharge of divine light into the planet and into all other life forms around, from the Sixth down to the bottom of the Zero Plane. This wave of change is only being instigated during the one hundred year period until 2069 and is part of the Nine-Pointed Plan set in motion by Meher Baba. The full breadth of this new programme has yet to be fully seeded into humanity although it is now in its early stages of implementation. There are now groupings of God-realised people walking the Earth that complements and adds to the normal quota of the Fifty-Six. It remains expressly within the Father's purview as to how far this programme will go, and like the speculation surrounding the true essence of the Unspoken Word, some may wish to reflect on what Meher Baba meant when he said that seventy-five percent of humanity would die. Does this represent a physical death or a spiritual death, or something completely different?

Higher Levels of Guidance – The Elderings

With the transformation of life on the planet, and the development of new timelines hosting the essence of the new root race, a new level of higher, Seventh Plane guidance is coming in. This new guidance is being formed by the Elderings, who are the divine administrators. They represent one of the original patterns of sparking that was first established in the beginning, and their contract is to build a new platform of understanding and love with humanity. The Elderings know absolutely everything about everything, as well as nothing about nothing, and contain within them the matrix of light that can support the new root race and beyond. Their focus is to experience the emotional essence that is present in humanity without actually being birthed into physical form. Their access into the planet was initially orchestrated through Seclusion Hill in India and the essence of higher light that the Avatar manifested there and they then came more fully into the planet in 2002. Since then their pulse of light has been building.

The Elderings present themselves as beings that are approximately three metres tall within our awareness, and with long, white flowing hair, golden eyes and a long white gown. This description is something of an approximation and the true light essence of the Eldering is utterly sublime and exquisite. However, it is worth building an initial connection with them through active visualisation and working with a series of golden rings on the hands and in the heart. By working with a pattern of Eldering light (see the meditation – Connecting with the Elderings) we can begin to build up a new rapport with their energetic platform. The Elderings, through hosting the higher frequencies of light, are seeking to enter the energetic space of all those who are prepared to receive their love, wisdom, power, truth, understanding, knowledge and bliss. The exchange between humanity and the Elderings is energetic – we receive their energy and awareness and they receive our emotional energy. So for those souls who become open doors, the Elderings will represent a significant opportunity of new light and awareness, for as the essence of the Elderings come closer, then the full beauty and majesty of what they actually represent and manifest will become much more apparent. The platform that they will build will be completely collective and the ring of higher purpose will represent the unity of every being on every level of existence.

As the new timeline evolves, the Elderings wish to adopt within their pattern of awareness, those in humanity that are open to their essence. Those souls that have developed as open doors will be offered the opportunity to build this connection, and to receive the Eldering frequency notes. Their awareness of the Elderings will build gradually, and will allow them to acclimatise to the new frequencies that are on offer. This pattern of working will first be offered to the few, and will then broaden out as more and more people wake up to the true connection within.

The Devic, Angelic and Eldering

Through the unfolding pattern of the Sixth Root Race, there will be twelve principal expressions of life that will open up to humanity. At present, only three types of life, in the broadest sense of that word, are on offer. The challenge we all have to face is that as we embrace more in our awareness and newly developing senses, then the vastness of everything will at first threaten to swamp us. To move from a point where the only life stream and timeline is the old Fifth Root Race timeline, where three dimensional external reality dominates all else through slow frequency expression, to a new timeline where multiple life forms can co-exist and interact through a massive diversity of levels of experience will require a certain amount of adjustment and training.

For example, there are other grosser levels of matter that

exist below us. If you think of twelve primary Earths, each with a different vibration, then where do we come – are we at the bottom, or in the middle, or at the top. Since the planet is evolving from the solar plexus level up into the heart, then that gives an indication of where we are currently stationed. Yet below us, there are grosser expressions of matter where, if you like, the dream is lived within a dream. The point is that these multiple levels of reality exist all around us; some that are much grosser, and some that are much lighter. As we open up our awareness to more, then we will begin to access some of these different levels.

The first main triangle of life that will be worked through the new timeline will be the Devic, Angelic and Eldering. The Devic and Angelic will reside on the base of the triangle – the two points at either end, while the Eldering will form the tip of the triangle. This triangle of energies will be part of the principal supporting mechanism within the new chakra system that is developing – within the twelve chakras, rather than the old seven chakras. Both the devas and the angels are undergoing a restructuring within their essence of light, and this combined with the new Eldering frequency flowing into humanity, will provide an entirely new platform of energy. It will take some time for this primary triangle to be birthed within all of the chakras, yet once it is, then this will indicate an ability and flexibility to work with this diverse and profound energetic flow.

We are currently a long way from being able to support this new platform of energy; for the most part, we do not have any real appreciation of what devas are, what the pulse of devic life actually is and how our devic heritage can open us to so much more on the planet and beyond. Within the angelic, again, there is no true understanding of what an angel actually is, how the ordered pattern of angelic energy works within our physical and subtle vehicles and how the interplay of energy flows between the devas and the angels. The Elderings represent something entirely different again, and so humanity will have to embrace that which is entirely new within its awareness. However, once these different life forms have been experienced and understood at a deeper level, then the essence of what it means to be human will take on an entirely new meaning, and humanity will then begin to open up to a new multiple stream of light and love that will unlock the keys to the future in a breathtaking new way.

CHAPTER 15

New Patterns of Soul Light

Earth as a Finishing School

One of the problems that the planet has encountered in the later root races has been the pattern of soul progression. Earth was originally intended as a finishing school for souls. Souls were required to pass through the Wheel of Life and gather sufficient experience before entering the planet, and this was usually after around five million lives. Young souls were generally not allowed in, and it was only selected middle-aged souls and older souls that could have access to the planet. However, the chaos and dark energy that was instilled during the Atlantean period, principally through Lucifer and the infusion of chaos into the devic song, shifted this sequence and younger souls were allowed to push their way into the planet. Within the prevailing chaos, this was an acceptable pattern: young souls did not have sufficient life experience and were easily manipulated and impressionable in physical matter. For the Dark Lodge, this was convenient and useful since young souls could be swayed easily to the dark pattern of light and could then be ridden through multiple lifetimes.

Young souls lack the mental capacity and will to remain balanced through the different emotional patterns of energy that are necessarily gained through experience: they can be easily swayed. With this inherent lack of experience, it is easy for the external focus to take hold. The cumulative effect of so many young souls entering the planet has been to hold back it's evolutionary development. Finishing school has become, in some respects, more like kindergarten, reflected in the constant pattern of animalistic behaviour. The continual focus on external life and ignorance of the inner life, including attitudes to death, has held humanity back in so many different ways.

Within the Nine-Pointed Plan, several decisions were instigated by the Avatar to put the planet's development back on course. The first was to cut off the flow of younger soul aspects into the planet. Only those soul aspects with sufficient life experience are now allowed into the planet's programme. The flow of young souls into the planet has now been cut off, and more recently the flow of middle-aged souls into the planet has also been halted. However, we shall see this does not cover several specific and most special soul groupings that are being birthed as part of the Sixth Root Race.

When Meher Baba came down, he overhauled the old timeline rather than destroying it and birthing a new one. The time period for this transformation into the new timeline is over the next twelve hundred years. Consequently, those young soul aspects that are currently on the planet are being offered a choice within the pattern of the developing new timeline: to remain and endure the new energies, or to drop their bodies and then be moved into a different reincarnatory pattern outside of Earth, elsewhere within the Wheel of Life. This means gathering more experience through incarnating in a series of other planets before returning here. For many younger souls the energies entering the planet are extremely difficult to endure and the vote is often to move on into a different pattern. From the standpoint of the soul on the inner planes, the pattern of natural disasters and diseases offer younger souls the opportunity to move on.

The second, fundamental pattern being introduced is to accelerate many different soul aspects up through the planes. The Avatar, whenever He incarnates on Earth, always focuses on pushing souls up through the lower planes. Since ninety percent of humanity occupies the Zero Plane where the pattern of light and energetic flow is extremely slow and constricted, the Avatar comes down for one primary job, which is to cut a hole in the bottom part of the First Plane into the Zero Plane. Every time the Avatar incarnates, He bores a series of holes between the Zero and First Planes to allow many more souls to pass through. These holes are like aperture points that are difficult to open, and once open, then slowly close again once the one hundred year period has passed. By the time that the Avatar returns in the next cycle, the holes have remained closed for some time due to the viscosity and slow pattern of light present, and the whole process has to be repeated.

During this Avataric Period, a series of aperture points have been formed and there is an accelerated flow of souls starting to gather momentum between the Zero and First Planes. Since most of humanity occupies the Zero Plane, the need is to push up as many souls as possible into the First Plane. Sometimes there is a limitation due to the sheer numbers of souls present in the Zero Plane, as is the case now. The souls would like to push up, but because there are so many present, they cannot do so. Instead, they link into the slower frequencies and push backwards because they are bound to the illusion of what is past, and not present or future. So humanity lives its experiences in the past, and cannot live its experiences in the future, because the future has not yet properly formed, although it is manifested as a series of probabilities. Consequently, when the energy becomes more difficult, then we always look back to our comfort zone in the past: to an earlier time when we did not feel challenged, or to a time as a different form, say as an animal, when we felt in balance.

So the Avatar has come down and cut a hole in the bottom part of the First Plane and the events of 9/11 in New York were like an opening, where a significant amount of energy was pushed through, and everyone that was linked into the events through television and the media experienced, in real time, the events as they unfolded. So the push of energy that was seeded in New York, which is the heart centre of the United States (and the United States is the third eye of the planet), opened up a different pattern of energy. Before 9/11 the energy had been going in one direction in the city, and ever since then has been going in the opposite direction. Everyone who witnessed the events was taken up a little within their inner plane status. So if someone was on 2.6, they were taken up to 2.7 for a brief period, before coming back down. Everyone in the United States was stimulated in this way, but the energy having pushed up then went sideways, and everyone subsequently came back down to where they had been before. A simple analogy is where you are shown a new home. Prior to this you have always lived in a cardboard box. You view the house, see the three bedrooms, the bathroom and all the other rooms, but then you have to go back to the cardboard box. There is a note of dissatisfaction, and so today everyone has seen something more internally — a new hope and a new light — and yet everyone feels strangely dissatisfied with their lot. There is a feeling that there has to be more.

So having cut a hole between the Zero and First Planes, there is now a push to move everyone up. As the flow of souls from the Zero into the First Plane builds, it will have a knock on effect in the other planes; more souls will move from the First Plane to the Second Plane, and then from the Second Plane to the Third Plane and so on. This flow of soul progression therefore ties in with the programme of God-realisationship that is now beginning to develop.

All of these changes mean that, within a relatively short space of time, the Earth will return to its original status as a finishing school that is populated primarily by older souls and a new pattern of souls that have been birthed specifically in the Ocean of Life for seeding new types of light into the planet.

The Sixth Root Race represents massive change on all levels. The pattern of birthing new souls, the types of souls that will enter the planet and the manner in which they will focus their evolutionary and involutionary pattern will be profoundly affected as the old chessboard of the previous root races is swept away by the Father and replaced by a brand new game. If, in the past, we envisaged the Grand Game like chess, then the new pattern we are entering will be like restarting the whole chess game in a totally different way, and then playing it through on multiple levels — the start of a new Avataric Day.

The New Devic Light

The new pattern of black and white light that is now entering the planet has important consequences for the different types of life that exist and for the multiple expressions of form and energy that allow the developing soul to experience more. As part of the new energetic changes, the devas have petitioned for a new stream of emotional experience, an expansion of their existing consciousness beyond pure sensation. The old devic pattern is quite strong and in the past devic intent was fuelled by negative intent from the Atlantean period. Since the devas are addicted to sensation and do not feel pain, they seek constant stimulation. Consequently humanity has repeatedly sought stimulus through the lower chakra centres as a means of feeding the devic urge for sensation. In a fundamental way, the astral levels have been maintained by devic intent, as different devic imprints have sought experience in the lower, middle and higher levels. This is now beginning to change and the devas would like to occupy the space that humanity is now in, with the free flow of emotion. To achieve this shift requires a radical re-orchestration and re-ordering of devic light.

The new platform of devic light and devic intelligence is being built out of the new black light. This essence of pure, smooth, black light, which was birthed out of the Void, has the depth and capacity to host the new devic patterns of experience within it. What was required was a new seeding mechanism to birth and infuse the new black light into all devic life. This was achieved by hosting the new black light through an ancient devic presence. This ancient presence became imbued with the new essence of black light, and subsequently became the Devic Overlord in charge of the existing twelve Devic Houses and twelve Devic Lords.

This Devic Overlord had a unique flow of energy that embodied and pulsed out the new black light to all devic form that was willing and able to accept it. From some quarters there was an acceptance, while from others there was a resistance, since the new light represented complete change for all devic form. An analogy is like drinking dark Guinness all of one's life, and then suddenly being presented with a much deeper and more potent version that makes you much more drunk in a shorter space of time. The taste is also much more pleasing and the net result is that the old version is quickly superseded by the new, more potent version. This was exactly the case with the new devic light — it was much more potent and blacker.

So, through the presence and substance of the Devic Overlord, all devic life on the planet was offered the opportunity to receive this essence of new black light. The old black light is being stripped away and being replaced by the devic light that is more potent and able to birth an entirely new devic intelligence, love and understanding. Those devic life forms that are not prepared to host the new pattern of light have been invited to leave. The net result has been a fundamental transformation in the devic light that now exists in the planet; all of the old, devic black light is being cleared out and replaced by the new, deeper essence of virulent black light. All of devic life is being offered this new essence and so now has the capacity to build devic light into something more.

With this new pattern of devic light, the new chaos is also being seeded into the planet and this chaos represents the new devic order, and the new living expression of devic intent. So from the standpoint of the devas, the new black light represents order, while to those who work with order, it is the embodiment of chaos. The devas have been given a new inner essence that will allow them to host and retain a whole new series of frequencies, so that they may experience and become more through sensation, feeling and emotion.

While this platform of new devic light is being established, further infusions of different types of devic light are also underway. In particular, the new pattern of chaos and order has allowed a further infusion of a new type of devic light that is now touched and seeded with an aspect of the new order. So while the new black light is the new chaos, there is also a new type of devic light that is being suffused with an aspect of the new order, or with an aspect of the new angelic light. This new type of chaos, which also hosts a small percentage of the new order, has birthed another type of devic light that is silver, rather than deep black. This silver light is of a higher vibration than before and presents the devas with a new opportunity to absorb and host an entirely new pattern of devic light. There is a special significance in this because it marks the initial steps in creating a completely different devic pattern based on the more dynamic interplay of chaos and order.

While the new black light is the manifestation of the new chaos, in which chaos has been stimulated by an infusion of order, so the new sliver pattern is a further stepping stone where there is a direct mixing of the new chaos and order. This marks a significant start to a pattern that will develop through the Sixth Root Race and beyond.

So, where souls entering the devic pattern, in the past, would work with the old chaos and light, they now have the opportunity to explore devic life through the essence of new black light, and through the potency of a new silver light. This silver light will provide the devas with entirely new levels of sensation and experience which before were never possible, and is also part of the unfolding dynamic between the devas and the angels.

The New Angelic Light

Just as the new devic pattern of light has been restructured and infused with the new chaos, so the angelic pattern of light has been re-orchestrated according to the new pattern of order and higher light. Angelic light has always been the living embodiment of complete order, although for each angel, as a living recorder of everything that takes place, a number of limitations have been imposed on their focus. Angels cannot see the face of God, and so can only experience the essence of God through all that takes place around them. At the same time, there has been a point of limitation within the flow of light between the devic and angelic. The chaos expressed through devic intent has been the opposite polarity of the angelic order.

Yet within this limitation, the new pattern of chaos and order has enabled a profound shift to take place in the angelic realms. Since the new order and the new streams of light are birthed out of the Seventh Plane, the new order that is being birthed will build in a step-like fashion. In the future timeline, this new order is the embodiment of the Cosmic Christ, yet before that is realised, the new order will evolve through several different streams of higher light to eventually become that which has been ordained. The new pattern of order is being orchestrated under this new umbrella of higher light frequencies, and as a result, new patterns of angelic light are being birthed. This has meant that wholesale change has taken place in the Angelic Realms.

The Head of the Angelic Hierarchy, Archangel Gabriel has ascended up into the Seventh Plane and has been replaced. The new Angelic Overlord has birthed new frequencies of light from within the Paramatma.   A new pattern of order and light has entered the angelic realms. The old order has been replaced by the new order, so that a brand new type of angelic light has been birthed out of the higher essence of the Seventh Plane, and then downloaded into angelic form. This new angelic light, like its devic counterpart, is much more vibrant, powerful and refined, since it has been seeded into the angelic from a point much higher up in the Seventh Plane than before.

The new order and angelic light has meant that angels have become much more than they were before. A new type of dialogue has been established between the angelic and the devic, originally though the new Devic Overlord and the new Angelic Overlord. The pattern of twelve, new Devic Lords and the twelve, new Angelic Lords can now negotiate, in a freer and more diverse way, a different pattern of interaction and co-operation. The devic and the angelic are deeply interconnected, and the new angelic essence, having been birthed out of the new order, has also been mixed with a small amount of the new chaos. It is like the devic and angelic are sampling small amounts of their polar opposites; for the devas, the new order, and for the angels, the new chaos.

At the same time, the angels have been gifted in a new and profound way and have been given back their sight. They can now look at the Father directly and can experience the essence of love and light in a much more direct way than before. This momentous change has signified the end of the old, and the start of the new angelic energies that will now grace the planet. Some of the existing archangels have also moved up into the Seventh Plane, while other angels are being offered the opportunity to experience the one life necessary to complete their cycle, through the essence of those already in living matter. This is like a deeper level of merging, where certain angels, rather than having to incarnate into matter for one life only, can actually do it through those already living, like riding their living awareness through an open door. The angels can then experience the physical play through this deeper level of merging. And those in matter who have the capacity to host and hold the angelic energies will receive the lived experience of the new type of angelic light and order.

Another aspect to the unfolding of new angelic light has been the birthing of entirely new types of angelic souls out of the Ocean of Life. Specialist, advanced souls have gone on poaching expeditions in the Ocean to seek out new souls that irradiate a new type of spark. These new sparks are untainted and manifest a new essence that has then been infused with the new angelic pattern in the shadow planes. Once birthed, these new souls were then taken down to the Sixth and Fifth Planes, where they were woken up on one or other of these planes, as either archangels or as angels. The new souls then went down through the lower planes, into the Zero Planes, and then back up the planes to be finally anchored on the Fifth or Sixth Plane. They have experienced a new pattern of angelic light and will, at the appropriate time, be born into physical matter for one life only. They represent the first in a new and developing breed of angelic life.

There will also be a major influx of angels into human form for their one designated life during the Nine-Pointed Plan. The aim is to infuse the planet directly with angelic light, to seed the new order into the physical vibration of form, and to build a new platform of angelic light that can broadcast the angelic signal to all those around. The angels will enter the planet in a wave of new births, and these new angelic children will require special care and attention to ensure that they can endure the grossness of the physical planes, and can survive the shock of slow frequency light as it comes into contact with their much more refined and ordered, angelic systems of light. The combination of birthing new angelic souls that have been called out of the Ocean of Life, along with the existing angels will create a wave of new angelic energy that will flow through the planet. The angelic and the devic will harmonise in a new way, and the new patterns of chaos and order will then be hosted and manifested through living form. The angelic pulse of light that will be expressed in human form, will give humanity a significant energetic push, and also infuse the physical vehicles with a new type of angelic light that will lead to a deeper merging of the angelic and devic patterns of expression. The human vehicle will become lighter and stronger.

The New Mast Song

The masts are also birthing a new type of light into the planet. During his life Meher Baba spent a considerable amount of time searching out masts in India and then re-wiring their physical vehicles in preparation for the new changes to sweep across the planet. The masts represent a level of purity and focus on the divine that is utterly unique and sublime. Being God-intoxicated means that their focus is exclusively on God, and nothing else. For the most part they have lived in the East, where the structure of society has been more accommodating of their inner focus. Through His re-wiring, Meher Baba focused on preparing the new masts for incarnation in the West. The masts will then irradiate, once they are reborn in the West, this new pattern of light that will be virulent and extremely focused, and will set a new standard of energy for those around to receive and to work with. The masts, with their complete focus and love for the Father, will show the way for humanity and will be a living example of how to love and serve the Father. As more and more masts incarnate in the West, the energetic focus will shift and those who come into contact with the masts will experience the deep purity of their light and begin to understand the true meaning of devotion and service to the Father.

Just as a new type of devic and angelic essence has been born, so new types of masts are also being poached out of the Ocean of Life. These new masts will embody a brand new type of mast light and there will be five principal types of mast soul that will enter the planet in the future. At the same time, those who are working as open doors and who have the capacity to experience the mast frequencies, will experience a new standard of light work that will be born directly out of the mast light frequencies. Through directly experiencing the new mast energy, they will then turn and look at the Father and all that he was, is and will be, in a brand new way.

At the same time, the mast and the angelic frequencies will combine to produce a new pattern of light that will retain the essences of both and set up a new triangle of energies between the mast, angelic and the devic, as well as establishing other, future triangles.

Birthing New Souls into the Planet

As these new platforms of light are brought into the planet, the combination of the new devic, angelic and mast light will imbue the new timeline with a brilliant new series of frequencies. These new light streams will then host the older souls returning into the planet after a long absence, and also play host to a whole series of new, special souls that are being birthed out of the Ocean of Life. Yet, as the new spark is reborn, and the new Avataric Day dawns, then the Ocean, too, will undergo something of a restructuring and re-birthing as part of the re-orchestration of the inner planes. As the old chaos is cleared away and replaced by the new chaos and new order, then the Ocean itself will begin to change and become more, and give birth to a different pattern of souls that will host a new spark inside, that will, ultimately, be able to ignite into a new type of flame, once the full circuit of 8,400,000 lives has been completed in physical matter. The re-orchestration of the inner planes will be an integral part of this. The focus of the planet will be to allow the old souls to complete their full complement of lives, without the active interference of the Perfect Masters ahead of each soul's scheduled ascendancy into the Seventh Plane. The new light of the Sixth Plane will ensure that the pattern of ascendancy will prepare souls for the new focus at the bottom end of the Seventh Plane, where the limitations of bliss will be superseded by the higher frequencies of the Fourth and Fifth Divine Journeys. At the same time, the new timeline will embody the essence of grace.

The Ocean of Life, as it receives a new and fundamental spark at the start of a new Avataric Day, will be infused with the new pattern of chaos and give birth to new souls with different potentials and abilities to house different levels of consciousness. The sparks of the new souls will, ultimately, become the new flames of more that will establish a series of different pathways and vehicles of consciousness within the different plane settings and manifest new types of experience in the unfolding pattern of the future root races.

The new angelic and mast souls that will enter the planet will host an entirely new presence of light that will allow an opening up of the new root race into a vast series of different timelines, and to open up and birth the new pattern of soul families. Until now there have been twelve principal soul families, each reflecting a distinct colour or dominant frequency. The new root race timeline will also birth a new type of soul family, the thirteenth, which will be like the colours of the rainbow and will retain the best of the preceding twelve families and embody more within their soul essence. This new soul family will capture a new, more dynamic pattern of light that will then gain, through experience, a new level of emotion and common sense that can be hosted within, and which will manifest the new living will of the five Perfect Masters, as they, too, in turn, become that which is more. The essence of common sense will then be fused with a new type of love and give birth to something more within the living moment of divinity.

So the new soul family that is being birthed has been formed out of the oversoul, where significant changes have also been invoked for the pre-existing soul families. New types of soul groupings have been created within each of the existing families and different soul exchanges have been worked through the Oversoul down into the lower planes where the illusion of separation has invoked a new pattern of soul interaction. It is a bit like taking all of the pre-existing soul families, and then exchanging different numbers of souls within these families, so that the new family members can experience their journey under a different umbrella of soul light and focus. This pattern of swapping different members between each soul family offers each soul a new pattern of experience that is not dissimilar to being adopted by a new family.

The newly poached souls out of the Ocean of Life all represent a series of new types of sparks, whether they be angelic, devic or mast and the new energies, like sparks, will imbue the different levels of existence with new essences of soul light that will be stunning to behold. The new Avataric Day will birth these new souls into a different arrangement of chaos and order, light and dark, and plane levels, so that the timeline of the Sixth Root Race will pulse in a new, dynamic way as it becomes infused with the light of a new Sun. The fabric of time, and the pattern of devic and angelic light will provide the foundations for a new pattern of life and Natural Law to be invoked.

As a finishing school, the Earth will then be able to evolve in a more dynamic way and host a myriad of different life forms and souls that have been awaiting the advent of a new age. The planet, and all life on it, will engage in a new dialogue of light, where time and timelessness will open up a new fabric of being and becoming, and the future timeline can be invoked so that humanity need no longer look to the past for artificial support, but be capable of embracing the present and the future in a new cycle of grace. The permanent atoms of all souls will pulse to a new type of light, and will support different patterns of soul growth and progression. The ring-pass-not will resonate to this new vibration of soul light, and enable new streams of other life forms to interact with the planet and the different life forms on it. The new sparks of soul light will play host to new levels of consciousness and give birth to new vehicles of consciousness that will then form the framework for future root race life to blossom and radiate out from Earth, first into the other two Earths, and then into the 18,000 Earths and ultimately to the whole of creation within the Wheel of Life. And the Wheel of Life will dance to a new pattern of light song that will form the seeds of the future in the now.

CHAPTER 16

Working in Shadowlands

Assessing our Plane Levels

Since May 2003 the astral levels have been completely open. This is only the second time that this has happened in Earth history; the other time was during the Atlantean Root Race. Astral light is now pouring into the planet and all life forms present on it or within it. Since astral energy includes all the feelings, thoughts, motivations of animal instinct and the habits and desires of the current and previous root races in a very total way, in practice it means that all of these frequencies are now fully accessible to humanity. And for humanity, this means an expanded sensitivity to all of the different astral energies, from the grossest to the most refined.

Astral light is also activating a lot of old memories, seed thought forms and other slow frequency energies that have been locked or dormant within people's energetic systems. Astral entities and other energetic patterns that have their own awareness, however limited or slow, are coming more into people's conscious awareness with predictable results. The rise in mental illnesses and other physical diseases such as cancer (which are lower astral viruses), are all part of the increased flow of astral light. For many people the problem lies within the past, where their old karmic practices and energetic training can come back to haunt them, and the old addictive patterns, whatever they may be, appear to take hold and lead to a downward emotional spiral. For some, the pattern of astral light feels too intense and the slide into depression becomes part of a negative feedback loop between the negative thoughts and emotions and the resultant energetic flow. Energy always follows thought, and if we think negative thoughts, then we will experience them within the astral flow of slow frequency energy. Astral light is also activating the old energetic patterns of energy held within the ground energies, or even within ancient buildings or ancient sites of power. The effect has been for all of the old astral thought forms and energetic streams that have been formed in the past, to be reactivated in the present; and humanity now has to live these experiences as part of the processing of the old root race energies. So, as a platform of thought, the old astral frequencies have to be re-lived to be transmuted.

In opening up to these different energies, and the roller coaster ride of emotions, thoughts and feelings that many people are now experiencing, it is becoming increasingly important to find an explanation that can help make sense of these experiences. And from this explanation, a new approach to working with these energies can then be formulated and implemented, with the principle aim of providing greater balance and a sense of inner calm in the face of the different waves of astral energy that are engulfing the planet.

The Unspoken Word, which was issued by the Avatar, has gone out to the edge of the Wheel of Life, and is now returning to the planet; as it comes back in, it pushes all of the old dross and slow frequency energies in its path back into the planet and humanity for transmutation. Consequently, wave after wave of slow frequency energy is now hitting the planet.

Whenever we incarnate in each life, we have to come down from the inner planes and take up position within our physical vehicle. The soul has to learn to harness the different levels through the physical body. We have to be fully present within our physical vehicle and as part of this coming down, we have to then create a series of forms that can act as a reference point within our specific planes of experience. For example, we create an astral body that has to sit inside our physical shell. Using these specific subtle vehicles, we then work the different sets of frequencies, starting with the lower astral first, followed by the middle astral and then higher astral. Once we have worked this astral light we are then ready to receive the mental instruction, initially from the lower mental level and then beyond. This lower mental instruction will tell us to let go, open up to divinity and to collective consciousness. We then have to earth these lower mental energies, so that the mental body can eventually reside inside our astral body. We can then effectively ground the different streams of energy into our physical consciousness. In doing this, we begin to build up a series of experiences which demonstrates that where we anchor ourselves will dictate the flow of information that we receive and download; principally whether we are focused astrally or mentally. So, while we may feel strongly that the lower astral manifestation of thought has to change, we have to rise up to the lower mental levels to receive the change. To bring in lower mental light is to invoke change. And to achieve this, we have to understand the way in which we focus our energy and how this focus can impact us.

The first point of reference in becoming conscious of the flow of energies within our different subtle and physical bodies is to understand the level that we are operating from. For example, if our energetic focus is in the lower astral levels, then we will feel the full force of the negativity and slow frequency energy; unpleasant and virulent thoughts will fill our awareness. If, however, we are working more in the middle levels, then we will feel less constricted and heavy, and the quality of our thoughts will improve slightly. We will still experience negative streams of thoughts and emotions, but they will not be as dense as in the lower astral. If we are working with the mental levels, then the flow of energy will feel entirely different – much freer and clearer.

However, there is an important difference between our inner planes status and the level at which our soul aspect is anchored for work in any particular life. This is all part of building up a picture of how we operate within the astral and mental levels and this can help us to understand the type of energetic work that we are doing, and also free us from the sense that we are at the mercy of the grosser frequency energies all around. For example, if a person's soul aspect has progressed to the top of the Third Plane, say 3.8, but that person has a contract of work down in the First Plane, for example between 1.2 and 1.4, then their energetic experience will be centred in the bottom half of the First Plane, rather than the top of the Third Plane. The plane level at which we are operating from will determine the type of energetic flow through our system. If we can establish the plane level that we are working from, then it is easier to negotiate with the energy.

It can take some time and practice to establish our precise operating level on the inner planes. There are several ways to approach this: the first is to look at it purely from the different astral levels — lower, middle and higher within the nine different levels. For example, if we intuitively come up with level 3, then we will be operating in the top end of the lower astral level. Alternatively, level 7 will be the bottom end of the higher astral. If we are in the lower astral, then it is easy to focus our awareness and push up out of these lower levels by allowing our intent to push us up. By simply focusing on going up, then energy follows thought and we will then move up out of the lower astral levels. By the very act of thinking and willing the action of going up, we will move up. The more focused we are about it, then the more effective we will be. Ideally, it is best to station ourselves in the higher astral, although most people will be working in the middle astral. Those who are prone to depression and repeated illness are invariably trawling the lower astral levels. A similar pattern can also be used for determining whether we are working in the mental levels, and if so, from which specific level.

In addition to this type of intuitive 'dowsing', it can be extremely helpful to build a sense of the plane level that we are working from. This can be from the Zero Plane, normally above 0.6, although a few souls will work as far down as 0.0, up through to the Sixth Plane to 6.9. It is extremely easy to introduce the element of bias into this process, because our ego will always want us to be in the Fifth or Sixth Plane, when the reality may be somewhat different. Requesting assistance from our highest guidance can be very useful and one way to build a preliminary feel for our own plane level is to open up in our heart centre, and then to see what number forms there, from Zero through to Six, or even Seven. So, if for example, in opening up, we obtained a number three, then this would mean that we are stationed on the Third Plane. Now, if we take this number and then place it in the heart centre again, if it grows, then it is likely that the figure is correct. If it fades and quickly disappears, then it is incorrect. Once the basic plane level has been ascertained, it is then possible to look at the plane sub-division from zero to nine. So if the figure five comes up, then we are operating at plane level 3.5. Now, just to complicate matters, this figure can either relate to our real status on the inner planes i.e. a direct reflection of our degree of soul evolution, or it can be related to the level at which we do most of our inner plane work. For example, as soul aspects become more advanced, they can be split between different plane levels according to the type of job they are doing: so one part of the awareness can be on the First Plane, another on the Second Pane and so on. And yet their real status is on the Fifth Plane.

It takes a certain amount of practice and a ruthless degree of self-honesty to ascertain the plane of work and inner plane status. Yet, where we work on the inner planes will translate into a variety of physical, emotional and mental lived experiences. If we are working on the Zero or the First Plane, then the energetic focus is extremely condensed, slow and heavy. It is like we feel heavy inside; as we work higher up the planes, the feelings of constriction, heaviness and emotional density gradually lift, so that by the time we hit the Fourth Plane and above, then feelings of expansiveness can be felt. When we are working in the lower planes, there is an emotional sensitivity that comes in, and a sense of sometimes being overwhelmed by small things, almost as if we do not have room to breathe. In contrast, if our awareness is anchored on the Fifth Plane, then minor inconveniences and emotional problems drop away much more easily.

The flow of astral energy through the lower planes can be especially unpleasant and virulent in today's energetic climate; negative seed thought forms easily take hold in our awareness, and what starts out as a minor irritation can rapidly escalate into incredibly powerful feelings, reflecting the negative imprinting in the first place. So, if the original emotional charge is based on fear, then if we give in to it, and give it importance and energy, then it will build and build. The same is true for any other emotion, whether it be anger, shame etc. The trick is to understand that these negative emotions are all part of the astral levels and that what we experience is what is held within the different astral levels. If we choose to focus on it, then it will draw us in, making it harder and harder to let go of. A recognition of the plane level that we are operating from and an understanding of how to remain balanced in the face of the different energetic streams can go a long way to helping us ride the waves of slow frequency energy flowing into the planet at this time.

Working with Different Levels of Guidance

Guides are separate beings of energetic awareness and intelligence stationed on the inner planes that can communicate with us directly, or indirectly through others, thereby providing assistance to us. Guides can be positive or negative, light or dark, and will work according to a plan of agreed outcomes and changes. Guides are rarely seen within the physical, and are more often felt as a presence or pulse external to our physical and subtle awareness. They can communicate in a variety of different ways and operate under the laws of karma and/or Natural Law.

Guides come in an array of shapes, sizes, forms and each with different degrees of experience and expertise. Each incarnating soul usually has a guide, although in rare instances people have been born without guides, usually as a result of a major disconnect from their previous lives. Each person will have a central doorkeeper who acts as the main guide and who oversees the dialogue with other levels of guidance. Guides may stay with a soul over many lifetimes and for each of us, there will be opportunities to act as guides during our various stints outside physical matter.

It is important to recognise that different guides come with a range of skills, and that guides, like humans, may make mistakes, or provide information that is not always accurate. It is therefore important to be mindful of the information that guides supply to us, and to take responsibility for that information: to test it and our guides, if necessary. Over our millions and millions of lifetimes, we will have worked with a huge diversity of guides, from the Mineral, Plant and Animal Kingdom, all the way through the different planes. Consequently, we may have had animal guides in the past, such as a wolf or other type of life form. Each plane level will retain its own level of guidance and expertise; so Second Plane guides will tend to give us a more protective function, and can be seen as Roman Soldiers or other types of warriors on the inner planes. More evolved guides may appear as Native American Indians or as Chinese Healers, while many of the more potent forms of new guidance coming in may appear in the feminine form, either in Eastern or Western dress, reflecting the pattern of work. Guides can also be crystalline, angelic, devic or extraterrestrial and will again reflect the pattern of work that is being undertaken. Ultimately, though, the highest levels of guidance are the Perfect Masters and the Avatar and eventually, evolving souls will come under the guidance of a Perfect Master. Sometimes the Perfect Master will only appear on the inner planes and until in the fullness of experience, a life will come when the external presence of a Perfect Master has been earned.

One of the key requirements in the new timeline is for all of us to communicate more directly with our guides. This can be achieved either during our waking hours or through dreams. The new levels of Sixth Root Race guidance are massive and are being spearheaded by the Elderings. The new guides are all working according to the new protocols of the new timeline and will provide, through a focused interaction, the precise knowledge and information that we need to manifest and to become the new essence of higher light. On one level, this means that all of the old patterns of guidance have to go, and for some, this is as painful as loosing old friends or loved ones. Yet, only through embracing the new levels of guidance, those from the lower mental levels and above, can we learn to host the new energies. The new Sixth Root Race guides will also make the necessary internal adjustments to our physical and subtle vehicles and will provide the means through which we can access and retain a greater degree of high frequency light. There is a need to embrace our highest levels of guidance and to invoke for that which is more according to the dictates of the Father's Will.

In addition to guides on the shadow planes, different levels of guidance exist in the Seventh Plane, and it is these higher levels of guidance that are being sought and brought through. Some of these higher levels of guidance will seek to provide an energetic understanding of how Natural Law operates, while others may seek to provide understanding and yet seek an alignment of their wishes over ours. Different guides also exist for working through the lower parts of the Seventh Plane, such as in the first three Divine Journeys. Ultimately, though, if we are ever in any doubt as to the focus and advice being presented by our guides, then it is always best to offer it up to a higher authority – whether it is the Father or some other higher authority. Nevertheless, the pattern of change being manifested in the new timeline will open us up to a stunning array of new guides that will show us a new roadway and educate us in a new code of conduct.

Earthing Techniques

As more and more high frequency energy flows into our systems, there will be a tendency to be drawn up into the light, and to disengage from full physical experience. The higher frequencies of light are extremely alluring, and some of us, when confronted between the alternative of working in slow frequency slime or communing with the delight of higher light, choose the latter. While there is always a time and a place for accessing the higher frequencies, it is also essential to understand that when we access such frequencies, we need to bring them back into our conscious awareness and ground them into our physical bodies. Many light workers suffer from being ungrounded, and in so doing, are failing to properly process the higher frequencies of light. By constantly being ungrounded and floating along, we cannot effectively fulfil our role as light workers.

To earth oneself means to align one's physical and subtle bodies in such a way that there is a direct connection from the physical into the etheric, and from the etheric into the astral, and from the astral into the mental. It also means that our astral body fully inhabits our physical vehicle, followed by the mental body, so that our awareness and consciousness is fully grounded. There may be a number of reasons why we are not properly earthed, some of which go back to the birth process, when there was a reluctance by the soul to fully engage in the physical body. In such circumstances, the soul has to come fully into the physical body, work through the different astral levels and then re-engage with the appropriate plane level of work. Once this is done, then the person will feel much more aware and connected to the world around. Being ungrounded also means to be disconnected from our immediate environment. More commonly, though, as light workers, we may feel the irradiation of higher light, and then find it so intoxicating, that we do not wish to come back fully into our body. By rooting ourselves into the earth, and by placing heavier patterns of energetic robes around ourselves, it can then be a lot easier to come back in. Ultimately, however, physical force, such as an accident, or pain through an injury will always force us to come back into our bodies. Indeed, for more advanced souls, the reluctance to come into their physical body can only be effectively counteracted by physical pain. Pain is often the preferred tool in matters concerning effective grounding.

Working in our gardens or walking in the countryside can help the process of grounding, and through meditation practice, it becomes easier to bring the subtler levels of awareness into our physical vehicle. The energies, as they become more virulent, will necessitate an active point of focus and will to ensure that we all remain effectively grounded. Shamanistic robes can also be very useful in the grounding process. Darker, heavier robes will help to bring back the subtle bodies into the physical.

Other grounding techniques involve effective closing of our chakras. When we open up to doing energetic work, our chakras will open. Different chakras will open to different degrees depending upon our energetic focus and once we have completed the work, it is always important to close them down. Ensuring that our chakras are shut down can take practice; sometimes a chakra will not shut properly or be held in a type of spasms where it remains only partially open or closed. In these circumstances, the chakra will need to be effectively cleared of the debris of the past.

Building Collective Unity

Above all else, as the new timeline unfolds, there will be a need within every fibre of our being, to embrace collective unity. Collective unity is the ring, the foundation block, upon which the new frequencies and emotions will be brought into full realisation. Collective unity will be the doorway through which humanity can move forward, out of the limitation of the past and off the ray of suffering, and onto the new ray of love and grace. Collective unity is not just conscious unity, it is also sub-conscious unity forged through understanding, love, tolerance, an acceptance of that which is different, and through embracing the pattern of diversity through unity. It can also work through multiple levels, from the physical right up to the soul and the oversoul.

Collective unity means that we have to work through all of our biases and our prejudices, both conscious and sub-conscious. In other words we have to work through our karma, finding ways to clear out all of the old emotions and traumas that keep us locked in a particular space. One of the most direct ways that this can be achieved is through energetic merging with another person. Most people will usually have personal karma with another person, unless one of the people involved is God-realised; then the individual who is God-realised will have no karmic ties with anyone else. However, it is pretty rare not to have karma with another individual, whether it is physical, astral or mental karma and the practice of merging energy systems can quickly clear the karmic knots.

This process is straightforward and can be done simply between two or more people: each person agrees with the other and they then open up to merging their respective energetic systems. So, for example, one person can remain passive while the other one projects their awareness into that other person's space. With some people this may be difficult, because of the underlying karma, while with others it will be easier. If two people can merge in this way, and they focus on merging into deeper levels, then the first steps have been made in experiencing collective unity. In a merging, the energetic systems of two people come together and a negotiation takes place; old patterns are brought up, and if allowed to flow up without attachment and are offered up to the Avatar, then slow frequency energy can be cleared. As this process builds, the two people may share similar experiences, feel past life associations follow through, and will ultimately come to a deeper connection with each other. The superficial, outer, physical shell will be stripped away, and each person may experience a more direct connection with each person's underlying essence. And within this essence they will find different qualities that were not apparent at first.

Merging can help to overcome superficial prejudices about how we look, because as we merge more deeply, then it becomes obvious that everyone is different, and the physical vehicle is just that – a local fashion that houses the soul and connects the soul through a series of subtle bodies. Through merging we can begin to connect with these subtle bodies, build up a new platform of energy and begin to feel the pulse of love that underlies everything.

By routinely merging, more profound levels of connection and communication can be opened up and with practice, can lead to a more unified connection with others around. If energetic merging is practised within a group of people, then after a time, it can become possible to feel the energy change within the group in many different ways. If everyone can merge with everyone else in a group, then there is considerably less bias and prejudice and the flow of energy between everyone is much clearer. Old cordings can be negotiated and cleared away and any points of pressure between individuals can be processed through the collective will and intent of the group. A group can considerably speed up the karmic process by working through the patterns of interplay between participant's different subtle bodies, and remove old thorns and seeds of negativity. A group gives greater flexibility to the pattern of energetic negotiation and also focuses a greater degree of electronic energy. Both can be extremely useful in removing old karmic patterns.

Ultimately, the aim is to have a clear flow of energy within a group of people. This flow should encompass each of the chakras, so if a group of individuals are sitting in a circle, then the flow of energy through, say, the base chakra is free and uninterrupted. There are no energetic 'spikes' or blockages. The same should be true for all of the other chakras. This pattern of collective merging represents the first step towards building collective unity.

Collective unity ties each of us into the ring of higher purpose, and allows us to be held within the support and love of the collective, while working according to the laws of faith and trust. It allows us to absorb and become much more than we can through the limitations of our individualistic bias. It frees us from limitation and opens us up to a new way of being and merging on all possible levels. Fundamentally, collective unity is an energetic expression of a shared, collective focus that can entertain change, banish the old, embrace the new, and forge a new level of light that ultimately, will play host to the essence of the Cosmic Christ.

To embrace this new pattern of collective unity means that we have to be open to more all of the time; we have to embrace change; we have to operate from the principles of trust and faith; we have to push past any personal prejudices and seek out the bigger picture; we have to look to the present and the future and let go of the past; we have to ignite, within our hearts, the flame of love forged through purity and innocence, which is then smelted down on the anvil of everyday experiences. Above all, we have to recognise that the focus of the Avatar is everything and that the one true marriage in all of our lives is with the Father, as manifested through the Son.

Collective unity means that we need to let go of ignorance and find ways to embrace common sense. Collective unity represents the spiritual platform for the future and ultimately is the expression of love that will be manifested through the Christ Essence in the future. And while we may experience the collective focus much of the time, there is always more to be found and more to be experienced. So, through the first steps of energetic merging, and then building this into a more collective experience of energy, this then has to be taken to a higher level of light and love through the focus of the Perfect Masters and the Avatar. Collective unity means unity on all levels, both seen and unseen; known and unknown; within and without; at a soul level and beyond, as well as on all levels of our subtle bodies, all the way down to our physical body.

Collective unity also hosts a spirit, or essence of divinity that is about manifesting and retaining higher and higher frequencies of light and love; ultimately to love that is unconditional, all encompassing and collective. Through embracing this collective focus, many of the slower frequencies and difficulties that we experience in our lives will drop away; they will no longer be important, for when set against the enormity of the spirit of collective unity are trivial. Collective unity will provide us with the means and the purpose to ride the waves of slow frequency energy that are now engulfing the planet. The new timeline *is* collective unity, and so will not allow any of the old astral frequencies of competitiveness, feudalism and mistrust to co-exist.

Clearing Past Lives and Karma

Collective unity also provides the foundation for speeding up our karma and for a much more rapid clearing away of both negative and positive karma. As we progress through our lives, being reborn and then dropping our body in countless ways, we seek to clear away our karma through the law of opposites. One life may give us everything material that we could ever want, while in the next life we are destitute. This playing out of opposites ensures that we do not become too attached to everything around us, although in truth, the process of detachment from the physical, astral and mental takes millions and millions of lives. With each life that we live, we leave a trail, a mark, which can be seen as a subtle representation of that life, like a living hologram. In some virulent lives, these holograms will be quite potent, and may irradiate a pattern to a future life that will lead us back into the old addictions of the past.

With the astral levels now fully open, we have access to all of the past holograms that we have ever been, in the sense that those still in existence means that we have unfinished business surrounding their energetic pattern. Imagine if you can, a series of subtle bodies that stretch up from your physical vehicle to your soul on the inner planes; and within this diversity of subtle bodies, each one represents a point of incompletion from the past. At first, it is extremely difficult to feel a pulse that comes down from the soul into the physical body, or from the physical body to the soul. The different subtle bodies are out of energetic alignment. However, the aim is to build up a clear flow of energy through the different subtle bodies by clearing away any unfinished business and karma associated with those past lives.

Another way of looking at it is to visualise our astral karma and to see it as a wall; if the wall is incredibly high, for example, over five miles high, then there is a substantial amount of karma to clear. If the wall is low, say knee high, then there is much less. Ultimately, the wall should be completely eliminated and the space where it was free of any objects or energetic patterns. The same practice can be done with mental karma. It is also possible to look at the walls and to see what the colour the bricks are; they will all be slightly different colours ranging from black to clearer colours; the colours will reflect the energetic focus of those past lives.

The burden of all of these past lives can be more rapidly cleared through the collective focus of group work. In a group setting all of the past lives of those present is spun through each person, and progressively stripped away. Of course, there has to be a focus and intent within the group, and the process will be amplified in the presence of individuals who resonate on the higher planes. In a group, the process of merging and working collectively will help to remove old karma, and other practices, such as rescue work, can also facilitate this process. The group offers greater flexibility to negotiate the old karma and provides the power to begin clearing away those aspects that represent unfinished business.

As the old energetic patterns are washed away, the flow of

energy between the different subtle bodies becomes progressively freer flowing until eventually there are no obstructions at all. The essence of the soul can then come down into the physical and touch the moment, and our physical awareness can also stretch back up into the inner planes through the perfect alignment of these subtle bodies. It is like feeling the beads on a string that stretches from our physical vehicle back into the inner planes. As more and more karma is stripped away, there eventually comes a point where a near perfect balance is maintained between light and dark on all the different levels. In progressing towards this point all of these subtle bodies become more condensed and are pushed into a compression of energy. At the point of God-realisation, all of these subtle bodies are compressed into a stream of energy that flows up into the Seventh Plane, which is absorbed as the ark of the moment by the Father. All that ever was and has been, through the millions and millions of lifetimes of experiences are returned to the Father. It is like all of those lives have been on loan, and when we become spiritually dead, through the process of God-realisation, then we offer back all of those experiences to the Father. We merge into a greater collective unity within the ever-refined levels of the Seventh Plane.

From what has been said so far, it should be clear that the frequencies of bliss do not represent collective unity. Collective unity is something much deeper and has to be found on the increasingly refined Divine Journeys that flow up through the Seventh Plane. The new timeline will reflect this collective unity in many different ways on the Seventh Plane; and these different layers of unity will then be pulsed down into the shadow planes first by the Fifty-Six, and then subsequently by those beings who act as open doors.

Invoking Change

Every aspect of the slow frequency energy that is being brought to the surface in our awareness, through the ground energies, the emotions and actions of the past root races, and the thoughts that flow through humanity, need to be cleared. This clearing is both an active and a passive process. Some of it goes on beyond our conscious awareness, while some of it takes place consciously. So, much of the slow frequency energy – the thoughts, the habits, the desires of the old timeline, as it flows through the lower astral levels, is unacceptable. The thought forms, the emotional and physical abuses all need to be transformed. This can only be done through an active desire, on the part of humanity, for change. At present, this desire for change is limited.

We are fed on a diet of misinformation and slow frequency energy which is, in truth, unacceptable to the new timeline and which has to be neutralised and cleared away. This can be done most effectively by invoking for change in our own lives, according to the greatest good and the Father, and through invoking change for all other life forms on the planet, and the planet itself. The process is like waking up to a different reality, where suddenly all of the grossness and negativity is revealed to us. In waking up to this new perception of a different reality, we are then presented with a choice – do we do something about it, or do we go back to sleep, as it were, and remain passive about it? If we are to embrace the new timeline, we have to invoke for change, through the laws of faith and trust, and without attachment to the outcome.

The Avatar has rewired everything for the next three thousand years. He has made all of the decisions necessary for complete change. Yet, we can choose to embrace this change and become part of it, according to the manifestation of higher will, or we can ignore it; in which case, then, the energy will make its way through everything according to the Father's Will, but will do so in such a way that we will be challenged by it in a more potent, and possibly brutal way. Change is already happening and if we embrace it, then we support it and become part of that change; if we ignore it, then energetically we are not aligned with it and are resistant to it. In this situation, the energy will always work through such resistances. These points of resistance will manifest in our lives as problems. So, whenever the Father gives us a problem, it is really an opportunity to work through the point of resistance, and come through to the other side to embrace more, not less. In embracing change, we align ourselves with the Will of the Father and then feel uplifted and happy in the energetic stream of change.

So the new timeline is about bringing something utterly new into our conscious awareness. It is about being happy and excited; it is about clear thoughts and clear virulent energy; it is about dispelling negative thoughts and believing that the planet is perfect and beautiful. In actively thinking this, then as energy follows thought, it becomes so.

CHAPTER 17

Working with Astral & Mental Light

Techniques for Protection

Astral light is diluted mental light and represents thought in action. In other words, mental thought drops down through the stimulus of energy known as emotion, and emotion has an active intelligence that has to be directed by the substance of form. Mental light is now flowing into the planet like a tidal wave and is spinning everyone around in their emotions, since as it hits the astral layers, it invokes a response and the emotions are challenged. The "we-focus" of mental light challenges the individualistic focus of astral light. The old negative energies have to be cleared away through crisis. The different tides of astral light will also expose different levels of astral awareness, and sometimes the grosser aspects of the lower astral levels will be pushed into our conscious awareness. So everything that has been suppressed is pushed to the surface and is in a state of activity. Emotions then get traded very rapidly through the lower, middle and higher astral levels and we sometimes feel the intensity of this. At the same time the astral levels are constantly replenishing themselves, partially through the recycling of old thoughts and emotions. All of this means that we live in an environment where we are constantly being bombarded by emotions and thoughts that are not our own, but which stimulate us according to the dictates of our energetic focus.

The multiplicity of energy streams within the astral levels necessitates the adoption of sound techniques for energetic management. The most basic of these is protection. Wherever we are, we are always bombarded by different frequencies; some may be more in tune with us, while the majority will be unsympathetic to us. Indeed, some will regard us as opportunities for stealing energy or imprinting their own energetic patterns into us. Either way, we need to recognise that thought forms, energy pirates, entities, and other astral manifestations, represent a point of pressure on our energetic systems all of the time. We rarely have an opportunity to rest, and what we would normally take to be a leisure or rest activity is not really so. Books all have cordings flowing through them, principally from the author, but also from all of the people that have read the book before us. Television sends out electromagnetic energy that interferes with our aura, just as all other electronic devices do. The constant barrage of news information stimulates emotional responses, while different levels of encodements within films and soap operas all target the emotions. If we go shopping in a large supermarket, we are constantly bombarded by the electromagnetic energy and the frequencies and cordings of all the produce carried by the store. Travelling by plane puts further stresses on our systems, since we are effectively sitting inside a giant electromagnet. At night, when we sleep, we are not really resting, since our system is clearing and processing the different frequencies that we have absorbed during the day, and all of our chakra centres usually release slow frequency energy at night.

With so much negative energy around, it is important to protect our systems, first through regular clearing of our energies, and second through sound protection techniques. Some of the meditations at the end of the book provide a series of steps for doing this. Clearing our energetic systems means not only clearing our physical vehicle, but also working on our etheric and astral bodies. Maintaining a clear aura is a significant challenge and requires constant attention. Pushing high frequency Paramatman light through our system and clearing out the older, slower frequencies will help to keep us in a pattern of inner and outer balance. Sitting in baths and taking frequent showers can also help to clear the slow energy frequency out of our bodies.

If we go into a space that is antagonistic to us, we do not want our chakra centres to be open. We should wear shamanistic robes that surround and protect our aura whenever we go out and about. The pattern of these robes should reflect the type of energy that we are working with. When working with the lower astral levels, they should be black to make us invisible, while in the middle and higher astral levels other robes, such as the artic owl can be particularly helpful. We should bless and dedicate the spaces that we live in, and we should also build protective patterns into our homes and cars. Any objects that have a negative feel should be removed and disposed of since it takes just one physical object to lower the vibration around us. Since our food has an energetic history, and will contain everything that has happened to it , then it too, should be blessed and dedicated. This is best done by offering it up to the Father and making an invocation to clear it. Since energy always follows thought, the food will automatically be cleared.

There are usually telltale signs if we are absorbing too much negative energy. We tend to become irritable, sometimes angry, have a constant flow of negative thoughts and feel heavily 'sludged up'. Our solar plexus may become active and we may feel like there are energies pushing into our auric space. In addition to being irritable and short-tempered, constant exposure to slow frequency energy over a period of time can lead to depression or physical illnesses.

It should be recognised, however, that negative energy will seek to enter our space from time to time in a more virulent way, and this is usually when we least expect it. A virulent telephone call from a family member or close friend can sometimes lead to a negative, downward spiral, as that person's energetic system becomes ridden by negative energies that are then downloaded into our space. All of this energy has to go somewhere, and if we do not clear it, by offering it up into the light, then our systems will vibrate at a slower rate and we will become more affected by it.

As we gather more experience through working with slow frequency energy, some souls choose to specialise in this type of work. Their role is simple: to absorb and transmute as much negative energy as possible, while remaining in a point of balance and harmony. This pattern of work requires practice, and may have been initiated many lifetimes ago. Individuals who work in this way may process the slow frequency energy physically, through illness or accidents, or emotionally, or in rare cases, mentally. Sometimes young children who are terminally ill may choose to absorb as much slow frequency energy as possible, as part of their tip to humanity. They may have only contracted to come into matter for a short period of time, and so will seek to absorb as much negativity as possible. They do this through terminal illnesses and by stripping away slow frequency, negative energy from all those people that they come into contact with.

When an individual begins to wake up to the different energetic streams, they may then gain impressions through their third eye. Slow frequency energy may appear as dark patterns of energy, like a mist, or as objects that move around. Sometimes it is more concentrated and virulent, such as in the more primeval aspects of the lower astral levels. There is then a need to give these impressions no importance, and just to let them flow through. As the inner sight develops, then more virulent entities may appear, such as gargoyles or other astral forms. Sometimes people will hold astral entities within their energetic fields that can appear as black snakes wrapped around them. These entities can present themselves in a host of different ways, and through working with these lower astral energies, the individual will build up a range of experiences that will provide a deeper level of understanding about the principles of energy management.

People's emotional energy will also have a flow of light and dark, although for the most part, it is usually dark. When a person becomes angry, or is about to commit a murder, it is like their system is overridden by something else – their own awareness fades away, they come out of their body for a split second, and the negative energy then has unrestricted access. If someone becomes angry with us, they are seeking ways to make us respond and react. If we react emotionally, then we become tied in with their energy; if we do not engage, then the energy that they are seeking to push onto us has to go back to them. And since energy always follows thought, whatever we think, will always have an impact on us.

Working with Emotional Energies and Thought Forms

All emotions have an energetic charge and are usually part of the astral flow of light. Lower astral emotions, such as anger, hatred, fear and terror, are often extremely virulent, and the slightest thought about them can very rapidly lead into full blown feelings of terror or whatever is the dominant emotion. This energetic exchange between ourselves and the thought form, or the emotion, often means that we have dropped down into the lower astral zone. If we stay in that space, we will become overwhelmed by many negative feelings.

To push through these emotions and thought forms requires an effort of will whereby we imagine our energetic focus moving up into higher frequency light, and where we can feel washed by different light streams, such as Paramatman Light. Sometimes, the emotions will be recurrent, and while we may push up into the middle and higher astral levels, we quickly find ourselves dropping back down. In these situations, there are usually other factors at work, such as past life habits and desires, where our old addictions may push us into depression, or we are attracted to slow frequency energy. In these circumstances, we should offer the pattern up to the Father or another higher authority of light that will enable a clearing out, from a standpoint of unconditional love. This process may have to be repeated over and over again, as the negative charge is slowly dissipated out of our systems.

However, within a spiritual context, there are always different perspectives, and if we do specialise in working with slower frequency energies, then we are working in a unique and powerful way. Through absorbing negative energy, and through feeling emotions such as despair, hopelessness, shame, sadness, loss, fear, anger, hatred etc. we are clearing and harvesting those experiences. The more virulent the emotions, then the more virulent ark that is being harvested, and this is ultimately offered up to a higher authority. By working in this way, we are undertaking acts of spiritual service. The three-dimensional experience may not seem like it, but from the perspective of our higher self, the work represents higher service.

Working with slow frequency energy builds spiritual muscle.

Rather than training with weights in the gym, a light worker will undertake to work with unpleasant, slow frequency energies. Once we have absorbed the living experience of some of the more slimy frequencies, we then build muscle. We find balance in a situation that previously would have pulled us off centre, and in maintaining this balance we can absorb the experience, live it in the moment and transmute it. A soul may spend lifetimes working with one or more frequencies, such as despair, until eventually, after a huge amount of hard work, he or she has learnt to master all of the frequencies of despair. That soul then becomes a master of despair, because it has lived all of the different experiences and permutations that despair has to offer, through the physical, emotional and mental levels.

In a very real sense, light workers today are learning to be despair masters. The amount of slow frequency energy that has to be cleared from the planet and all life forms on it is huge, almost immeasurable. By volunteering to work with it, we are building spiritual muscle that will then give us the right to work with the higher frequencies of light, and as we work through the slow frequencies, we burn off more karma, and so can then absorb the more delicious frequencies on offer. Despair becomes a tool for success because once we have endured it, and mastered it, anything else that gets put in our path will have a limited impact. It is like having learnt to master all of the weights and machines in a gym, so that we are super fit and ready for anything. So even when a new type of exercise machine is brought in, we have an underling level of fitness that will allow us to work that machine without becoming exhausted. And so it is that through working with frequencies such as despair, we build the stamina, love, flexibility and understanding that can allow us to become much more. As light workers, we will not just be able to host and hold the higher frequencies of light; we will also have the capacity to work with the slowest and grossest frequencies without falling apart or becoming emotionally overwhelmed by what is presented to us. In this way, we can then build up balance through experience and can open ourselves up to a new way of doing things where, irrespective of whether we are working the higher or slower frequencies, we can feel balanced, centred and happy in ourselves. At the same time, our energetic systems will have become sufficiently developed to endure whatever comes our way.

Clearing Ground Energies

The Earth has hosted five root races and within each root race there have been millions upon millions of cycles of life. Billions of lives over many millions of years have left their mark in a variety of different ways. Within each root race, different groupings of organisms have left energetic imprints on the land and in the sea. Even if we consider a small piece of land, in any country in the world, many generations will have left their signatures over the last two thousand years. For example, in Britain, the land has multiple layers of energy that have been laid down by the different populations that have lived and died. Their emotions, physical acts and even thoughts have been recorded in the rocks and ground energies all around. In any country in the world, it is possible to walk around and gauge the energetic level, whether it is positive or negative, and the virulence of the thought forms and emotions held in it. There have been so many wars, natural disasters, famines and other devastating events, that the ground is filled with all these different vibrations. These retained energies are then either amplified by the subsequent actions and events that have superseded them at any given place, or diminish through the passage of time.

The planet is also a network of interconnecting energetic lines. The more obvious ones, called Ley Lines, criss-cross the surface of the planet and provide interconnecting pathways of energy, either positive or negative. Deeper patterns of energy also flow with the different elements, as well as with other energetic holograms that have been created in and around the planet. Elements such as water also retain strong emotional pulses and so the planet is a complex maze of superimposing energies. The various subtle bodies of the planet also contain the different flows of astral and mental light. For some considerable time the planet has been entirely open to lower astral intent; the different devic presences have tended to concentrate in the lower and middle astral levels.

A large percentage of the land mass retains slow frequency energy patterns, and even those sites that are supposed to house a specific pattern of energy, are too slow by today's standards. Old temple sites, such as Chichen Itza, which were originally light centres, have been turned to the dark. Old battlefields, concentration camps and other negative placements of thought forms and emotional energies, all impact the flow and patterns of light and dark. Areas where the land has been heavily deforested, or where extensive mining takes place, all leave physical and energetic scars that need to be healed.

All of these patterns of energy are now in need of transformation and purification. Higher frequencies of mental light and unconditional love are now streaming into the planetary essence. Mental light is activating the astral energies at old energetic sites and is also flushing out of the ground many previously dormant, energetic patterns. Wherever we walk or rest on the land creates an energetic interplay, and if we walk around areas of slow frequency energy, then we can play an important role in clearing the ground energies. There are different ways in which this can be done, and the very act of being present and irradiating our inner light, will create a change and an effect. However, more active patterns of working are helpful, and so bringing down the Paramatman Light in our awareness and then projecting it into an area of land can create a shift and raise the vibration. This can be done remotely, by sitting quietly, and picturing the ground area within the inner eye; and then projecting high frequency light into that spot. There should be no attachment to the outcome, and as the high frequency light flows in, there may be subtle or occasionally more dramatic energetic shifts. The effects can be amplified if this is done through a group. Focusing on areas where significant traumas have taken place can therefore be extremely beneficial.

In working with the ground energies, the depth and type of energy that is retained also has to be taken into account. Places that we visit, and where we feel inexplicably tired and heavy, usually retain a heavy, negative charge, and the tiredness we experience comes through the processing of the slow energy. Just as we can work with the retained energies in the land, we can also work with pollution in our rivers, through tuning into the river, bringing through the Water element, and then offering an invocation for clearing and purification. Similarly, areas where trees and the land have been devastated by human intervention can be worked on, by bringing through different devic patterns to clear and birth a new pattern of harmony. In all of these activities, it is important to recognise that the planet, and every part of the land, is a dynamic expression of life where the consciousness and awareness flows through different physical and subtle structures. Negotiating with the ground energies, working with the devas and offering our love and light in a balanced and ritualistic way can help bring about profound change.

Rescue Work

Another integral aspect to raising the vibration of the planet and to the complete cleansing of the old astral energies is through rescue work. Rescue work is the conscious or subconscious act of finding souls that are trapped close to the physical realms, usually following a traumatic or emotional death, and then helping them to return to the appropriate level on the inner planes, where they can then continue their ordained pattern of reincarnation. In some cases, the work done during the life in question, or the nature of the death, may require that soul to rest and recover for a particular length of time. In such cases, the souls then go up to a holding place on the inner planes, and may spend the equivalent of many Earth years resting, before reincarnating.

Again, if we look back at all of the wars that have taken place across the planet and the many different ways in which people have dropped their bodies, then there remains a vast reservoir of souls that have not properly passed over. Some souls can be held back through the emotional ties that living family members may exert. In clinging on to the past, we can often make it more difficult for our loved ones to pass over. This reservoir of trapped souls needs to be shifted as part of the planet's evolution, and part of the programme has been to undertake extensive amounts of rescue work.

Efficient rescue work requires that the trapped soul is persuaded to let go of his or her current point of reference, and to be offered a route back up into the light. For traumatised souls this can be difficult, because they may believe that they are still alive. Different methods of persuasion have to be utilised, such as spending a period of time with them, before suggesting that they might like to move on. Once one person has been focused on, it is possible to use their energetic systems to trawl for those who have died in similar ways and are also trapped. So, in cases where people have drowned, dead sailors represent a focal point to call in all the other souls nearby that may have drowned. The trawl for lost souls can be pushed out many miles from the central focus. What usually happens with this pattern is that our own astral body will represent a point where other trapped souls can attach to it, and then other trapped souls will, in turn, attach to them. Once a large grouping has been built up then all of the souls can be taken up the inner planes in one go.

As each soul passes through our energetic system, they take a small portion of our karma as payment for the service. Rescue work is therefore an efficient way in which light workers can clear their karma through active service.

It is also possible to use collective group work to enhance the focus of rescue work and to magnify the number of souls passing through at any one time. Specialist guides are always present to help in this process and sometimes the rescue work can be seen as large groupings of trapped souls going through the group up into the light. A small number of people, such as three or four, can with a specific focus on rescue work, make a substantial contribution to helping trapped souls move over. In consciously undertaking this work, we have to absorb the emotional flow of energy, and so at times, the fear, despair, sense of loss and confusion can be quite powerful, as the older frequencies that have held that soul in bondage are stripped away. Rescue work can also encompass many different life forms, not only on Earth, but also from other star systems and planets.

New Patterns of Mental Light

All of the above patterns of light are firmly anchored in the astral, and as light workers our focus, of necessity has to be in the astral. However, as we build up our light and different levels of experience, we can then earn the right to work with higher streams of light. These higher streams encompass the flow of mental light. The opening up of the astral levels has also meant that mental light can now directly enter the planet, and the initiation of the new Sixth Root Race timeline has been accompanied, first, by a flow of lower mental light into the planet, followed by middle mental light and then higher mental light. All of these levels will be initiated by new streams of unconditional love that will flow down from the new platforms of energy manifested in the Seventh Plane. As the mental planes are overhauled, then the knock-on effect will flow down into the astral planes.

The Nine-Pointed Plane provides for a step-wise orchestration of different levels of light. The initial flow of lower mental level gives us access to the collective and to all of our previous lives. Through connecting with mental light, we can push up out of the limitations of astral light, and embrace a new level of light and understanding. Each step or gradation into a plateau of higher light is accompanied by a series of effects that reverberate back down through the different light levels, as a new type of balance is demanded. For example, widespread flooding is one of the effects of lower mental light entering the planet. Flooding represents clearing and the new mental light is orchestrating a vigorous pattern of clearing across the whole planet. Lower mental light also represents the forerunner of new patterns of emotional energy that are part of the new timeline. For example, the life and work of Princess Diana invoked lower mental light, which in turn led to an emotional response at the time of her death.

By graduating into the higher flows of mental light and building up a pattern of direct access with mental light, light workers now have the capacity to work with higher levels of guidance, and to access higher information, mental concepts and seeds that have been placed specifically within the mental light streams. New ideas and concepts are birthed in the mental planes, and can then be stepped down into the astral levels for greater access. The frequencies of light in the mental planes are extremely brilliant, and the new timeline of the Sixth Root Race is predominantly focused on these light streams. As the older astral frequencies are cleared out, then the planet can receive a more direct irradiation of mental light, which in turn will open up a new level of stability, hope and reality in those who absorb the new light.

A whole series of new holograms have also been placed into the mental planes as part of the new timeline. Principal among these are the crystal skull frequencies, which are a collective hologram of higher frequency light that was originally birthed on the Seventh Plane. The probable reality that is now being manifested through the essence of the Father's Will, and the specific crystal skull frequencies that are being chosen, are creating the new timeline and future probable reality.

Integral to this pattern of crystalline energy is the placement of mental holograms at different points on the planet. Giant crystal skulls have been placed at a number of sites around the world, including Switzerland, Mexico and in the Indian Ocean and are forming a new grid of mental energy that is beginning to replace the old, lower astral grid and bring through an entirely new pattern of light. This new grid will support the new infusion of Sixth Root Race concepts and ideas, emotions and thoughts, and the new physical vehicles that will be needed to support the new type of soul light that will grace the planet.

At the same time, new levels of Sixth Root Race guidance will also be formed, and these new guides will form the advancing tide of new information and concepts. They will offer new types of healing that will supersede the older patterns. Our patterns of DNA will be re-orchestrated and will capture a new series of harmonic frequencies of light. New ways of artistic expression and creativity will be accessed through mental light, and new forms of telepathy will also be birthed. A new understanding of whom and what we are will be opened up, and a whole new emotional pattern of experience will be birthed. The dynamic interplay between masculine and feminine will be completely overhauled, so that the feminine energy base will truly come into its own. Higher intuition will flow more easily so that each soul will be able to build up a direct connection between the higher and lower, and with the essence of God, the Father and the Son. This new level of access will provide a new level of conscious awareness of our true divinity, and of the interconnectedness of all life, and all form, in a new and dynamic way.

New levels of information about the past, present and the future will also be entertained, as veil after veil of illusion is stripped away to give a higher level of knowledge and truth. A completely new level of understanding will flow into our consciousness about different co-existing life forms, such as the Devas, the Elderings, the Angels and the star beings that are waiting to come into our consciousness. Different types of mineral, plant and animal form will be birthed, in some cases replacing the older models that have now completed their work on the planet. All of this will be pushed through the new mental grid of light. New types of frequency holder will be unveiled that can host the multiplicity and diversity of new levels of conscious awareness from the higher planes up into the Seventh Plane. Completely new types of soul will incarnate into the planet, hosting a stunning new series of light energies.

New levels of information about the creative flow of everything will become available and new patterns of love, power, wisdom, bliss and knowledge will form. The new mental grid will support the older souls coming back into the planet, and will also provide a higher pattern of light that can help to provide balance to the entirely new types of soul coming in for the first time.

The mental streams of light will manifest much more than before, since they will encompass the first three Divine Journeys that will have been shifted from the bottom of the Seventh Plane into the top of the Sixth Plane. The Ocean of Life will have been cleared out and replaced by a different Ocean at the bottom of the newly restructured Seventh Plane. This will mean that the new platform of mental light will be as brilliant as what used to be focused within the unconditional pattern of love on the lower portion of the Seventh Plane, so that souls who have yet to become God-realised can sample an entirely new pattern of higher light within physical matter.

The changes to the top of the Sixth Plane and bottom of the Seventh Plane will have a dramatic impact on the types of new souls that will be birthed out of unconscious bliss. A new Ocean of Life will replace the old one, which will have been cleared out before the patterns of plane restructuring are implemented, and the new Ocean of Life will manifest an entirely new pattern of divine light. The old level of unconscious bliss that was birthed out of the old dark bliss will be replaced by something completely different — a series of higher frequencies of divine light that will produce a brilliant new type of spark.

Body form and the various subtle energetic systems will undergo significant changes to accommodate the successive patterns of increasingly virulent light. The bar or standard for God-realisation will, if you like, have been raised, but at the same time, the newly formed Sixth Plane will give more advanced souls an entirely new level of experience in matter focused through the essence of bliss and grace. Experiencing new levels of bliss will become part of the shadowlands experience and as the new mental frequencies suffuse down into the lower planes, the whole planet will undergo an energetic transformation. The older patterns of lower astral light will be comprehensively cleared and a higher form of astral light will be birthed which, ultimately, will be replaced by mental light alone. The planet will then come to host metal light and the emotional focus that used to be pushed through the astral levels will then come to be worked through the mental streams of light in a much more potent and powerful way.

In short, the brilliance of the mental frequencies will ensure a brand new pattern of life experience in human form, as the mental streams of energy provide an entirely new grid of love, light, information, understanding, healing and power to all those who have the capacity to access and absorb it. Physical form will change, and the structure of our subtle anatomy and chakra systems will also change to reflect this new grid of energy. We will come to be the new living sparks of light that are imbued with grace and which can irradiate a unique new pattern of virulent light on Earth and out into the Wheel of Life.

This new grid will be a prelude to an entirely new pattern of higher light that is being birthed out of the Seventh Plane, and which the Sixth Root Race will act as the preparatory system of experience and the testing mechanism for this new light flow. This new light flow will manifest the essence of the Cosmic Christ.

CHAPTER 18

Working from The Seventh Plane

Building Collective Experience

The accelerated pattern of involution through the inner planes is all part of an experiment that has been ordained by the higher Will of the Father. It is also an integral part of the Nine-Pointed Plan. The end of one Avataric Day requires a final accounting before the new Avataric Day can get underway. These changes present a series of challenges that have never been encountered before. Many souls are being taken up to a new platform of experience when they have not gathered the sufficient number of lives in matter to normally support that status.

The accelerated changes are collective in nature, and the only way that developing souls can gather more experience is to act and become collective. So, if a soul aspect is originally stationed on the Second Plane and is accelerated up through the planes to the Seventh Plane, then that aspect will lack millions of lifetimes of experiences. The dramatic shift will require that all karma is balanced but also that the soul aspect gathers what it lacks; and what it lacks is experience. This experience has to be supplemented from somewhere; and this somewhere is the collective experience of the group. All of the frequencies that the soul aspect is missing can be downloaded from the collective awareness of the group, and by doing this prior to God-realisationship, then the soul aspect will build up its strength and baseline of frequencies in matter. For those souls that stay in matter once they have become God-realised, lived experience in matter is still extremely important to their future trajectory and development.

Once a soul becomes God-realised, the previous lived experiences are like a currency. They give that soul the ability to work with those original frequencies and to build them up through the new platform of the Seventh Plane. It is like that soul has built the muscle and expertise to work and further amplify those frequencies. However, if the frequencies were donated to that soul by the collective intent of the group, then those frequencies will remain present but cannot be amplified and worked in quite the same way. Nevertheless, these donated frequencies are extremely important because they give that soul the necessary flow of experiences that will give balance and stability to their working pattern. For example, if a soul has worked multiple frequencies of despair in previous lives, but has never experienced terror, then once it has become God-realised, the despair frequencies can be further worked and amplified, while the frequencies of terror cannot.

Similarly, once a soul has become God-realised, it can also absorb anything it lacks through the platform of collective experience that is the sum total of all the souls that are gridded into the collective. So if, for example, one million souls are gridded into this collective and have an average of four million lifetimes in matter each, then the collective and accumulated experience available would be four trillion lives. This gives a great deal of flexibility. At the same time, the God-realised soul could access all of the collective frequencies that are part of the collective experience within the Seventh Plane. Consequently, the need to become collective is paramount in the new accelerated pattern – both for souls that are accelerating up through the planes, and also for those souls that have ascended into the Seventh Plane.

Balancing Bliss and Despair

The new programme of God-realisationship requires, within those who have crossed into the Seventh Plane, a new type of understanding and balance in everyday physical life. At the point of God-realisationship, when the physical vehicle is normally dropped, adjustments have to be made to it to ensure that the soul can continue to inhabit it. There is a split moment when everything drops away and has to be replaced by something new. The one, true, spiritual death leads to a complete detachment of all cordings and karma within the physical, astral and mental realms. All past lives are condensed and released from the ties of karma. All subtle bodies are absorbed and so the soul that has become God-realised irradiates a pattern of light from the Seventh Plane. Consequently, whenever the soul now drops its consciousness back into the lower planes, it has to borrow either an astral or a mental body to do this. To remain in the physical state, the God-realised soul has to borrow karma and this can be done within the collective focus of group work.

The normal stage of experience within the early stages of God-realisation is bliss, since the soul enters the bliss of the First Divine Journey[1]. This has to be balanced within the framework of physical existence; all of the chakras are now clear, balanced and open, and in particular the aperture in the crown is completely open – where before it had a been only a pinprick of light, in the God-realised being, it is usually fully open – about several inches across. This has profound implications for that individual since it is now much easier to drop the body and entertain physical death. The human body was never designed to host such a high light vibration and any weaknesses within the physical structure will potentially become points of pressure.

The God-realised being is presented with an entirely new energetic dichotomy – entertaining the new pattern of bliss while being held in lower frequencies of light that hold no interest at all, on any level. The analogy is a bit like being dressed up for a wonderful ball in stunning clothing and feeling on top of the world, and then being asked to go down into the sewers where all you have to eat is a packet of old sandwiches. The sewers represent the energetic focus in shadowlands, and the sandwiches are the frequencies that have to be absorbed down here. The challenge for all people who become consciously God-realised is to remain in their physical bodies. The frequencies of higher light are so delicious and constantly call out to the soul to come back home into the light. An active point of will is required to remain in the physical body; and since energy always follows thought, if a thought about going home is emotionally entertained with real meaning and force, then that will actually happen – the person doing the invocation will drop their body and return home.

The main point of anchoring is, however, provided by the slower frequencies around; by the despair and suffering. Through living the moment in every day, the God-realised person can experience and live this despair as a counterpoint to the higher bliss. The despair acts as an earthing mechanism. From the vantage point of the Seventh Plane, the God-realised person becomes detached from everything around; all that previously would grip his or her attention, externally or internally becomes irrelevant, so that the emotions, physical pleasures and mental stimulations of everyday life become trivial and almost pointless. This state of detachment represents the true detachment from the everyday world; and the God-realised being is therefore a living whim of the Father. He or she is in physical incarnation yet is not of this world and not of the shadow planes. His or her vibration transcends and is beyond all that is present in the shadowlands. The past, present and future are of little interest and so to remain in the physical world with such detachment requires a focus and effort of will.

Physical and Emotional Changes

At the point of God-realisationship, the physical body undergoes a subtle, yet profound shift. All of the karmic lines of bonding are removed and the physical body has to host an entirely different vibration of light. Typically, a variety of physical symptoms can arise shortly after God-realisationship, including an initial tiredness. This relates to the physical vehicle having to process the new energies. The three atoms in the heart centre have now merged to become one, as all of the past masculine and feminine lives become balanced and return back into the one permanent atom. The one permanent atom pulses to a new light frequency and sometimes it can feel like there is a gap in the heart centre, almost like a vacuum there. This pause can also relate to the eighteen pulse beats per day, which represent the alignment and focus of higher energies. The heart centre, which hosts the one permanent atom, also becomes transformed in the God-realised being. The centre becomes much larger, and ideally should become several feet wide and build in size continuously. The third eye is also usually activated in a new way, although certain veils will remain in place to ensure that the nervous system does not become overloaded. The third eye will also host a more direct connection with the heart centre. All of the old cordings that were present within the different chakra centres and those around are also stripped away and cleared. Eventually, the aim is for a borehole of light that is many inches across to run from the crown centre to the base centre. This still requires some energetic work to achieve it and forms part of the ongoing energetic transformation of the God-realised being.

There is also a tendency for older physical ailments to re-emerge as part of the clearing process of the physical body. Old operations, old sports injuries, and other old illnesses will appear out of nowhere, rather like the ghost of that which has passed. This is part of the flushing out of all the old frequencies. At the same time, bizarre new ailments may also pop up and just as quickly disappear. This is all part of the pattern of collective karma that is being worked through. Eventually, however, over a period of months, and usually within eighteen months of becoming God-realised, the physical body should begin to change and stabilise. The glandular system will become more balanced and the nervous system should have become more adapted to hosting the new patterns of energy. Nevertheless, any deficiencies within the DNA and in the actual make up of the physical body will probably have been uncovered – consequently, if a person's genetics will give a predisposition to some sort of disease or syndrome, then if that person goes over their threshold of tolerance to high frequency light, then they will probably be brought back down through the limitations of their genetics.

Exposure to too much light means that the physical vehicle and the emotions all 'burn' – rather like becoming sun burnt, the physical body can be burnt by too much high frequency light. A balance, therefore, between absorbing high frequency light and remaining earthed and not overstressing the body has to be found and maintained. Just as the body can burn, and in particular the nervous system, so can the emotional system. Too much light will also affect a person's emotional balance.

During the burning down process, the personality also becomes smelted down. All personality patterns will be worked through the collective karmic pattern, and if a God-realised soul progresses up through the First and Second Divine Journeys, then he or she will begin to move out of the flow of bliss and begin to work with other frequencies. With time, the initial feelings of total detachment may fade away, and be replaced by a heightened level of emotional sensitization. Sounds, sunlight and noise can all become more difficult to endure, as the senses of the physical vehicle become more acute. Different emotional streams of energy will run through the body, and such emotions have to be lived in the moment, while at the same time giving them absolutely no importance whatsoever. The personality will be tested time and time again by the presence of slow frequency energies – some people may react positively to their energetic systems, while others may take an instant dislike to them, recognising subconsciously, that their energetic systems represent, on one level, complete change. The personality has to endure the flow of all these energies through the lived conscious awareness of shadowlands life. The sensitisation of their energetic systems make these experiences more intense, and yet each emotional experience has to be lived through a point of giving it no importance or ownership juxtaposed against allowing the flow of emotional energy to pass through. This in itself can be a challenge as the personality can endure the extremes of anger, loss, sorrow, or whatever other emotional pattern is passing through.

All that the God-realised being has is memories and so the emotional flow of energies may anchor itself to the past memories, thereby further amplifying the experiences. At the same time, the new sensitisation may bring through a whole range of new emotions that have never been experienced before. All of these will form part of the lived experience. These emotions will intensify if any feelings of ownership are placed on them, in the sense that they are taken "to be mine". And very quickly the person will begin drowning in them. Maintaining a position of balance as these different emotional streams flow through is extremely important.

Learning to navigate the different emotional streams is all part of the personality burning down; any negative thought that is entertained will become amplified out of all proportion to the original thought or feeling. Consequently, absolute responsibility has to be taken over every thought, emotion and feeling on a continual basis. Once this discipline has been found and is built up, then the personality, within its point of limitation will have found a point of balance. At the same time, focusing on the collective is extremely important. Souls that have become God-realised after fewer lives in matter may find it harder to maintain a point of balance, since they lack experience in matter. Embracing the collective flow will help to counteract this perceived limitation. This again goes back to the points made at the start of this chapter about building balance and experience through collective focus and intent.

For those beings that have become consciously God-realised, in the sense that they recognise or know that it has happened to them, a further challenge often presents itself: to work through the limitations of the mind. The mind is a tool and as such, acts as a point of limitation. Once a soul becomes God-realised, then it has direct experience of the everything and the nothing: both states are beyond what the mind can comprehend or hold onto. The state of everything and nothing is so far beyond the limitation of the mind, that the mind will always struggle to accept its reality. The mind, as a tool for processing our experiences and as a means to make sense of the world we live in, will always operate from a point of limitation. Yet, the everything and the nothing are beyond limitation and so the mind will never accept it as a reality. What this means is that God-realised souls will experience feelings of doubt and disbelief about their status. The reflected pattern of what they are will not necessarily feel very different from before they were God-realised, and this in turn will feed the mind and give rise to doubts about their energetic status. The mind will seek to bring conscious experience back into the normal, secure realms of the external three-dimensional reality that was part of the past.

However, in the moments of stillness that then become the silence, it becomes possible to transcend the limitations of the mind and move beyond the artificial limitation that it seeks to impose on the conscious awareness of the God-realised being.

The Open Door to Everything and Nothing

The God-realised being has access to the everything and the nothing. In one moment it becomes possible to experience everything, to have access to all different types of knowledge, information and different levels of higher guidance, and then in the next moment, to be in a state of nothing, where absolutely nothing exists. This state of the everything and the nothing is the experience of the "I am God" state. When residing in the nothing state, the God-realised soul experiences just that, the true silence of the divinity within the nothing. In the everything, the God-realised soul can bring focus and intent to bear, to access that part of everything that is calling. Within the everything, the flow of light and information is always present. The God-realised soul will also feel the flow of black and white light and will experience being ridden by different presences and awareness within that moment.

One of the side effects, if you like, that impacts those who have become God-realised is a loss of memory. Merging into the nothing means that everything drops away, and through living in the conscious moment, then memory also drops away. Being in the everything and the nothing means that each moment is always lived in the present and so what has become the past, ceases to exist and to be of no real value. The physical body may retain memories of its dominant habits and desires, but the mind and the conscious recognition of where we are and where we have come from can drop away, leaving the residue of emptiness, where previously our memories had held the pattern of everything that was in place.

Yet within these different states, there are deeper and deeper levels that can be accessed, as expressed through the different Divine

Journeys that can be touched in the Seventh Plane. The frequencies of bliss that a God-realised person in the First Divine Journey will irradiate differ from those of the Second Divine Journey and so on. Since all of the centres in a God-realised person are open and clear, the internal space is much larger than in an individual that is still in the lower planes. Each of the chakra centres has to be balanced and worked together in harmony so that a flow of energy can be maintained between the base chakra and the crown chakra. Yet to remain in physical existence, the God-realised individual has to connect with the physical and has to resonate with the other plane levels. In so doing, through borrowing different subtle bodies, and in transmuting and transmitting a whole host of different energies, the God-realised soul becomes an open door in the truest sense of the description.

An open door means that the individual in physical matter has access to everything and nothing, can host energies from the Seventh Plane within the limitations of the physical vehicle and can also radiate different patterns of energy across all of the shadow planes. The open door embodies the everything and the nothing; it retains the flexibility to allow much larger energetic presences to flow through the energetic system, and also has the flexibility to ride within the overall patterns of energy, from the Zero Plane to the Seventh Plane. An open door will allow the energy to flow, without hindrance from the individual's mind, personality structure or ego, to the designated point. This could be anywhere, from a particular person that is encountered in the street, to different levels of life within the planet; or to the stars and other planets in the Wheel of Life. The God-realised being that is the open door in the moment allows the flow of energy to pass through him or her freely without judgement, or active interference.

In addition, as the God-realised being begins to work through the different Divine Journeys, then there is the scope for bringing through much more powerful patterns of energy. Sometimes the God-realised person will be overshadowed by a Perfect Master, either living, or from the past or the future; sometimes the Avatar Himself will overshadow that individual, or at other times, different Divine presences will come through, such as the Cosmic Christ.

At the same time, the open door will work with the slower frequencies, including clearing and absorbing slow frequencies from the astral levels. The capacity of an individual who is an open door is much greater than a person anchored to one of the shadow planes. So souls that have become trapped in the lower planes after death will be pushed through such beings and, like pulses of energy, many souls that have become trapped within the old addictions and emotions can be moved through more effectively into the higher flow of light, to engage once again in the pattern of reincarnation. By connecting with different people, and places, the open door will absorb and transmute energy as either a conscious or unconscious pattern of work.

Consequently, the soul that is a true open door also has direct access to the oversoul, and those people fortunate enough to come into contact with such beings can register, within their awareness, a different energetic pulse beat of divinity. The open door represents direct access to the divine, and the doorway through the physical vehicle can open in both directions; either to allow the flow of light out from the inner essence, or for the flow of energy to be absorbed and flow in from the physical into the higher levels within. The needs of the moment will dictate the pattern of energy that is required.

The open door will also host multiple levels of inner guidance, each with their own speciality mix and skills. In particular, Seventh Plane levels of guidance will work specifically through the energetic systems of God-realised beings. Such beings will be able to host, with practice, the different patterns of Devic, Angelic and Eldering light that are now opening up in the planet. Yet each God-realised being will have a specific role, or series of roles, within the context of being an open door. Those that are part of the Fifty-Six will have one or more of the five Perfect Masters working through their systems; they are detached from humanity and work as open doors that are total generators of spiritual energy. Those that are part of the different groups of one hundred and forty four will have their specific Perfect Master pulsing through them; and those souls who have become God-realised consciously, but outside of the pattern of the above, will work according to patterns of energy that will be focused first through the

Five Perfect Masters, then the Fifty-Six and then the Spiritual Hierarchy according to the energetic platform that has been established. Finally, the souls that are God-realised, yet are unconscious of their status, will work according to the different levels of intuitive guidance within, which will ultimately flow from the Fifty-Six.

Building Common Sense

Those souls that become God-realised and are part of the Fifty-Six, will either live this consciously or sub-consciously. There is usually a split within this, and up to now, the Fifty-Six have been largely unconscious of their status. The exceptions are the five Perfect Masters and a specific number of the spiritual generators. However, this is all changing during the current Avataric Cycle. The aim is for all of the Fifty-Six to become consciously aware of who and what they are, and to be conscious of their status of God-realisationship. The extended programme of God-realisationship, as the one-off experiment of the Father, also embraces those who are conscious of their status, and those who are not. Generally speaking, the vast majority of those who are God-realised are not consciously aware of it.

The pattern of experience within the dichotomy of either being conscious or unconscious leads to some marked differences. If a soul becomes God-realised, and is not aware of it, then that individual will continue with their lives as if nothing has changed. There may be subtle differences, like some of the old habits and desires will drop away, and will become replaced by a different focus of interest. Some relationships will come to a natural end, while others will continue. Such individuals will be living out their divinity while still acting within the three-dimensional world. Their intuitive powers may increase and their perception of a different reality that intermingles and builds on their normal life may also increase. They may experience moments of bliss or despair, but will view this within the context of their old life. Everything will appear the same.

In sharp contrast, the individual that becomes God-realised and is made aware of this has a rather different programme of experience.

To be and become consciously God-realised requires entering a whole new pattern of experience, where all existing preconceptions about God-realisationship have to be stripped away. The mind, personality and ego all have to adjust to this new status, and yet each individual will not have the experience or the understanding to absorb the enormity and impact of what has happened. Sometimes the information will lead to denial and disbelief, and the subsequent search for proof. Yet this will not help, because the higher principles of light and love operate according to the principles of trust and faith. Others will go through a pattern of difficulty and despair, as they struggle to come to terms with the momentous change. It is like everything from the past has been stripped away, and above all, the old human part has now gone. Such individuals are no longer human, in the normal sense of the term, and so there is often a grieving process at this loss of the human inside. Everything from the past is now gone, and nothing is really of interest. The most effective way to counter this is to gain a deeper understanding within the heart, of what being God-realised actually is. Neither the emotions nor the intellect will supply the appropriate answer, and it is only through the heart, that a true connection can be found. The heart will open the door to experiencing the everything and the nothing.

There is also an ethical obligation to give those that are consciously God-realised as much knowledge and information as possible. This will assist in the transformation process. If we look at the pattern of energy that flows from information, through knowledge, to wisdom and ultimately common sense, then common sense is the ideal set of frequencies for the God-realised soul to work with. This is often difficult to absorb at first, and so different mixes of the three other patterns will usually be entertained. On one level, though, information is useless, while knowledge can help but may be distorted by bias, while wisdom along the old guidelines is not relevant, and so a new wisdom of the heart has to be found. Ideally, then, the frequency of common sense, which is usually earned through the pattern of 8,400,000 lives, is an inherent knowing about that which is the appropriate course of action or way to think or be.

Common sense is an inherent knowing of what needs to be done through the collective framework of balance and higher recognition of that which is more. For the most part, though, those souls that have become God-realised under the current pattern of change, have not had sufficient experience to absorb common sense, and so will have to access it through the collective experience of the group. Common sense embodies the right balance of how to live in a God-realised state of existence; it will provide a living, dynamic, knowing reality of what needs to be done and when, to ensure that the individual has the maximum point of balance and advantage within the constant flux of energies. For example, common sense will dictate what is the right type of diet, what is a good balance between work, rest and play, and how to ride the different waves of energy that will flow through the energetic systems of those individuals. In short, direct access to common sense will bypass all the other frequencies.

Passive and Dynamic

Within the pattern of existence in the god-realised state, the soul will work according to different energetic patterns. The first, and most fundamental state of being is the passive state. This begins within the point of nothing and then flows into the polarity of everything according to the dictates of energetic flow that have been invoked and brought through ultimately by the five Perfect Masters and the Fifty-Six. To be in the passive state, means to be in one's silence and stillness, and to embrace the essence of the nothing. There is no directed focus using the thought or emotion. In this state, it then becomes possible for higher energies to flow through; there is no attachment by the individual, and the flow of energy is experienced as a pulse of energy in the different chakra centres. Sometimes this flow of energy will be exciting and uplifting; at other times, it may feel slow and heavy, and will vary according to the dictates of higher purpose. Whichever it is, the key is to allow it to flow through by first acknowledging it, then living it, and yet not owning it. As this takes place, the flow of energy may become more intense and it may then shift. Within the passive state, different impressions may unfold either in the heart, third eye, or in the other chakra centres, and greater understanding of the energetic flow can be gained through recognising which chakra centres are active, and whether the flow of light is light or dark. However, throughout this process, the focus is passive and like flowing with the ocean and the waves. The awareness rides the wave of energy and at all times flows with it, rather than directs it. Any focus on directing or changing the energy is like an active point of interference.

The passive state therefore represents the fundamental and primary state of being within; it is the nothing that flows into the everything, and then back into the nothing like a pulse beat of energy. The eighteen pulses a day will ride the passive awareness and experience of all those who are God-realised. Tuning into those pulse beats will heighten the awareness and consciousness of what is taking place; yet it does not interfere with the process. So the flow of energy moves from unconscious passivity into conscious passivity, and the more conscious the God-realised person becomes of the flow of energy, then the more awake he or she is, and the more able to work the energetic focus that is demanded at any one time.

From time to time, as individuals become more aware and more focused in the passive state, then the flow of energy can, ultimately, build into the dynamic. However, the dynamic flow is different and at its source, requires a point of active intent to establish an energetic flow that is then directed through the conscious living will into a particular outcome. In the dynamic, the wave of energy is not just experienced; the dynamic being becomes the wave and directs the flow of energy in a conscious and living manifestation of will. Normally only the five Perfect Masters are truly dynamic since they create, direct and control the flow of energy as ordained by the eternal Will of the Father. Yet, those God-realised souls that are seeking more, and wishing to evolve into dynamic open doors, may slowly begin to work with dynamic energy and its flow through and at the command of their own will. This, of course, requires a perfect alignment with the will and desires of the Father and the five Perfect Masters, although free will may come in to play from time to time. The remaining Fifty-One spiritual generators are primarily passive, although can shift a gear to become passive-dynamic. Those other souls that have become God-realised, either under the direct umbrella of a Perfect Master, or as part of the broader programme, may experience glimpses of the dynamic mode, depending on how awake and conscious they are of the dynamic and constantly changing moment.

Consequently, it is possible to talk of being either passive-passive which means being passive one hundred percent of the time; or passive-dynamic, which means that the soul is often passive, but will shift into dynamic when being overshadowed by the presence of a Perfect Master, while dynamic-dynamic means to be fully dynamic at all times. It is this latter state of being that is usually only experienced by the Perfect Masters and, of course, the Avatar. To be dynamic-dynamic means to be fully conscious and awake to the essence of everything and nothing within the constantly changing eternal moments that flow in and out of time, and to be able to initiate, direct, regulate and control the flow of energy on all levels, through the dance between the nothing and the everything.

So the flow of energy starts within the nothing, and then flows out into the everything, like a pulse, and then back into the nothing. The majority of God-realised souls will then experience this flux of energy as their systems being ridden by higher streams of light and intelligences, and through the laws of faith and trust, can then hold, within the eternal moment of the ever-present now, the pulse of energy as it embodies the passive. To move from the passive to the dynamic means that the flow from nothing into everything becomes dynamic and directed through the living will and intent; the energetic system is no longer being ridden, but is the actual prime mover or creator of that which flows out from the point of divinity. To be truly dynamic means to initiate, generate and direct the energies.

Time and Timelessness

The God-realised being has also to work in and out of time. Since their essence is anchored in the Seventh Plane, and is merged in the oversoul, their focus and experience of time is totally different from an individual that has not been God-realised. Life in the physical planes is bounded by time, and so the God-realised soul experiences life in and out of time. When their awareness is focused in the physical, then they may be working in time; yet, at another level, another part of themselves may be focused out of time. This all relates to the amount that our awareness can be focused externally or internally. For example, in the shadow planes, those souls that we call masts are focused almost one hundred percent inside; a young soul will be focused almost exclusively one hundred percent externally. The God-realised being is usually focused ninety-eight percent inside and only two percent outside, and yet may flux, depending upon the flow of energy through them, into one hundred percent internally, for the briefest of moments, or out into fifty percent or more externally. When the focus is almost exclusively inwards, then the external holds little of interest and the challenge is then to remain rooted in the external while holding the deeper dialogue internally.

This presents a number of different challenges. The first is that the God-realised soul has to balance their awareness between the external and internal. The call of the inner light may far outweigh any interest in the outer world, yet they have to maintain a connection with the outer through their focus of will and intent. And this requires an emotional desire to remain connected to the external world, which is an integral part of the work focus down here in physical matter. The second difficulty is that the true focus of their work is always initiated out of time. To access the higher frequencies from the Seventh Plane, these beings have to move out of time, in order to receive the downloading of that which is demanded. Outside of time, everything is clear and yet, moving out of timelessness back into time, requires a capacity to recall what has happened out of time, something that is not easy. In coming down from the higher focus of the Seventh Plane, because grosser and grosser layers are encountered, then the high frequency energy tends to dissipate and this leads to complete memory loss of what was entertained and experienced out of time. In other words, there is a real difficulty in bringing this flow of energy back into time while retaining an understanding of what happened out of time.

To overcome this active point of limitation requires focus and trust; it is also something that can be developed through dreams where the attention of the mind is distracted and where the innate resistance of the physical to absorb such higher frequencies is, to some extent, bypassed. The spontaneous birthing of ritual, through rhyme and the poetic word, are ways in which the flow of higher energy can also be accessed and pulled back into matter. This again requires practice and focus, but once achieved, can bring through a flow of high frequency energy that can give birth to an entirely new flow of light.

Working out of time also means that the past, present and future timelines can be accessed and brought together. The only limitation to this is the mind and the resistance of the physical to such frequencies. Yet, through working with future timelines, it becomes possible to bring into the present that which is to be birthed in the future, such as a future, more evolved aspect of ourselves. If we go forward and then connect with our future aspect, then we can access all that we currently need to evolve into that which is in our future. We can become more and can retain a higher degree of light and order that will ensure we become that which we have invoked out of time.

In short, the pattern of energy that is now being birthed in certain people through the God-realisationship programme is helping to seed an entirely new hologram of light into the planet. By cultivating open hearts and empty minds we can begin to build up a new focus of unity and love within the collective harmony of that which we call life. This in turn will quicken and lock in our transformation from the old Fifth Root Race timeline into the new, super light, timeline of the Sixth Root Race.

CHAPTER 19

The New Energetic Hologram

Holograms

In modern physics a hologram is defined as a three-dimensional image formed by the interference of light beams from a laser or other coherent source of light. Holograms have a number of unique properties: they are always three dimensional, and every part of a hologram contains all the information possessed by the whole. So, if a hologram of a rose is cut in half and then illuminated by a laser, each half will still be found to contain the entire image of the rose. Further subdivisions of the rose will always yield the same result: a smaller yet intact version of the original. The complete whole is therefore found in every part. This view of reality is now being explored in modern physics where the possibility of the whole Universe being a hologram explains the experimental evidence that subatomic particles, such as electrons, are able to instantaneously communicate with each other, irrespective of the distance separating them. It does not matter whether they are five feet or 100 billion miles apart. Each particle knows what the other is doing and is therefore connected to the whole. While this observation appears to violate Einstein's long-held belief that no particles or energy can travel faster than the speed of light, the potential that we live in a rather different Universe, as compared to the old reductionist view raises intriguing possibilities for modern science. Under this old view everything has to be broken down into its component parts and contrasts markedly with the new scientific theorizing that concepts such as time and space may not be so fundamental as we think, and how absolutely everything is interconnected – from the neurotransmitters in our brains, to the scales on a fish, and to the stellar furnaces in space.

The new Sixth Root Race timeline is also based on a hologram, one that is not created by normal physical light, but is generated from higher aspects of light that flow down from the Seventh Plane. Nevertheless, having a parallel physical description can be helpful and the principles of how holograms behave in the physical realms also have similarities in the higher planes. The new hologram of light has a limitless capacity to retain information and knowledge; it is multi-dimensional, flowing in and out of time; and every part of it contains the essence of every other part so that access to one portion of it will allow access to all of it. The template for everything within it is contained within the smallest portion of light that is part of it.

The new hologram represents the essence of the Father, and embodies the full diversity of His Essence within an unconditional, limitless, eternal and fathomless expression of love. The new hologram is a timeless aspect, or series of aspects of the Father that are being captured by the Son in the dawning of the new Avataric Day. So, the old hologram of the Fifth Root Race, which held a particularly slow flow of light, is being replaced by a much more dynamic and potent light flow that is being birthed out of the Seventh Plane. But it is not like there is just one hologram; there are multiple, interconnecting holograms, each one being expressed as a different aspect of the Father, and each one birthed out of a different level depending on which Divine Journey, or cluster of Divine Journeys it embodies. This new light then flows down into the mental planes where it forms a new hologram of light that can then be accessed by humanity and other life forms. So, for example, one hologram could be formed out of the Fourth Divine Journey and would then irradiate a representation of it down into the shadow planes. The hologram would present a copy of what the Fourth Divine Journey is within the mental streams of light, and so would be diluted, yet would provide a living version of reality within the illusion of the shadow planes. The same could also be true of the Third Divine Journey – a holographic representation of what grace is could be captured and formed in the mental planes, providing a diluted hologram of what actually is the embodiment of the Third Divine Journey. So the hologram of the Third Divine Journey would host everything that ever was, is and would be in this Journey, and would then present this pattern of information and light in the lower planes.

The new hologram of the Sixth Root Race is a bit like this, although it will embody multiple, living holograms within its essence that could be said to capture a series of different Divine Journeys within it. So, if we attempted to bring through a hologram that captured the essence of the refinement of the first Twelve Divine Journeys, then those realities would be captured and would then unfold along the new timeline, and give increasingly refined versions of what the Father is.

Another way of looking at the new hologram is to say that it is a new, fundamental spark that has been ignited from the Father, and which is then creating, within the flow of the multiple sparkings that are birthed out of it, a series of multiple holograms capturing the higher aspects of the Seventh Plane, which are then brought together under a new unified hologram that will, ultimately, push down into the lower part of the Seventh Plane and into the mental planes below. This new hologram embodies the Essence of the Father and also is the manifestation of the new Son. This new hologram, as it becomes manifested, will present an entirely new version of reality and understanding, and a completely new stream of love that will, eventually, embody the essence of the Cosmic Christ.

The challenge for all light workers is to find ways to access this new hologram so that all of the information, tools, physical and subtle modifications necessary for change, along with the direct manifestation of higher light, and all that it embodies, can be efficiently captured and downloaded into their essence. Access to one part of the hologram will give automatic access to everything else contained within the hologram. The hologram will be a lived experience, or series of experiences, of what it is to be more within the new frequencies of higher light. Yet, because these higher frequencies of light are from the

Seventh Plane, we will have to experience them within the limitation and the imperfection of our physical vehicles as we go about our daily business in the shadow planes.

As this new hologram is birthed in the Seventh Plane, and then brought down into the mental planes, all of us will be able to access it and then undergo a series of profound changes as we absorb the living hologram into ourselves. All we have to do is to wake up to the possibility of this new hologram, and then invoke its presence and light into us.

The New Chakra System

The new chakra system that is being developed is really a mechanism that can hold the new Primary Spark, the new essence of the Father as part of the dawn of the new Son. The chakra system has to retain the vision that the spark has, the need that the spark has to remember and, of course, the capacity to return. So our chakra systems have been upgraded to hold twelve principle chakras and each chakra will then host the new hologram of light according to what is required. The chakras will each be like new primary sparks, pulsing in attunement to the one Primary Spark. These sparks will then spark out and touch all those around, invoking a pattern of change, and banishing the old dark. So, with the addition of two new chakra centres adjacent to the third eye and a second heart chakra, then the new timeline will introduce a series of new senses and awarenesses that have never been experienced before. The challenge for us all will be to first recognise that what we experience is new, and then to assimilate the flow of information in a way that makes sense to us. The simple analogy between black and white vision and colour vision is helpful here. In the old timeline, everything was black and white, while in the new timeline everything is in colour. Yet, as we begin to see everything in colour, we do not yet have a language to describe it. How would we describe green if we had never come across it before? How would we describe indigo or pale yellow? The new sensations will give us an entirely new field of experience, sensation and emotion.

The new emotions will challenge us on every level. The intensity of the new experience that is brought through, in say, the transition from black and white vision to colour vision, will give us an entirely new level of emotional experience. We will experience entirely new emotions while the backwash of old emotions that flow through us will take on a new potency and virulence. The emotions will span the full range of frequencies, including pride, shame and suffering; we will work between the polar opposites of bliss and despair, anger and calm, hatred and pure love, cruelty and compassion, and so on. The old emotions that will wash through us will take on a new potency as we ride the living moment of the experience. Another way of looking at it is to say that rather than looking at something from the outside, such as a rollercoaster in the fairground, we are offered the opportunity to go on the ride, and experience first hand what it feels like. The contrast between the two stances could not be more different.

The new chakras will be formed as vortices of light, through the balance of new order and new chaos, and the new black and white light. The different expressions of multiple, dimensional life will work through the new chakra system and will give each of us a new bandwidth of understanding and a new capacity to feel and connect with different energetic streams that previously had been beyond our sensory range. Those individuals who will become the new open doors, playing host to the true diversity of life within their conscious and unconscious awareness, will have to work their chakra systems with a new level of focus and understanding. Each one of us radiates an energetic pulse from each of our chakras, from the base to the crown. If we focus on just our base centre, then we will experience our reality from that centre. Similarly, if we do the same from the sexual/creative centre, then we will explore a different reality. As the new levels of light enter our systems, we will be challenged to retain these new patterns and to absorb the essence of the living hologram into each of the twelve chakras. The living hologram that is absorbed into the base chakra will be different to that which is absorbed by the sexual, heart or third eye. The new hologram will first push us up into higher streams of light, so that the focus will initially be in the higher centres, but as we then earth this new light, we will have to bring it all of the way down into our lower centres, so that there is an expanded space within each chakra that can house the new frequencies. In coming down to the lower centres, we will also have to push out sideways as part of the earthing mechanism.

As this new hologram comes in, there will be other changes. For those people that become open doors to the new energies, the one permanent atom that is housed in our heart centre will be drawn up into the third eye for a period of time; the heart chakra will also be energetically pushed up into the third eye, so that everything will be felt and seen in an entirely different way. Those individuals that are still working through their pattern of involution in the shadow planes will receive a diluted version of this according to what their systems can absorb and retain. So they will experience in a similar way the living hologram of feeling and seeing everything as one. This may be a temporary manifestation as the individual experiences a new level of seeing reality.

This shift will reflect the pattern of light manifested through the lower Divine Journeys as the different pulses of higher light are absorbed. With the restructuring of black and white light, the one permanent atom within us will also be remodelled and for a split point in time, will be taken out of our physical vehicles, and then replaced according to the new pattern of light that is required by the new hologram. This will be like crossing an abyss, living through another spiritual death, as all that was ever stored in the one permanent atom, is stripped away and replaced by a new pattern of soul light that will be the essence of the new spark. This pattern will start in only a few people at first, before spreading out.

The presence of the heart in the third eye will open up a new way of experiencing and seeing. The love of the heart will wrap around all that we see, so that we can experience love from within a different space inside of us. This will not be intellectual or emotional love, but a purer love that is felt within everything that we see. At the same time, we will experience emptiness in the old heart centre, where there will only be space and nothing else. Physically, this may manifest as a physical gap, almost like the physical heart missing a beat.

But this change will only represent the beginning, because the other, existing chakra centres will undergo profound changes. The old solar plexus will be expanded to host new levels of information and experience, while at the same time supported by a new platform of love. Our emotions will be suffused with a different level of love.

In the sexual centre, older frequencies of light are being harvested, dating back to the Lemurian Root Race, when the creative play reached a level of intuitive harmony that has not been achieved since. The sexual centre will be infused with the higher frequencies of light that were created in Lemurian times, and will allow an entirely new creative approach to be born in the new timeline. This is just beginning to manifest.

The New Light Body

For those souls that are progressing through involution, the ability to function on the astral and mental levels is facilitated by the presence of an astral or a mental body. These bodies are formed of particles of astral or mental light respectively, and resonate at different vibrations. The astral body vibrates at a slower frequency than the mental body. The structure of these different bodies has meant that they could be used as vehicles of consciousness and awareness within the particular plane levels that they were designed for. So practices such as astral travelling required an astral body, and more recently as the pattern of mental light has built, then opportunities for using the mental body as a vehicle of awareness has also presented itself. Yet each of these different bodies is limited and is unable to pass through the ring-pass-not. They cannot access the different streams of light that exist beyond this blue band of light.

The new hologram of light that is being birthed in the Sixth Root Race will bring though an entirely new type of body, a new light body that will allow an entirely new level of conscious awareness and creative flow of energy. This new light body is neither a mental nor an astral body and is formed from the new light particles that are brought through from the Seventh Plane. The new light body is the living embodiment of the new hologram and is, itself, a part of the new hologram.

The light body functions as a hologram, and contains within it the light and informational flow of everything within the Sixth Root Race. The frequency of this light body is much higher than anything that has ever presented itself before, and the trick will be to find ways of consciously accessing it and then begin to use it in a creative way that allows us to live the essence of the moment within the creative flux of everything that is. For example, the new light body will give us access to that which lies beyond the ring-pass-not, so that all of our old and future memories will become available to us. The light body will also give us a different experience of merging, so that as one light body merges with another light body, then a new stream of light can be activated within the new, living hologram. We can begin to experience someone else's reality as our own, as we feel the pulse of everything flow between our light bodies.

Our new light bodies will also give us a different level of conscious awareness of everything that we are and that we will become. It will give us a much greater degree of flexibility as we explore new ways to access the higher energy flows of the Seventh Plane, and to merge with new levels of divine guidance. The new light body will be like a new doorway to another series of dimensions within our own awareness, and as we move beyond the limitations of the ring-pass-not, we will begin to communicate with a broader array of life forms. Some of these life forms will be from the stars and beyond.

In connecting and beginning to feel the presence of the new light body, it is necessary for us to connect with the new hologram of light that contains within it the essence of the new stream of light. This stream contains within it the full and complete imprint of the new light body, so as the new timeline unfolds, and more and more people connect with it, then the higher light particles that create the new light body, will become accessible and will flow in. The new light body will facilitate, in time, a whole new level of conscious experience, both within our waking life, and also through our dreams. We will be able to consciously live in our dreams and to learn how to direct the flow of energy and the different outcomes.

The new light body will allow us to merge with the ring-pass-not in an entirely different way. The pattern will involve a fusing between the light body and ring-pass-not so that gaps or small holes appear in the living fabric of the ring-pass-not, and which will then allow new levels of light to flow and to permeate into the light body. Once the flow of energy has been completed, the light body can then disengage from the ring-pass-not.

The new light body will give us all access to entirely new streams of higher light, and as the multiple holograms of the new root race are birthed, then our light body will continue to evolve and grow, each time reflecting a different pattern of the living hologram that is being played through at that particular time. It will also give us access to different streams of time, so that we can work backwards and forwards down different timelines.

The essence of the new light body will be brilliant; it will be the living hologram of the essence of the Father and the embodiment of the Primary Spark and will bring through a new cycle of experience and understanding, as the flow of higher light will be captured and absorbed through its structure and form. It will birth in each of us a new type of consciousness that will be an integral part of the new hologram.

The Ring-Pass-Not

The ring-pass-not has maintained a protective envelope around the planet and has acted as a filter for different frequencies and timelines. All incarnating souls have to pass through it, and always undergo a stripping away of past life memories. While resting out of physical matter or carrying out other duties on the inner planes, each soul will leave their one permanent atom in the ring-pass-not. This permanent atom acts like a CD disc and contains all of the data of everything that has been experienced by that soul while in physical matter. The whole of the ring-pass-not is composed of all of these existing permanent atoms and is therefore connected to all of the souls that are currently working through their own reincarnatory cycle in the planet. The colour of this collective vibration is blue and so the ring-pass-not is always seen as a band of blue light.

The ring-pass-not represents a point of limitation where patterns and frequencies can be filtered out, and other points of limitation contained beneath the ring-pass-not can be explored, to allow the effective flow of natural and karmic law to unfold. The frequency of time is held beneath the ring-pass-not and for a considerable period of time, arrays of different life forms have been prevented from accessing the planet. This in part goes back to an old pattern of segregation that was necessary to allow the karmic flow to unfold, and also to allow humanity a sufficient amount of time to evolve without the interference from other life forms that would seek to impose their own particular stamp or essence on the creative play on Earth. This point of segregation is now coming to an end.

Within the last couple of years, all restraint has been removed from humanity in a number of ways, and part of this has included renewed access to the planet from those outside of the ring-pass-not. At the same time, there will be a fundamental restructuring of the living essence of the ring-pass-not. At present, the flow of restructuring the permanent atoms within each individual physical unit is taking place in only a few, but as this spreads out to more people, then there will be a shift in the vibration of the ring-pass-not. The electronic essence of light that was housed in the old permanent atom will be completely overhauled and the new permanent atom will be rewired according to the new pattern of chaos and order. The new hologram of light will be placed within the one permanent atom, and with time, this will mean that the ring-pas-not will begin to vibrate in a new and more virulent way. Natural Law, as it changes, will be reflected in the pattern of energy in the ring-pass-not, and the new permanent atoms will pulse a different sequence of light into the other, old permanent atoms. A tidal wave of change will flow through the ring-pass-not.

With the new swirl of permanent atoms beginning to flow in the ring-pass-not, then new rules and regulations according to the demands of the new chaos and order will come in. The old restrictions will be lifted and different levels of light will then be hosted in it. Old memories will be reinstated, so that Meher Baba's prediction that all saints and sinners will remember who they were will come to pass.

With time humanity may also be given the opportunity to work with another ring-pass-not, the galactic ring-pass-not, which contains everything to do with the galaxy and the souls contained within it. Just as the planet retains a ring-pass-not, so does the Wheel of Life, reflecting the pathway of different energy streams that can flow in and out of it from the different plane levels.

Working In and Out of Time

All of these changes that are being brought through on the new timeline, will also open up a new level of growth and opportunity for all life. If time is an illusion, then it follows that if we go outside of time, then we can access the future and connect with the different probabilities that have yet to be manifested in physical time. So, if we push down the new timeline, there will be a variety of probable outcomes or probable futures. Out of these different probabilities, there will be some that may be more preferable than others. It is similar to looking down our own personal timeline, and seeing different, probable futures. In each probable future, we embody a different stream of light and consciousness. Some may be slower, while others will be much more refined and vibrating on a higher level. If we wish to accelerate our growth, and find a way to vibrate on a higher level, then we can focus on that timeline which will give us that probable outcome. For example, if we have nine possible time lines, with each one vibrating on a level from one to nine, where one represents the slowest and nine the fastest, and under our current timeline we are pushing along on level five, then we may choose to accelerate our development and shift our focus, to say, level eight. This will automatically mean that we are pushing into the future, to find a different probable reality of what we can mutate into, and to bring it back into our present, so that we can become more.

The same type of pattern of becoming more, of seeding a more refined and potent hologram into the new timeline is possible through working outside of time. So, if we look down the different timelines of the future root race, there are a series of probable outcomes. If, in one of these timelines we see the presence of the Cosmic Christ coming in, and on another competing timeline, we see the Cosmic Christ more in the distance, then we may wish to focus on the timeline that brings the Cosmic Christ through much more quickly. The same principle applies if we wish to speed up change and decide to focus on the Seventh Root Race or even the Eighth Root Race. The probable timelines for these root races are not so well formed, but we can still focus on one or more timelines, pulse down them, and focus on invoking and bringing through that light and energy from the future into our present. By focusing in this way, we can begin to speed up change, and we can also invoke more within each root race, and within the different holograms that are being birthed.

Each timeline that we look down will also have a probable percentage outcome. So, the most likely timeline to manifest may have thirty percent likelihood, while other timelines may have only a five to ten percent likelihood of outcome. Yet, if we focus on these less probable outcomes, then we can manifest change according to free will and from the perspective of what is the most desired outcome. This energetic flow can be enhanced, however, if we choose to place our awareness at a point in the future. For example, if we place our awareness at a point in time in the future where the Cosmic Christ will become manifested in physical form on the planet, to the time when He appears as the living Avatar, then we will focus on making this outcome a reality. The timing for this could be at the end of the Sixth Root Race, or at some point during the Seventh Root Race. If we selected the most probable, current timeframe, which is the Seventh Root Race, then if we placed our awareness into that future point, and felt into what physical form and the essence of light on the planet was like at that time, then we could bring back into the present, the flow of light that will be present. In doing this, we can seed and make the probable timeline for the appearance of the Cosmic Christ more substantial, and can also engineer the necessary karmic and physical changes that will be required to bring this through into our conscious awareness in the now.

Working outside of time, and bringing back the flow of the future, can help us to become more in the now. The main hurdle to achieving this is the limitation of our mind; our mind is always linked into the past, and does not entertain the future. But what if we could go forward in time, recover the energetic excellence of the future and bring it back into the present and merge it into our awareness and physical timeline. We would be invoking and bringing through a new pattern of order, and would be enhancing the chances that we will evolve into that which our destiny has entertained from the start.

The pattern of collective unity that we are seeking to build is working to a future timeline that is, initially, about twelve hundred years into the future. By pushing forwards to this point, and then bringing the living essence of what that is into the present, we then pulse a new series of frequencies that are part of the new timeline. This focal point of twelve hundred years into the future is a stepping-stone to that which is more.

Meeting our Light Twins

If we look backwards and forwards down our timelines, then we will meet different aspects of ourselves in separate realities. In the past, we will have worked through the pattern of experience that is known as our dark twin, which represented the total and full pattern of our dark karma that needed to be played out according to the existing pattern of rules and regulations. For many light workers, this current life has been about meeting, and then facing our darker twins, and then absorbing the essence of that dark, and then moving through into a completely different pattern of light. Indeed, for most of us, the dark twin has been the manifestation of our old negative practices, particularly our Atlantean experiences, which have needed to be cleared.

However, if we look forward down our future, probable timelines, then we can begin to see our light twin, or our future aspect.

This light twin represents what we will evolve into in the future and is the full embodiment of our experience earned in matter that is then expressed through the evolving pattern of progression on the Seventh Plane. So, if we look beyond the First, Second and Third Divine Journeys to that point after which we have become God-realised, and have travelled through these Journeys, then we may see our light twin in the Fifth Divine Journey. As we look at our twin, it may then turn to look at us, and send us a pulse of light from the Fifth Divine Journey that will then infuse us in the present physical timeline. Of course, we may not be able to absorb all that is held within that essence of that pulse, but it will, nonetheless, act as a standard or point for our focus.

Yet, what would be the outcome if we were to look down a number of our timelines and see our light twins present in a number of different ways? These different twins, different aspects of our higher twins, may irradiate a series of different frequencies. One of the twins may appear gold in colour and look like a baby that we will become; another may appear blue and may be more or less adult; another twin may be green. We can then choose to merge with one of our future twins, one of our future probabilities, and we would become the essence of what we would be in the future, and then bring it back into the present.

Our light twin represents the essence of our destiny, in one sense, and yet can be segregated into different aspects or streams. For example, if we had twelve, probable, future aspects or twins that we could work with, would we select just one twin, or would we work through all of them to bring through the sum, total manifestation of all that we could be and could become. By merging systematically with each different twin, we could then become and bring through in the present, our full manifested essence of the future. In one very real sense, that is what we are trying to do in the new timeline: to push through into the future and to bring back that which is highest and most light, and bring it into our living conscious awareness. This pattern of working requires courage and discipline, and also a programme of increasing energy management where the physical body can absorb, bit by bit, the essence of the future into the present. If we were to try it all at once, there would be a strong likelihood that we would drop our bodies. So, the pattern of future merging with our twins has to be done bit by bit: first a glance from our twin, then a stare, and then an ever-building level of merging; until we can support the level of light from our future twin in the present.

So our twins are our future essences, what we will become, and each colour that we work with will signify a series of different frequencies. Yet our future twins give us access to more, and in merging with them, we can begin to build a pattern of energy where we can begin to work directly with the future manifestation of different light holograms and different, future Avataric presences. For example, if we merged with the future aspect of the Cosmic Christ that is now beginning to push down the new timeline, then we would begin to irradiate, in the present, the essence of the Cosmic Christ. We would live the future in the present in a very dynamic way.

CHAPTER 20

The New Creative Hologram

Artistic Creativity

In one sense, humanity has come full circle since the Lemurian Root Race when the creative and intuitive flow of light was explored in multiple ways. Today, the excellence of the higher Lemurian frequencies are now being re-birthed into the Sixth Root Race as part of a new creative hologram. The focus of this creative flow is the lived experience, where every piece of creative expression can be experienced by another person within the full totality of what was originally intended by the creator. In one sense, this is a way of creating something entirely new, and yet allowing those who come into contact with it, a means to experience in exactly the same mode, the full force of that creative flow.

The platform that was created in the Lemurian times, which was then held within three crystal skull frequencies – two larger skulls, and one slightly smaller – contained the living hologram of all that was most beautiful and creative. The skulls were and are the living hologram of the Lemurian times, and by directly accessing them, then we can begin to receive the downloading of the Lemurian creative experience. This has now started, and over the coming years, will flow out in ever expanding circles to those who are ready to access these new frequencies.

The platform of collective unity that we are building in the new timeline is part of the new creative hologram. Through constant and direct merging, we can begin to build a new pattern of unity that will come to be a part of the living hologram. A range of different frequency notes – music, art, creative writing, theatre and film, drawing, painting, photography, sculpture – will be contained within the new hologram, and the creative pulse will highlight new ways in which we can give expression to different sorts of radically new experiences which are beyond our current description. So, in the example, from the previous chapter, where we talked about describing new emotions, we will not necessarily have to come up with a descriptive language, but instead we will be able to capture its essence through artistic means, and then relay that to others as a direct, lived experience through a given artistic medium. For example, an individual has a direct experience of the new streams of light at the top of the Sixth Plane; the direct infusion of higher mental light into their system cannot be put into words, yet, if they painted this experience in brilliant flows of light, and in the very act of painting captured the mental frequencies that they had experienced, then anyone who later came to look at the painting would receive a direct downloading of what the artist experienced. It would be like they were standing there themselves having the same experience as the artist did at that time.

This type of creative hologram will allow all of us to access the massive diversity of the new collective frequencies, and will enable all of us who have the collective focus, to experience a series of living multiple realities that will all be part of the living hologram.

If we wish to experience at first hand the creative flow of light from the Lemurian times, then all we need do is connect with the crystal skulls within the appropriate chakra centre, and then experience first hand the Lemurian frequencies. The creative hologram means that not only do we have access to all of these new frequencies, but that when we access them and experience them, and then capture the moment within which they are presented, then others can live that moment as we do. If Meher Baba were to walk in through the door and stand in front of us, how would we describe the experience? Could we describe the experience? Or would it be beyond our capacity to describe it? Similarly, can we capture a deva through photography and what would the different devas look like? For all of us, the creative moment, the pulse, if you like, is that point where the essence of the experience is captured and then re-lived by others in that same moment.

The hologram gives us access to absolutely everything – we can access the skill base to express our creative flow through any medium we choose. It is like having a specialist teacher who can direct and explain everything that we need to know in the moment to express what we wish to capture. So, if we are trying to express something entirely new, then we capture the moment and then download the essence of that moment into an artistic medium that others can experience. So, if an author writes a new novel which is infused with the new telepathic and creative frequencies of the new timeline, then the person reading the novel can be transported into the book to experience, at first hand, the adventures and stories that the author accessed in the first place. It is impossible to imagine anything that isn't there and so when we imagine something, we are accessing something that is happening in a particular space or place, whether it is in our dimension of thought or an entirely different one. Each and every thought we have, and that which is created through the process of capturing in our imagination, has a focus of energy and therefore has an existence. By bringing through the different streams of energy, and by giving them artistic expression within the living hologram of the new timeline, we are birthing a new type of essence and experience into our reality. We are 'capturing' the new frequencies and allowing others to share in their expression.

The new creative frequencies will allow us to feel and live a huge diversity of experiences, from what it is like to be a deva on another planet, to a pulse of starlight, to the wind thought the trees, to the experience of being born out of the Ocean of Life as a soul in unconscious bliss. If we could give expression and call in the pulse of the moment, of that one unique moment where we captured something entirely new, such as a shaft of new angelic light, or feel into what the huge essence or presence of an Eldering, and then live the moment, we will then be unfolding the new creative timeline. To be able to show this to others, through the lived experience of the moment, will provide them with an utterly life transforming experience as well.

All of the different realms on the inner planes, including the Seventh Plane, shadowlands, and throughout the Wheel of Life, will provide a massive source of creative resources for us to capture and then bring through in a variety of ways. What would it be like to paint the future in terms of timelines and different frequencies? What if someone could look at a painting and then experience the different timelines in that one unique moment? They would experience a part of the new hologram. The new creative hologram will allow a different creative access to absolutely everything that is being birthed in the new timeline. By capturing the creative essence of the moment, we are not limiting it through the mind, we are not judging it; we are living it. So, connecting to this new hologram means that every bit we touch, we can download and access everything within it. The flow of energy will be limitless, and we will be spoilt for choice in how we bring through into the living experience, that which we choose to focus on. And as more and more people begin to capture and live different parts of the hologram, then we will have the opportunity to live and experience different aspects of the hologram as lived through their experiences, yet which become our own experience through deeper and deeper levels of merging. The hologram will become a living kaleidoscope of multiple dimensional living that will touch the very essence of who and what we are, and which will, quite literally, transform our view of reality and what it means to live in the moment in more than one place at a time.

Apart from bringing through new techniques for painting and writing, there is a need for new music to capture the higher frequencies and to allow us to live the new feelings and emotions in a profound way. The classical music of the great composers was birthed to allow people to feel different emotions within the constraints of their physical lives. Some of the great composers were ahead of their time, and the music that they brought through was from a future timeline. All of that was preparation, just as the new music of the 1960's brought through a new stream of light.

It is now time for another leap in musical expression, where the flow and rhythm can capture and hold the new frequencies of higher light, so that we can dance at every level, from subatomic through to the physical and subtle, and up to our collective expression. We can become the musician and the music as we experience the interchange of energy; we can feel the flow of energies within the music and, as these new sounds build, they will begin to open us up in new ways. In the past, some of the ancient traditions focused on sound to open up the chakra centres, such as in Tibetan chanting. Today, we need a new source of musical expression that has the potential to awaken us to a new level of consciousness; for music that can then resonate in our multiple levels of conscious, physical awareness and build a new platform of experience. The NASA tapes that capture the sound of the Voyager spacecraft passing through the solar system bring us a new type of experience, as we begin to hear multiple levels of sound within each of the notes. The new music will do this: it will house multiple levels of overtoning from a variety of different light streams that will allow us to merge in a different way with that light. The new music will capture the higher frequencies of light and usher in a profound new level of lived experience. What if our music could resonate with our soul and bring through a different kind of expression, where we felt our very essence dance to the new frequencies? This type of music could bring through deep layers of experience and open us up to what we truly are inside. For this to happen requires that only one person lives this type of experience and imprints and creates the music to capture this.

The new creative hologram will therefore allow us to access so much more in the new timeline; the flow of creative spontaneity will transcend our own perceived levels of limitation, and allow us to bring through something entirely different; a new artistic experience which is lived in the moment, and which captures the essence of the moment. The vast array of new, higher guides is ready and most willing to assist us in this process.

Ritual

The spontaneity of the creative flow also requires a ritualistic focus; yet, this is not going back to the old, outdated rituals of past religions, or ancient tribal practices. This is to invoke a new ritual of the moment, to find a new way to give expression to the higher frequencies of light. Ritual is constantly changing and is an honouring of the moment in a spontaneous fashion. Ritual helps to provide a focus for something new and dynamic. It allows us to recognise and to experience in an original way, that which is being energetically offered.

To work with ritual means to open up in the moment and to feel what needs to be done or said. Each of the different life forms that have been described, such as the devas, the angels or the Elderings, have subtle ways of working and communicating with us. Through ritual we can find avenues to build up a stronger dialogue. So, at its simplest, our ritual may be to sit in silence and become still, and then to open up. This simple act is a ritual and from it can flow a whole series of other rituals. So a ritual is about the moment, about focus, about accessing something unique, and about giving and receiving. Ritual is not about the past, or about following old energetic flows, many of which have long outlived their usefulness. Ritual for ritual's own sake, where the original energetic pulse has been long forgotten, does not add more; empty ritual is always less.

True ritual is always about more. Meher Baba used to wash the feet of the masts that he met. This simple act, like a spontaneous ritual, carried a significance way beyond what was recognised in the physical. Similarly, when we open up to the process of ritual, we are always invoking for more from a position of harmony, balance, love and recognition of what the moment demands. The moment and the flow of energy will dictate what needs to be brought through; it is by being open and in one's silence and then pushing up into the higher streams of light, that we can begin to bring through the living will of what is called for at that precise moment. A ritual on one day may have great significance beyond what is seen; yet if it is done on another day, the energy may not support that which is being invoked. Ritual never stays the same: it is constantly changing and evolving to reflect the more that is demanded in the moment.

So when we open and push up into higher streams of light,

ritual can help to bring though and earth the new energies in a meaningful way. When we invoke in ritual, we may have no idea of what will come through, but as the momentum develops, we can begin to experience and feel the pulse of the moment coming in, which will then direct us in the appropriate way. So the moment always demands more, and in that birthing of more, we can invoke a new level of love into our lives, built upon the foundation of collective harmony that is the lived expression of what is being offered. Through ritual we can experience giving and receiving and see how the flow of energy can manifest great change.

Ritual, at its purest, is a direct expression of higher purpose. By invoking the ritual of higher purpose we can begin to align ourselves with the new timeline and the living Will of the Father. There is always ritual on the inner planes, and so it is by reflecting this in our daily lives that we can begin to live and become aware of a new dynamic flow of energy as it is given expression and focus in the moment. Ritual also requires focus – focus on the streams of energy that are calling to us; focus to stay in the moment, and focus not to allow distractions or thoughts to block or pull us to one side or the other. So, for example, if we use poetic verse and rhyming to help capture the essence of the higher energy of the moment, if we let go of the thread of energy that we are focusing on, or if any distracting thoughts come in, then we can be pushed to one side and loose the thread of higher energy. It can subsequently be very difficult to recover that original thread since these higher streams of light are always subtle. So in focusing on that rarefied stream of light, it is essential to keep our focus and to remain relaxed in the moment, yet intent on what we are bringing through. Following the stream of energy then helps us to open up and be at one with the higher streams of light, so that we move beyond the mind and access something that is much higher frequency and which can be birthed into our awareness in our timeline.

Ritual through spontaneous invocation of more is a way to move in and out of time; it is a means to recognise the moment, and to then push up into the higher light frequencies in our awareness, and to then call through and bring back into time, the specific light frequencies that need to be birthed at that time. Ritual helps us to honour the moment, and in honouring the moment we can allow the moment to become more and become the lived expression of the now supported by love, power and wisdom and much, much more.

The New Telepathic Flow

The new hologram will also unfold a new type of telepathy that will open up an entirely different level of communication between us. This telepathy will also bring through a higher level of communication with an array of different life forms. The frequencies that made up the pattern of Lemurian telepathy have been accessed and are being used as a basis for developing a more robust form of telepathy that will allow the collective flow of energy to build. Higher mental light will allow this new type of telepathy to unfold and it will be entirely different from the emotional telepathy that we sometimes feel.

The Lemurian telepathy required the stripping away of fear, and although this was partially successful, humanity has now come through a series of cycles where every possible permutation of fear frequencies has been experienced. Since we have become saturated with fear, it is now time for the pendulum to swing in the other direction and for the fear frequencies to be banished from the planet. Fear undermines unity and harmony. To push through this fear in the current sequence of development, has necessitated the birthing of a higher level of purity and innocence, and these twin frequencies are being used to build a robust platform of unity. The new purity is virulent and brilliantly light, while the new innocence embodies a magnificent degree of love never before seen on the planet. These twin frequencies are then combined with unity to build a new triangle of attributes that can then support the new telepathy that will come in. Purity will ensure that there is no pollution or contamination; innocence brings through virulent love, while unity is the focus required to birth the new telepathy. Until now, humanity has lacked the unity and focus to hold the new telepathic frequencies.

In 2005 a series of Lemurian frequencies were resurrected

in the Indian Ocean and manifested through three, primary crystal skulls. Each of these skulls supports the old Lemurian frequencies, but also gives access to the flow of telepathy that was present at that time. By merging with these frequencies and building a new light body, it is now possible to take these Lemurian frequencies and use them to birth a new form of telepathy that is not limited by the past, and not constrained by any imbalance between chaos and order, and which is not tainted by fear.

This new telepathy will be based on an inner knowing, and also through a variety of different mediums of expression. One of the main frequencies of telepathy is the colour silver, and this will be used in the higher mental planes to build up the new access required. And if we recall the new pattern of devic energy that was being birthed, silver, then this will remove the need to focus on older, dark desires such as fear and other forms of negative intent. So, in other words, the energetic programme for humanity is allowing a stripping down of the old, and a replacement by something new that can then support a new pattern of unity. As unity builds, all of the older, subliminal frequencies will be stripped out of our energetic systems to allow a purity of vibration that will then give the energetic access that will form the telepathic flow. Mental telepathy will supersede the old emotional telepathy and will be experienced in so many different ways: through our creative work, through dreams, through moments when we can feel the essence or someone that we know enter our space; through an intuitive knowing about something or someone. The feeling will bring with it an inner certainty or knowing. The new telepathy will not be about being able to read the mind chatter of other people; it will be about experiencing the new, living hologram in a deep and profound way. It will be about communicating with all life in many different realities and about feeling the pulse of unity that lies behind all life.

To bring through telepathy is really to see Natural Law unfolding. In the past telepathy has been seen as a magical quality, but really magic is Natural Law and an expression of more. So those who are fearful of the new changes and the higher energies coming in are really going back into their past and seeking out the older darker frequencies that were their old comfort zones. The new frequencies of telepathy have nothing to do with the older darker practices; they are all about invoking a new platform of love, bounded by unity, purity and innocence and forged through the collective experience of the group.

The telepathic flow will first start off as a small pulse, like a momentary knowing of something for certain. It will be a lived moment of recognition. Bit by bit this pulse will build, as more and more telepathic fragments of intent come into our consciousness. They will be like shards of consciousness that give us a knowing. As they accumulate, we will then experience the flow of telepathic experience, as different presences and essences dance in and out of our conscious awareness. Those individuals close to us will be within our awareness; it is like a computer screen, where different software programmes remain dormant, yet can be easily activated; we only have to shift the focus from the exiting programme on the screen to another one to re-activate them. This shift in focus is our intuition. With each telepathic pulse, we will not be presented with a superficial perspective of life, or its representation. Rather we will feel the underlying essence of life, or the essence of someone we know and love. Similarly, it will be our focus and intent that will allow us to feel the telepathic flow more powerfully, between different people's essences and light streams.

It is also important to recognise that this telepathic flow will not just be between one individual and another. Since the platform of support is based on collective unity, then we will experience collective telepathy. So many people may experience the same energetic pulse simultaneously as the telepathic stream flows within the hologram of our living experiences. We become the living hologram, and so live every moment of every part of the new timeline within an enhanced awareness, with access to everything that is contained within that hologram. So like pulses of higher light and unity, the new telepathy will give us a living knowing of that which is unfolding at precisely the point at which it becomes manifested in the new timeline.

Those individuals who are open doors and have access to the Seventh Plane will experience the new telepathy in a more dynamic way, since they will be able to access the higher streams of light in a less diluted form than is present in the mental planes. Since they have access in and out of time, they will be able to feel the telepathic flow out of time and work with those frequencies in a more profound way. The sense of flow will be more all encompassing and more virulent and will support a different level of communication. The challenge will be to bring that stream of energy back in through time, so that the platform of light in the newly formulated part of the Seventh Plane, can hold and host the new telepathic streams. The telepathic light essences will, at their source, resonate to a series of different frequencies, which will then be stepped down into the mental planes.

So, the living experience of the new telepathic flow will not be what we expect, and the lived experience of the new telepathy will challenge us to accept the energetic flow, to push beyond the limits of our mind, and to embrace something uniquely different yet collectively refined.

Triangles of More

The platform of energy entering our new timeline is based on the triangle. This is also a reference to higher purpose, and the triangle will be used to present, offer and download a whole series of new Sixth Root Race frequencies. The first triangle to be formed, at the creation of the first spark, was the Father, Son and the Holy Ghost. This triangle represents freedom on every level. Yet as each spark gave off more sparks, then a whole series of triangles was formed. In the new timeline, the Father has ordained that a sequence of new triangles hosting a plurality of attributes needs to be birthed and absorbed within humanity, other streams of life, and the planet.

The different triangulations of energy will be unveiled in a specific sequence. As we tune into each of them, they will be like a reflection of the original Trinity, but will represent the different segregations and birthings of the new energy streams in the new timeline. We will then absorb these different triangles according to the sequence that we need. For example, a fundamental pattern is love-love-love, and one of the main Sixth Root Race triangles is power-power-power. This represents the flow of energy that is being manifested by the Perfect Master of Power. Each of the other Perfect Masters will embody their own attribute – knowledge-knowledge-knowledge, truth-truth-truth, wisdom-wisdom-wisdom and bliss-bliss-bliss. Whichever three Perfect Masters are in dominance at any one time will then be reflected in the triangle of energies that is being worked. For example, power, wisdom and knowledge will form one triangle, and then at another time it will be power, bliss and truth, or whatever combination is in ascendancy.

There are a series of other triangles that are key to the new timeline. The first of these to be unveiled is purity, innocence and unity. The other triangles will follow as the new frequencies are invoked through the Father's Nine-Pointed Plan and the new timeline. These will include the new light frequencies such as light, hope, common sense, compassion, magic and others. With every triangle that is formed, there is a flow of energy in a particular direction. It can be either clockwise or counter-clockwise, and it can start at any point on the triangle. For example, it may start at the top and then flow down to one of the other points in a clockwise or counter-clockwise direction. The attribute may also shift position, so at one time unity may be at the top of the triangle, while at other times, innocence or purity may be at the tip, depending on which flow of energy is dominant at that time.

The pattern of energy will also be reflected in whether the triangle is pointing upwards or downwards. The six–pointed star of the Sixth Root Race is formed out of two triangles – one with the tip pointing up which hosts the new platform of white energies, and another triangle with the tip pointing down which reflects the new pattern of black light. Together, the six-pointed star hosts all of the new frequencies of the new root race and each triangle can then be worked to include a series of different attributes at each of the points.

The orientation of the triangle can relate to whether the pattern of energy for that individual is in or out of balance. People who have health problems may have specific triangles in different chakra centres pointing down rather than up. Ideally, the dominant triangle of energies that anyone is working with will be in a state of harmony and balance in each of their centres. However, this is very often not the case and further energy work is required to absorb the energies present within each triangle of energies. So, to build the telepathic flow in our systems requires that we host and absorb the frequencies from the unity-purity-innocence triangle. If any of the triangles are upside down in our centres, then the flow of energy will be distorted and will not function properly. By the right use of the will and with a proper focus, it is possible to turn the triangle back to the right orientation and thereby shift any underlying energy blockage that may be present.

In addition to the above, there will be a series of other types of triangles that will house the diversity of different life forms: the first to be worked is the Devic-Angelic-Eldering. And within the Devic and Angelic Realms, different triangles will arise to represent the different types of frequencies and life forms. Within the Devic Kingdom, the four triangles of Fire, Earth, Air and Water mark the beginning, where each triangle can be formed of each element, or can be a combination of different elements. A variety of other platforms will be birthed into existence once the Angels and Elderings come more into our consciousness.

Ultimately, there will be one hundred and forty four triangles of frequencies, each one to be hosted within all of the chakras of all those who work under the umbrella of each of the new Perfect Masters. The one hundred and forty four triangles reflect the number in each Perfect Master's circle. The one hundred and forty four triangles will make up the complement of new frequencies that will constitute the basic platform of energy for the new timeline. Those who can host all of these different triangles will then be utterly unique in their ability to radiate the new frequencies of the new timeline.

CHAPTER 21

The Devic Pulse

Devic Streams

The focus of development has been astral in the previous root races. The Sixth Root Race is the first where the mental platform is being invoked. This has major implications for all life forms on the planet, especially the devas. In one sense, devic life originated in the mental, since it is a structural thought form that is mentally expressed, but then coated in the astral ways of energy according to its need. It imbues form, around which experience is gathered. Devic form inhabits multiple modes of expression, such as the roots, flowers, bark, branches, leaves, sap and all the other beings that go over it, such as the fairies, the gnomes, the elves and the stick people. The devas pervade our physical bodies at every level – they are in every organ, tissue, system, cell and atom. We are a living collective of different devic life forms and when we tap into the higher mental, then the structure of our bodies will hold a series of different frequency notes. This means that the devic pattern in our systems will have to change. The same is also true for all other physical structures that are imbued with the formless essence of devic life: the devic pattern of expression will need to change. As we have seen, a new devic light has been birthed into the planet and this is forming the basis for a new archetypal devic pattern on Earth, which will then be exported to the eighteen thousand Earths in the Wheel of Life.

Up to now the astral levels have been maintained by devic intent, expressed through different patterns of form, resonating at the atomic, mineral, plant, animal and human levels. The Mineral Kingdom occupies the lower astral levels with the slow movement of energy, the old dark light and the retention of basic substances through a feudal, yet collective pattern of intent. This pattern is now changing as the new dark light is infused into the Mineral and other Kingdoms. In the old pattern, devic experience is through sensation, and so if we experience everything in one type of reality, where we see in colour and hear sound, then the devas do it differently: they hear colour and see sound. They assimilate everything through a veil, where they receive the afterglow of the lived experience.

Devic expression is always seeking diversity and something new, and so has always focused on going backwards or sideways, rather than up into order and higher streams of light. While devic purpose does seek to cultivate order through time, it is always within the context of devic knowledge: to become more and absorb all in its rhyme. Thus, the old, chaotic imprinting has ensured that constant experience generates never-ending variation. The devic path has focused on experiencing everything possible over and over again. It is important to understand that our concepts of chaos and order are different from the devas. So for example, what we take to be order in our gardens, through mowing the lawn and constantly cutting everything back into a neat and tidy format, is almost the antithesis of devic expression. It is limiting and the embodiment of devic chaos. In contrast, a garden where everything is allowed to grow unhindered and free is the living manifestation of devic order. The devic note will always seek to express more through diversity.

The devas have explored multiple streams of old dark light and white light. Devas have not just worked with the slow, darker frequencies, but have also embraced the higher light frequencies in the higher astral realms. Different types of devic life have been anchored at higher points of understanding and intelligence, and have allowed the diversity of experiences to spark different types of life patterns. As the form builders, the devas are everywhere, and it all depends on how we focus our intent and will. If we look in one way, then we may see one type of devic expression; and yet if we look in a different way, we may see something entirely different. The two are connected but are differently presented. If we focus on the subatomic structure of matter, then the devic presentation will be very different to us looking at the devic expression in flowers, where higher frequencies of light are birthed through a more ordered presentation in matter. Similarly, the various elements will present different levels of devic awareness, from the small to the large and collective.

The underling devic essence may manifest through a whole range of different physical forms. In the past the old type of devic light flowed through the Mineral and other Kingdoms. Old devic light can be felt in the forbidding presence of a mountain, or in a dark and thick forest. Both types of form house a similar underpinning of devic light, although each devic pattern will be experiencing different sensations. So while the grosser manifestations of devic life will exhibit the old dark frequencies, the higher patterns of devic form can manifest lighter frequencies. Through experience, the deva will slowly tend towards a different level of awareness and intelligence, and in some cases, this may mean bringing through white light as opposed to dark light. Thus, the underlying essence of devic life can be dark or light, where the light focus represents more order and is usually earned through the long march of experience, from initial chaos into order. The different devic streams will not always follow this route, and the various patterns of devic expression, a few of which are now coming to our attention, will be manifested with time. For now, it is worth recognising the different levels of devic expression, from the lower astral to the middle and higher astral, the various patterns of devic light, which are predominantly black but sometimes can be white, and the massive diversity of structure that can accommodate devic life through the different Kingdoms, and manifestations of the minute to the large.

The devic streams are therefore like seams of experience that flow through the different devic patterns of life. Some seams are always dark, while some may evolve out of dark into light; others may explore different types of physical and subtle form, according to the different local fashions that have been birthed as the living vehicles of awareness. So higher devic forms, such as fairies will manifest magic and love, while planets and stars will host a devic intelligence that is vast, powerful and brilliant.

To attempt to understand devic life from an intellectual perspective is doomed to failure. Devic life cannot be captured in this way; it can best be experienced in the living moment where the devic pulse catches us and calls to us and opens us out into something more. The diversity and magnitude of the devic programme can only be experienced.

The New Devic Path

Higher purpose is now demanding change in the devic form. And this change is fundamental. If we go back to the description of the sparks and how life was formed through the various different planes, according to the dictates of limitation and experience, then if we think of the Mineral Kingdom, and the different life forms, such as the fairies, and the vibratory pattern of form that associates with minerals, then the mineral down here has a loose dialogue of energy and vibrates in a particular way. It has a certain, fundamental series of sparks – atoms, neutrons – all coming together and creating a vibratory dream going above it. Within this vibratory pattern there are other life forms present that give credence to themselves as they start to develop according to the rules and regulations and the stimulation that they receive from the input of the soul as it comes down. So devic form is primarily formless but exists in multiple and different levels of lived reality according to its own dictate and need for experience. Thus to conceive of devic life within a traditional, three-dimensional format is limiting and inaccurate: devic life is the essence that imbues the substance of form, and provides the vehicle of awareness through which the soul can gather particular types of experiences. These experiences may start off very slowly, like in the devic night of everything, where the soul progresses through the multiple levels of different aspects of the Mineral Kingdom. Yet through this experience, the soul will touch the higher notes of mineral light, such as in the fairies, where a different stream of light can be entertained.

In our human forms, these multiple levels of devic expression co-exist, from the very small, to the overall gross, human form. So our bodies contain many different devas, all vibrating as different sparks - but they have a general management focus, where the initial impulse of the atomic vibration, as it comes down, will bind our devas into a sort of superglue which holds the dominant thought form which is humanity at the moment. In this way, we can talk about the devas as the superglue that holds all form together.

The larger, collective expressions of our devic essence can vibrate on a number of different levels. Lower devic presences in our physical bodies appear rat-like, with dark-coloured fur, whiskers, teeth and tails. They come up to the top of our chest and the tail can be long or short, according to the degree of lived experience in matter. The eyes are piercing and intelligent. Higher vibrating forms can appear white, with the fur appearing snowy. This higher-vibrating devic presence is known as 'white rat'. Once an individual expresses this type of collective devic presence, it indicates that they have pushed out of the lower astral focus of devic intent and are embracing a higher pattern of light that is more collective. There is another pattern beyond the white rat, known as 'star rat', where the devic presence becomes a deep black. Points of light can begin to form in this complete blackness, reflecting different streams of stellar light. As more and more stars form, the devic pattern may change from deep black to a much lighter colour.

Finally, the devic presence may turn a golden colour, what can be termed the 'love rat', where the vibration of light flowing through is from the Seventh Plane and is hosting the unity and diversity of unconditional love. In one sense, the love rat is what humanity is striving for through the realisation and cultivation of a higher devic presence within our own awareness. So each of these different devic patterns are an expression of the light pushing up through the lower astral notes, and into the middle and higher astral, and then into the mental streams and beyond.

The recognition and manifestation of these different devic

presences all relate to the type of light that is hosted within our systems. Ninety-eight percent of illnesses are from the astral levels, and as the higher streams of mental light flow into us, then our physical vehicles have to change. And this has to start at the level of devic awareness first, rather than in the physical shell. If our devic presence is vibrating too slowly, then when the new light streams in, there will be the inevitable 'punch-up' between old and new, as the old light is pushed out through illness. So, there is a need to raise the vibration of our devic essence in each of us. Yet, the old devic presence is tenacious and strong, and up until now has been ill disciplined. Our bodies do not control the devic presence; it is the other way round. So, in opening up to these new devic expressions, there is a need to control the devic presence; to imbue it with discipline through our intent and will, and to then invoke for the higher streams of devic light. In particular, we need to call in the new devic light that can give each of us a platform of new love and devic power within the context of our physical vehicles: the old focus of the square is replaced by the new vibration of the triangle. The feudal and dark seeds of old devic intent have to be replaced by a new level of devic collectivity that is seeded through the higher frequencies of love and light. Once this underlying platform has been established, then the physical substance of our bodies can mutate and form in a new way. For example, our DNA is highly fragmented and splintered. If we can manifest and bring through the new devic light into our systems, and then balance this with the new white light, then our DNA frequency and structure would be utterly transformed and re-balanced. One strand of the DNA would be utterly black in frequency, representing the new devic platform, while the other would be brilliant white, embodying the new light platform.

The devic path is long and arduous; experience is gained through the different levels of light and the different substance of form that is called in to give that which is formless form. In the Mineral Kingdom, devic awareness builds from the microscopic into the macroscopic; from the subatomic to the mountain range and the ice sheet, and as the collective focus of devic light builds through experience and sensation, then information and knowledge is gathered. Through collective aggregation of awareness, the deva builds intelligence flowing through the various streams of devic light. Slowly, devic energy builds through the lower parts of the Mineral Kingdom. Once souls have experienced the grosser forms in rock, mineral and metal, they may experience the higher vibrations of elemental life, such as water sprites, fairies and elves. These life forms host a different pattern of devic light from the slower frequencies, and manifest more order within their pattern of existence. Collective love frequencies build through the lighter streams of light, and devic experience can be gained through light streams other than the pure black that forms the primary platform. With time and experience, different, higher frequencies of light can be utilised in the devic pattern, with access building from the Zero Plane into the First and Second Planes. Higher devic presences such as Pan are manifested on the Second Plane and for humans to access some of the higher devic notes requires an anchoring at this plane level of awareness, as well as in the Third Plane. Souls that are working exclusively with the devic pattern of light will work through multiple, collective frequencies of higher devic light, and after aeons of experience in matter, will eventually graduate into a higher, regulatory focus of energy known as a Devic Lord.

There are twelve, principal Devic Lords that oversee and experience the total flow of devic experience in the planet and the Wheel of Life. Each Devic Lord has a speciality note and represents the different aspects of devic life. The Devic Lord is the expression of devic order and will live the flow of different devic streams in matter. The twelve Devic Lords are overseen by a thirteenth, Devic Overlord. As described earlier, the pattern of devic light has been completely changed and is now flowing from the Devic Overlord into the twelve Devic Lords, and then into all devic life below.

Just as the old timeline is being overhauled, so the old devic pattern of life is being re-orchestrated. As the old black light is replaced by the new pattern of black light, so the focus of devic intent and power is changing. The new pattern of black light and the new deva has been brought in, and has been anchored from the Zero

Plane to the top of the Sixth Plane. This new deva is more primeval or primordial, but currently lacks the empowerment of the old devas. It is almost like they have been starved of desire in the way that we have it, and so once they are fed with desire, then they will come into their own power and grow very quickly. In one sense the old devas have been too ill disciplined and we are now seeking a pattern of greater co-operation with the new devas.

The underlying platform of love is building something much more into devic experience; the devas want to experience more than the afterglow – they wish to experience life more directly through emotions and feelings; and to feel the underlying pulse of light directly, without any veils. All the old patterns of devic knowledge, power, wisdom, bliss and truth are being stripped away and will be replaced by new types of devic power, wisdom, love and knowledge. Higher light frequencies will give the devas a new tier of understanding and the time has come for the devas to receive external recognition, from humanity and other life forms, for their true role in the physical world. Humanity, with the odd exception, is currently oblivious to what the devas are and what their roles are. It is time for this to change and over the next six years a new pattern of devic access and interpretation will be established, which will then allow people to see what was not accessible before: to experience, at first hand, the pulse of devic light and power, combined with a new type of devic knowledge and wisdom. The old will be combined with the new to make more, where the knowledge and wisdom can support the new template of common sense.

So, the new pattern of devic light is manifesting a new type of chaos and a new purpose. This new purpose is embodied through devic intent, knowledge, power and wisdom. The old feudal patterns have to go and are being replaced by a collective pattern of devic unity that can host the essence of new chaos, and the different degrees of order as they become birthed in the new timeline. Devic awareness will build into something utterly unique, where a new presence, strength and power will form a new platform of consciousness. Devic experience will evolve into something much greater than it has been, where the devas can absorb a greater diversity of light streams, and can host a new level of truth. Devic truth will then dance to the call of higher purpose in the silence of the moment. All life will then mutate and change as the new essence of devic light imbues all physical form with its new energetic platform.

Working with Devic Energies

To work with the different types of devic energies requires that we focus and capture the devic pulse within the essence of lived experience. The devas are everywhere, yet our prejudices and misunderstanding ensure that we very rarely see them. The reason for this is simple: we are reluctant to embrace a space where we can feel the diversity of life, and where things can exist in the realms beyond our physical sight. The more direct physical structures always capture our attention first, and the slow frequency education we receive at school combines to ensure that our openness is shut down from a very early age. Consequently, young children can see many things, yet if the parents or adults reject these intuitive experiences, then the children will close down. Children can see and feel many of the different devic presences and with attunement and practice, it is easy for us to recapture our lost intuition and subtle focus of awareness.

One of the easier ways to focus on devic life is to use photography to capture the moment. Taking pictures of trees, rocks, flowers, fires, waterfalls and many other natural phenomena can open new doorways in our awareness, because the photograph can capture a moment. If we photograph trees, it is often easy to see faces peering out of the leaves and branches. The faces can be quite large, up to many feet in size, or smaller, perhaps only inches across. The face may appear with eyes, nose and a mouth and the shape may vary: however, the underlying devic presence will be very obvious in the face. It is also possible to find different faces overlapping one another, or to see different shapes in the tree bark. With practice, the actual photographic act becomes a case of waiting for a pulse or presence to build up in the photographic field. By waiting for the devas to come into our space, by waiting for their timeline to manifest, then it becomes easier to photograph them. So, rather like tuning into the new timeline, we can tune into the devic timeline and ask the devas to come through. By waiting for this devic pulse, we can begin to access a whole new realm of different devic presences. The same is true for flowers and rock formations, and other types of physical structure. Waiting for the moment when intuitively it feels right to take the picture will open us up to the essence of the energy flow as it is presented to us.

The photographic medium has great potential in demonstrating the different devic life forms around us. Another way to experience the devic pulse is to tune into the different trees, flowers and rocks everywhere. Building a pattern of communication with the different devic presences requires practice and an innate respect for the devic presences around. Through opening up to a tree, and standing at a distance away from it that feels intuitively right, we can begin to feel its presence build up. At first we may engage with different levels of feeling, such as sadness, happiness, grumpiness or just a general resistance to communicate. If we empty our minds of any thoughts and just open up to the tree, we may begin to access different impressions as the energy between the tree and ourselves begins to flow. In our emptiness and silence, different impressions may build and we may feel that an actual dialogue is building where we can send out a question to the tree, and then an answer will form spontaneously in our awareness. This pattern of communication is like opening a new door on a different world where the main obstacle to success is our mind, and its pattern of rigid thinking that will say that trees cannot communicate. Once the mind is superseded, it can become much easier to communicate with the different devic life forms around us.

To push into a deeper devic interaction requires that we embrace a deeper level of merging with the devic presences around us. For example, to merge with the sky and clouds gives us a focal point of recognition with the element Air; or to merge with the essence of a stream of water or a blue sea, can give us the feeling of what it is to be like the element Water. The process is not difficult and again requires that we are open and can project our awareness in silence into a bank of clouds or into a stream, and to then open up to whatever impressions we get. Sometimes this process will feel natural, and may reflect our past life patterns of devic work, while at other times, it may seem harder to establish a dialogue. Whatever the case, there is a necessity and need for all of us to connect with the devas, and to honour their request for more, and to provide a focus that will allow our lives to be imbued with a different way of experiencing life, one that is much closer to us than we think.

Communicating with the devas is also about negotiation and working with the different patterns of energy all about. Connecting with the ground energies around our homes may give us an indication of what energetic streams are present. If the devic presences around our homes are unhappy, then this will be reflected in the energies around us. The food we eat is all devic, and depending on how the energy was used in the growing process, then the different devic streams will be present. A fully-grown carrot may contain mental light while it is in the soil; yet by the time that it has been harvested, packaged and distributed to our supermarket shelves, any last vestiges of mental light will have drained away. The vibration of our food always reflects the underlying devic presence, and if the food is more vibrant, then we will benefit from this. We will absorb the higher focus of devic energy.

So, when trees are cut down, and food is eaten, it is not that we are killing off the devic energy around us; we are changing its pattern. So when a tree is cut down, the devic life in that tree will seek to find somewhere else to live and will occupy other structures around it or go into the ground. The same is true for food – when we eat our food, the devas come into our own systems and merge with the different devic levels inside us. If the vibration in our food is low, then we will absorb this slower frequency light. If it is higher, then we will benefit from this. This is all part of the change that goes on continuously and the diversity of experience that the deva seeks.

Communication with devic life goes on at many different levels and is often subconscious. When we go walking in the hills or the mountains, there is a communication between us and the devic life all about. It may be that the devic energies are hostile and make us feel uncomfortable, and for some people, the devic expression can be extremely strong. So mountaineers who fall or die in the mountains are experiencing a pattern of devic energy that is overpowering them and through which they have no means to communicate effectively. All storms and weather patterns are the product of devic intent and purpose. As the devas grow stronger and more focused, then the patterns of devic expression will build and become more powerful. It is therefore important to be mindful of how we communicate with the devas around us; effective communication can open up brand new vistas of experience, where the pulse of devic light will imbue us with a deep, inner knowing of devic life; where we are at one with the devic expression at any one time, and where we can feel everything that the deva feels in that particular instant. It is like experiencing in a second what it is to be a mountain deva in the Himalayas looking out over the vast, snow-capped, mountain ranges and high plateaus; or to be a huge thermal circling up through the atmosphere; or to be a flower essence that dances to the rays of the sun. All of these different experiences are open to us, and with practice we can access the different levels of devic knowledge, wisdom, power and light that are ever present around us.

The Darklings

With the new stream of devic light and the birthing through the Devic Overlord of the black essence of love, new opportunities are being unveiled. One example is the new role being taken on by an ancient devic grouping that was one of the minor devic houses, and which is now embracing greater responsibility. This grouping is known as the darklings, and they have taken on the role of translators and communicators between humanity and the devas.

The darklings are devic guides and can be presented in our awareness as being quite short in size, black and with bald heads. Each darkling has a proper name and once given to an individual, can then be used by the recipient to build up a deeper level of understanding of devic energy and protocol. The darkling, when called, will come in and give advice on how to work with different patterns of devic energy, and will also provide a means of working with different streams of devic energy on the inner planes.

Devic information and knowledge is not easily accessible to us due to the way that our minds have been wired up. The darklings can provide the necessary energetic translation to help us understand, in more detail, devic protocol and their methods of working. The darkling, then, is our guide and translator, and can with practice, give us unique access to deeper levels of devic awareness and expression.

The darklings are seeking more within their focus of intent, and through this manifestation of desire, will help to give us the necessary experiences for uncovering successive layers of devic life. Since there are so many different vibrational streams of life in existence, from the slowest and grossest to the lightest and most refined, the darkling can help attune us to the different frequency notes that the devas manifest. They can show us the slow groan in rock, where the devic pattern is extremely slow; they can help us dance with Air, rushing through canyons and gulleys. They can also educate us in the ways of the different Devic Lords and how each Lord works the different streams of devic light. In this way, the darkling can become our constant guide and companion in the devic realms.

At the same time, the new devic frequencies are building a different pattern of unity and presence. One such unique frequency is the "flower that never dies". The flower that never dies is the manifestation of an essence of love that can grow in any conditions. This flower grows in situations that could be called desert-like, where the focus of light and energy is not always favourable. And yet the flower that never dies can grow anywhere and can seed the new frequencies of love to all that is around. This undying flower is therefore a new devic expression that is the focus of more and which will build, in time, into a unique pattern of devic energy that will host something utterly exquisite and sublime. And just like in deserts, where flowers can bloom for no apparent reason, the flower that never dies will maintain its own flowers all the time, irrespective of the surrounding conditions. It is the manifestation of a new type of love that can endure the harshest of droughts and which can survive any and all conditions.

The time has therefore come for humanity to open up to the new patterns of devic light with a new level of understanding. The new black light that has been hosted into the planet is the start of something entirely new and will be built upon in the future, by different waves of devic light. These waves will open up new vistas of chaos and order, and entertain new levels of awareness that will harmonise and vibrate in unison with the potent and higher frequencies of light now coming in. While the initial platform of light will be lower and middle mental, soon the devic essence will support the higher mental platform where everything will change and be unlocked into the physical manifestation of life all around.

The old devic patterns of existence are now flowing away, and those old devic patterns that are resistant to change are being ushered out of the planet. Once the new devic light has taken root in Earth, it will then be offered out to the eighteen thousand Earths as part of the new seeding of the Wheel of Life. Another way to feel this transformation is to sense a new level of creation coming in, like a new Wheel imbued with the new black essence, which will lock into the existing Wheel of Life and then merge into something completely new where the new black light will flow within the Wheel and balance the new light frequencies coming in. So like the two halves of a giant Wheel, the new platform of black and white light will completely transform the existing creation.

The new platform of devic light will therefore embrace the new mental focus of energetics, and be able to house a collective unity supported by the excellence of the new white and black light. Devic life will be transformed into much more, as the formless expression of everything will hold and sustain the new emotional platform that is being birthed on the planet. The devas will no longer be limited by sensation; they will experience much more through the new streams of emotional energy coming into the planet.

At the same time, humanity will have the opportunity to work with a number of different groups in the Devic Kingdom. Until now, the focus has been very limited with access to one major group;

that is about to change as other devic groups mutate and evolve into more. Ultimately, the devic flow of life will be pure light and embody a vibration that will bring through a new pattern of order birthed out of the chaos. Out of the new dark, new light will evolve which will be the manifestation of a new type of order, and this new stream will be like a new platform that will push out into the new timeline, and which will then split and birth a whole series of new devic frequencies in the Seventh and Eighth Root Races, and beyond. The devic frequencies will be utterly beyond comparison and will host an entirely new level of devic consciousness, a consciousness that ultimately will be able to accommodate the frequencies of the Seventh Plane in a direct and undiluted way. This process is just beginning.

CHAPTER 22

The Wheel of Life

Sparking the Wheel

If we go back to the start, when the Primary Spark dropped down through the Seventh Plane, and then into the shadow planes, all possible forms of life were birthed out of the multiple probabilities that were latent at that time. In the Seventh Plane, different tiers of Creator Gods were sparked and then sought to replay, in a slightly different way, the experience and understanding of the Father and the Son. They sought to create that which was more. And as the Primary Spark continued to give off multiple sparks, then all that was birthed out of these different sparks became manifested. So, for example, the Earth was a spark that was birthed by a dream of Macheldavek. And in that dream, Macheldavek sparked Gaia, which was a spark of himself. Similarly, all the eighteen thousand Earths were created out of sparks. So in the ebb and flow of different vibratory patterns, life was created in all its forms.

If we think of the Primary Spark as resembling a comet which dropped down, sending out millions and millions of sparks, then some of these sparks lasted longer than others and were less diluted than others. All these different sparks then sparked more and so the whole fabric of creation and the creative play was formed through this process of multiple cascades of sparking. Everything comes from the Primary Spark, and ultimately, everything will go back into this Primary Spark, as it seeks to become more in the everything and the nothing.

While the myriad life forms were created out of these millions and millions of sparks, then the thought and intent that was invoked through the different tiers of Creator Gods that were descended from the Primary Spark, gave birth to a whole series of life forms that inhabited the developing stars and planets. So each manifestation of creation, each new life form, was like an experiment, where the local conditions and the predilections of those who did the creating, invoked a pattern or form that could explore and gather experience. It is a bit like having thousands of different directors and each one is putting on a play with a cast of characters and a story line. Each play is uniquely different and has the potential to create totally different characters and expressions of life. So, some directors may choose to direct the play according to the dictates of local custom, where the local form would be used as a vehicle of choice in the story line. In other plays, some directors chose to invent entirely new costumes and characters to tell a very different story line.

Another way of looking at it is to see that the multiple sparkings gave rise to a series of massive wardrobes that were latent and then activated within the process of creation. Each wardrobe contains millions and millions of possible clothes; each set of clothing is uniquely different, with some being small, say only 2 feet high, and others being much larger, at around 6 feet high. So each set of clothing is unique to a given life form. Each set of clothing represents a different life stream and was formed within the intention of the type of manifestation of will that was developed at that time. The different sets of clothes can then be used to form a story line where the life form invoked could accept the bondage in matter, the spiritual permutation of energy and the rich language that would form through experience on the inner and outer planes. So each play established a story and series of experiences, latent and active, that could then be manifested through the selected wardrobes and clothes worn on the set.

As this massive array of plays unfolded and were birthed in the different life streams and dreams of the Creator Gods, then under the principles of Natural Law, all of the developing thought forms that became infused with their life energy and became different vehicles of expression for the sparks that were souls to manifest in, then allowed a whole dance of life to unfold in spectacular fashion. In some cases, it was like each play had a series of shadows, or alternative realities, where the wardrobes and events could be played out slightly differently. So, for example, one play would be worked through at a higher vibration than another, so that multiple plays could be explored in the different currents of energy that were part of the manifested dream at that time.

If we think of this plane of thought at this time, is this where the vibration of the Father ends or are there other layers underneath us? In the case of the Earth, and if we focus on the twelve primary Earths, is our Earth at the bottom, at the top or somewhere in the middle? Now, if Earth is evolving from the solar plexus into the heart centre, then there are other Earths beneath us with other vibrations where the spark is less dominating and where the afterglow is reflected down there as a rhythm of energy that is starting to wake up. In other words, as our level of experience begins to mutate into a higher stream of consciousness, then the slower levels beneath us do the same. It is like a dream within a dream, or dreams within dreams.

So as the galaxies of different planets and stars were birthed through the multiple array of sparkings and creative fluxes of the in and out breath of the Creator, then all of these different solar systems held different patterns of energies and birthed different forms, each one vibrating according to the potency and focus of the initial sparks that created it. Some were slower, and others quicker. At the same time, the different streams of creative energy also opened up different probable timelines of expression. So in one timeline, one outcome could be played through while in another, a different set of outcomes could be entertained. And as these timelines gave birth to more, through the flux of life on the inner and outer planes, so it was that the full majesty of the Wheel of Life was born. In a unique and sublime way, the Wheel of Life was created out of all of the sparks and sparkings that originated from the Primary Spark, as light and dark danced to the orchestra of the Father's Will.

The Wheel of Life is not just a three-dimensional description of life, the Universe and everything. It is a multiple-dimensional, living hologram that houses multiple levels of existence, and which has the capacity to allow souls to explore different pathways in form through the subtle and physical realms. The Wheel of Life contains all of the possible life forms and vehicles of existence that were birthed out of the initial creative impulse, and which were then given form through the different types of sparking. Some life forms within the Wheel vibrate very slowly, while others dance to a higher frequency. The Wheel contains everything within the everything and allows multiple streams of existence to unfold within a dynamic and directed pattern of energy. This energy is the manifestation of everything that was invoked by the Primary Spark. In one sense the manifestation of the Wheel is like the out breath of the Creator that simply goes on and on. As the different Avataric Days come and go, so it is that the Wheel will pulse in and out, or breathe in and out, as a reflection of the fundamental change that is ordained at that particular point in the cycle of creation.

So if we imagine for a moment, a massive wheel that is spinning slowly and which houses millions and millions of different planets and stars, and also contains the multiple life forms that were birthed out of the various patterns of creation, then within each particular soul, as it drops out of the Seventh Plane, and into the shadow planes, has a diversity of choices. Young souls may start off at the edge of the Wheel where the diversity of life is more limited, and where the substance of experience can give a particular focus. Like actors in a series of different plays, the souls go through different wardrobes and sets of clothing gaining more and more experience of all that life has to offer. Each stage is a new opportunity to explore different patterns of life, and to sample the different offerings from the creative directors and the retained structure of local thought. So one play might be like the vegetable patch, while another may be a world full of grasshoppers and crickets.

Yet within all of this diversity, it was recognised ultimately that there was a lack and in the dream of Macheldavek, a new possible expression of life came to be manifested through free will and choice. Each soul, as it progressed through the Wheel of Life, gained experience and one of the founding concepts behind the planet Earth was the opportunity to give those souls, in the fullness of time, an opportunity to experience all of the best and most interesting bits out of all the local plays under the direction of one star director. Thus Earth was birthed as a melting pot for all that had been the best and possibly the worst of what had been formed in the Wheel itself. So, developing souls could go through millions and millions of dress rehearsals, learning their lines on different stages, until eventually they could graduate on to the Earth stage, where the flow and intensity of experience was like nowhere else; where the diversity and array of frequencies could be experienced all in one go, and all that had been learnt could be put to the test in a brand new production that was open ended, and which had no pre-ordained outcome. Souls could learn to become their own creators within the creative play on Earth, rather than being directed in one of the local plays. It is like having been an actor in a local repertoire, moving from town to town for many years, and then eventually ending up on Broadway where the play itself is open ended and where the actors get to choose all of the best bits from all of the plays that they have ever done, and to mould all of these bits into one huge creative play that goes through a series of major acts or root races.

Earth therefore gave developing souls an opportunity to reprise the experiences gained from the Wheel of Life in a unique way. And for this to happen, Earth itself had to be seeded with many of the different life forms from the millions of solar systems. Life on Earth was donated or inherited from different patterns in the Wheel. So, for example, the stage itself was inherited from one solar system, and this represented the old devic pattern; the mix of elements was also taken from different systems, and then the actual wardrobe of life was the donated DNA that was gifted to the planet to host, within its own diversity, the new physical vehicles. Millions of different types of DNA were gifted according to the local body plans or fashions of each selected star system. So the streams of physical form that we would call bacteria, viruses, worms, insects, jellyfish, starfish, amphibians, reptiles, mammals such as primates and elephants, and so on, were all donated from different planetary streams. The different life forms were the different local variations and were either inherited or representative of the different flows of life. The planet itself was anchored on a vibratory note that could sustain and support these different uniforms of life, and then other patterns of life were created on the other, parallel Earths that were birthed and created to explore the different vibratory signatures.

The eighteen thousand Earths formed the template or substance of the Earth experiment and were like the arteries or tributaries of lived experience and form that streamed into the central Earth. Not only did all souls usually come through these eighteen thousand planets, but the flow of frequencies and experience were all directed into the centre, where the experiment allowed diversity to unfold against the backcloth of light and dark, and chaos and order.

The arrays of different life forms that have and are present on Earth represent the procession of diversity that was birthed out of the Wheel of Life. Earth has witnessed a procession of life, some of which is captured in our geological record, and which has manifested a series of major flora and fauna shifts according to the requirements of that time. So, the early Cambrian fauna with its huge diversity was a manifestation of one series of donated keys to the planet; later infusions and radiations of life around central body forms, such as the fish, amphibians, insects, reptiles, birds and mammals provided different central themes around which form could dance and evolve.

The dolphins and whales all came from a particular array of stars, just as the different patterns of DNA were donated from the planets and stars. Our inherited DNA is an ancient pattern of physical expression and the different life forms that we see are all part of this inherited pattern. There are planets where the insects dominate, or where spiders exist; where elephants are the dominant life form. On other planets, the carrots are the dominant life form, and within their vibratory universe see themselves as the masters of all that they survey. So the huge diversity of life, and all that we see in the fossil record, despite its incompleteness, is a reflection of the procession of life and the structure of DNA that has passed through the planet.

And in keeping with the succession of root races, life on the planet has formed, flourished and then become extinct according to the timeline and pulse of energy around which each root race was formed.

Frequency Holders and the Living Library

Once the Earth was formed and the unfolding pattern of root race expression was underway, certain souls, who had progressed through the Wheel of Life in specific ways, were given access to Earth to experience, more directly, the flux of life. These specific souls came to be known as frequency holders since they had experienced sufficient diversity within the Wheel of Life, through the different types of form and body plans that were available, to give them a different access note or recognition. These souls were offered an opportunity to reprise or re-experience in a different way everything that they had been through during the journey through the Wheel itself.

Each soul had been through a certain trajectory in the Wheel, sampling the different living forms, some of which we would recognise today, and some that we would not. Once on Earth, these souls then worked through the different donated physical vehicles present to give a different type of experience, and to recall, at a deeper level, memories of what they had been through before on distant planets. These ancestral memories gave them sufficient energetic flexibility to become the planetary frequency holders. Their role was to reprise and experience all of the energetic streams of life on Earth through their living vehicle at that time.

So, for example, in a lifetime, a particular soul may incarnate in Lemuria, and host a multiplicity of animal frequencies that were present then. Through their earned experience they could hold these frequency notes, and then broadcast them to others who were prepared to listen and absorb, and so could gain, at first hand, the direct experience of being a dinosaur, or a small mammal, or a frog or whatever particular animal frequency was flowing through at the time. The concentrated essence of the animal form that was present in the frequency holder could then form the lived experience for others to tap into. In a given life, the frequency holder would then shuttle through a proportion of life forms on the planet in his or her lived experience, and so gain a unique experience, rather like a replay of what that soul had experienced on those planets that originally hosted the life forms that the soul had connected with this time. Since telepathy was present at that time, others who were not the primary frequency holders could communicate with the frequency holders and experience the pattern of life form shuttling within their awareness, and so experience, in a direct way, the substance of what was to be a frequency holder.

The focus of the frequency holder was to gather and live the experience through the essence of love where a recognition of unity and diversity could be experienced. So some frequency holders might specialise in animal form, while others would focus on trees and flowers. And within each grouping, some lifetimes would be more specifically focused. For example, a frequency holder might work the pattern of reptilian and dinosaurian energies, where the old notes from the Wheel of Life would cord into their lived awareness, and they could then sense the origins and expression of the current lived forms. They might merge with a pterosaur and feel the freedom of flight, and then feel the essence of the donated DNA from the original planet in the Wheel where the pterosaurs were first birthed, and then resonate in and out between past and present. In this way, connections that are more direct could be built up between Earth and the other planets so that a two-way exchange of energy could speed up the pattern of development on the original planet.

As more and more streams of energy were built up in this way between the original planets and architects that donated the DNA, and the frequency holders, then the different streams of energy began to pulse and flow in and out of the Wheel. The frequency holders then worked through series after series of life form, retaining as a genetic memory, all that they had been and were.

The frequency holders could also store all of their experiences for the future, and as root races came and went, then the different frequency holders had various opportunities to experience the breadth and diversity of living form that was present at any one time, and to merge with the underlying pattern of DNA that hosted each form. Each frequency holder became adept at shuttling backwards and forwards through these libraries of lived frequencies, mastering the reptilian, mammalian, amphibian, invertebrate and so on. Each frequency that was lived was stored and an essence of the DNA hologram was downloaded into their systems, rather like a filing system. With time, these frequency holders then became the librarians or the host for all of the frequencies that had been through Earth. They became the living librarians of the total diversity of all life, as lived through the energetic hologram of the living DNA. Since all DNA on the planet was donated, then working directly with any aspect of living DNA allowed the frequency holders to access those original doorways in the Wheel.

However, during the later root races, the extensive tinkering with human DNA, both by the inhabitants of the planet and others, contributed to a significant energetic and physical pollution of our DNA. With this pollution came a loss of access and ability to flow in and out of the living libraries of DNA frequencies. There was a lack of stability and harmony in the DNA. Today, our DNA is heavily contaminated and has represented one of the major hurdles in the rebirthing of the new root race with physical vehicles strong enough to absorb and retain the new light frequencies coming in. As our DNA has been repaired within the subtle levels, this healing has started to flow down into the physical pattern of our double helix. The old pollutants are being stripped out and will eventually allow us to recapture a more refined and harmonised pattern of DNA expression. And with this new pattern of DNA vibration, we will, once again, be able to access the living libraries through our physical vehicles.

The original DNA matrix was birthed in a platform of mental light and then worked through the different permutations of astral light. Today, the constant manipulations of DNA has invoked a response in the astral, where our DNA is breaking down and malfunctioning more than ever, as part of the karmic response to what has taken place. These old DNA manipulations are being cleared out through various genetic disorders, cancers and other genetically-based diseases. At the same time, our DNA has been stripped down to its bare essentials. With only two physical strands of DNA, there is limited scope for housing the higher streams of light and in the future there will be some adjustment to our physical genetic make-up.

On the subtle levels, our DNA also has to be strengthened with an expansion to the full complement of twelve pairs of DNA now being demanded. This pattern of twelve will give greater balance, flexibility and scope. Each of these pairs will then provide a platform that will work with the different chakra centres, so that each DNA pairing will reflect a series of higher or lower energetic streams. On a basic level, the current structural pattern of DNA of two strands per helix represents the old pattern of chaos and order, light and dark. With the new pattern of light and dark, angelic and devic, and the new platforms of life being established through the different triangles of higher purpose, it remains to be seen whether the double helix will evolve into the triple helix. This would then embody the new triangle of energies.

Before some of the higher frequency changes to our DNA matrix can be introduced, the actual harmonics and frequencies contained within our genetic make-up need to be completely changed. The lack of harmony and imbalances within our DNA, and the subsequent physical expression through our cellular machinery, needs to change; the fundamental vibration of our DNA has to move out of the bottom half of the astral, into the top half of the astral and ultimately into the mental streams of light, where the hardcore re-wiring that is so necessary can take place according to the information and light that is waiting in the higher streams of mental light. Our DNA will become more crystalline and will host the higher streams of light and the new love vibrations that need to form the basis for our new physical vehicles. These will be seeded from the Seventh Plane. Higher guides are waiting patiently to assist with this process.

The living librarians hosted all of the different energies and DNA harmonics within their lived awareness; on one level they were like prototype donors that could allow other life forms to flow through them, and who could also allow the original donors, or planetary frequencies to flow through them as well, thereby establishing different links to the other solar systems that had become karmically involved with the planet. They were open doors to the lived diversity of frequencies that had been developed in the Wheel of Life and which were ultimately gifted to Earth. As living librarians, others could key into their energetic systems and access their frequency notes according to need, seeking the diversity of experiences that the librarians had to offer through lived experience.

In another way, the frequency holders were like doorways that offered the means for other life forms to experience more and to speed up their timelines through an active engagement of their energetic systems in matter. The living library, apart from being the unique energy systems of these frequency holders, was also the planet itself. The librarians, as frequency holders, allowed guests and visitors to experience, at first hand the uniqueness and beauty of all that the planet had to offer in any one cycle of thought. Today, the role of the librarians and frequency holders is changing. The old frequency holders that are still on the planet are now remembering who and what they are, and are beginning to pulse in unique ways again. Yet the new energies coming into the planet are demanding complete change, and in this change, many of the older life forms are now being offered the opportunity to go home.

So the librarians need to mutate into something different. The new timeline is bringing through new streams of light, and this means that the older frequencies will be stripped away. The platform of energies that the librarians have maintained will be overhauled and restructured to accommodate the new, higher frequencies. And within these new light frequencies, the pattern of DNA and its interrelationship with energetic expression in matter will be re-orchestrated. The old DNA patterns of energetic expression are tired and the pulse of light that flows through the current DNA is weak and has been heavily tampered with in the past. The original purity of the DNA has been lost for some considerable time, and all of the older negative frequencies now contained in DNA need to be removed. The living template that the librarians need to utilise has to be dramatically enhanced to support a new type of library of frequencies and a new type of librarian.

The new librarians will become more crystalline, as the human form slowly evolves into a more crystalline pattern of energy, where purity and power can combine to produce something new. The new librarians will then become the frequency holders for new holograms of light that will contain much more than was ever possible in the past. The librarians will host the huge diversity of new holograms of life that will be birthed in the new multiple timelines that are now forming. They will begin to vibrate to the new harmonics of light that can be captured within their essence, and with time, the frequency holders will learn to pulse in and out of time, and to move backwards and forwards in time, learning to feel the lived experience of past, present and future life forms. The living library will therefore become a multiple-dimensional series of portals to all of the planets and stars within the Wheel, as well as contain the different time streams of those life forms that have yet to be birthed on the planet.

New Patterns

What takes place on Earth will ultimately be seeded out into the Wheel of Life. This means that, like Earth, the Wheel has to undergo something of a clearing and cleansing process. The older astral frequencies will be removed, and those extra-terrestrial souls that have become locked into the physical planes at the point of death, will also be moved on through a pattern of extra-terrestrial rescue work that will complement the work now being done on Earth. Simultaneously, as more souls are waking up, there is a grand shuffling of frequencies and sparks; the sparks that have gone out into the shadow planes are all manifested in the Wheel of Life. New sparks are forming in the process of re-igniting established by the Avatar.

Like sparks flowing through multiple streams and levels, the new patterns of change are manifested in every stream of thought and existence within the Wheel of Life. The eighteen thousand spokes and the three primary Earths in the centre host the different pulses and streams of energy, like principal regulators. As Earth evolves, then the other two Earths change, mirroring the central Earth, and obeying the law of opposites. The three Earths also collectively mirror the pattern of change within the soul's three permanent atoms, where the one central atom is reflected in the other two atoms through the focus of masculine and feminine, while all the time reflecting the law of opposites and the vibratory laws therein. Change is therefore manifesting on all levels, from the fundamental level of the primary permanent atom through to the planet, and then into the Wheel of Life. The new pattern of black and white light and chaos and order is being woven into the very fabric of the Wheel to bring about a profound change in its entire substance and focus.

The new beginnings on Earth will be transferred first to the eighteen thousand Earths, and then into the outer hub of the Wheel where all the other planets and stars reside. This in itself represents a break from the past where the outer hub has not always received the frequencies that were originally birthed in the central Earth. The new birth of Gaia and Macheldavek on Earth has brought about another birthing, where Gaia has given birth to Macheldavek. And this new birthing has been seeded into the Wheel of Life, so that each planet now has a twin of the new Gaia and Macheldavek. The brothers and sisters of Macheldavek and Gaia are also coming into a new pattern of energy and focus, mirroring the new energetic platform that has been birthed. All of this represents massive change within the Wheel and the beginning of a brand new stream of energy. Similarly the pattern of soul involution has been speeded up, and on each planet in the Wheel, one soul has been accelerated to host a new type of frequency that can act as a catalyst and beacon for those other life forms to focus on.

The energetic changes that are being birthed on Earth in the new timeline will be pushed out to the Wheel. The new timeline, as it is birthed on Earth, will then pulse to the other Earths and set up a resonant harmonic where the other Earths will begin to resonate to the new timeline. This will invoke wholesale change, and like wildfire, the Wheel of Life will pulse to the new timeline and give birth to itself through this new stream of consciousness.

Death

While the Wheel of Life provides every soul with an opportunity to experience multiple frequencies, the new timeline will also demand a dramatic change in our understanding about death. In the West there is a widespread belief that we have only one life and that after death there is nothing. In the East, it is recognised that we reincarnate many times although the precise mechanism and focus of this pattern is not always understood. Physical death and the actual process of dying is one of the major areas where misinformation has been keyed into our systems. The old dark frequencies closed down our capacity to understand death. We now retain so much fear around death and if fear is to be banished from the planet, then the fear of dying will also have to be removed. There is little or no understanding of what our physical death represents and no concept that the process of death is just a transition stage between one level of awareness or being and another.

Death represents a point of change where we drop one body that has been borrowed for a set period of time, and then return to the inner planes where we digest and consider the lessons that were learnt during our life, and then plan for the next incarnation. When we die, it is like we are leaving one harbour where our loved ones and friends bid us farewell, and then head directly for another harbour, where another group of our friends are waiting to welcome us back home. The actual process of dying is the mechanism through which all cordings are cut between our higher vehicles of consciousness, such as our astral and mental bodies, and the physical body. When we drop our body we enter a different state where we vibrate at a different level and where our ability to interact with the physical is removed. The soul aspect will leave the physical vehicle through the crown chakra, and in the minutes before death, each of the chakras will slowly close down as the life force energy drains out of the physical body. The process of death is like an in-breath and an out-breath that gets weaker and weaker, as the soul essence severs all its physical ties.

The process of death arises when the soul turns its focus away from the physical vehicle and so the focus of energy is removed from the body. It is, however, the devic presence in the body that concentrates so keenly on surviving and continuing to live at all costs. This is why the physical drive to survive is so prevalent and strong. Yet the actual process of dying is simple and straightforward and is like adopting a change of clothing or uniform. If the actual process is accepted through surrendering, then it becomes easier since there is no resistance.

When a person dies, they will usually hang around the vacant, physical shell for a few days afterwards, before moving up into the different light streams. It can take many months or years in Earth time for a soul aspect to find its resting position on the inner planes. However, sometimes when the death itself has been traumatic, or old emotional attachments from those still alive call out to the departed soul, then it can take much longer to move on and souls can become trapped. Young souls will often be more confused than older souls, since they lack the necessary experience to find their way home and to recognise the various transition states.

Where an individual has suffered a traumatic death or a life of great pain and difficulty, then they will be taken to a holding plane where they can rest and sometimes enter a state of slumber where the memories of the previous incarnation can fade away. Similarly, if a soul has been actively involved in great patterns of destruction and death, then they will be left to rest and recover for many years before incarnating again.

In normal situations though, the soul aspect will push up through the astral layers into different streams of light. As it does this, it will systematically shed the different layers of its astral body, thereby seeming to reverse the aging process and becoming gradually younger. The different astral experiences may be replayed back to that soul and in circumstances where a life has ended prematurely, then the remaining portion can be played out on the astral levels.

Unfortunately, many people grieve the death of loved ones

to the extent that their emotions act as a binding mechanism to the departing soul. Often a person will hang onto life because those around him or her do not want to let go. This is a point of limitation. Rather the attitude should be to rejoice that the soul has the opportunity to go back home and actually to move back into a different stream of existence where they are eternal. And given that we have so many millions of lives to practice everything, then the actual death should be of no great consequence. However, in the current climate of our conditioning, this is a difficult view to accept since people have no understanding of what is experienced in life after death.

During our life, we will have certain points where we have probable deaths. These are like exit points in our contract where the soul can opt out. Some newborn babies, when they incarnate, find that the physical vehicle is not to their liking, and so drop their bodies almost straight away. Consequently cot deaths and other unexplained causes of infant death are part of this process. However, if we die at our appointed time, as specified in our contract, then we are usually met on the other side. This can be by old loved ones, or the Angel of Death, or some other level of guidance. If we successfully complete our contract then there is plenty of celebrating. In situations where we drop our bodies prematurely, then there may not be anyone to meet us, and this can be where confusion arises.

Premature deaths also release certain amounts of electrical energy. This applies to all physical form, be it human, animal or otherwise, where the physical body will hold a specified quantity of electrical energy necessary for that individual or organism to live to old age. If the life ends prematurely, then this electrical energy is released. Consequently, the huge number of deaths during the 1st and 2nd World Wars released massive quantities of electrical energy that helped open up a new pattern of energy that was used as part of the invocation of the new timeline by Meher Baba in the 1920's.

Today, as the new energies are building, more people are going through near-death experiences, either as a means of shedding karma through crisis, or as a way to show them that life, and the after-life, are separated by a veil, and that after dropping the body, then the soul aspect continues to exist as a vehicle of consciousness.

As the soul aspect goes through millions and millions of deaths, diversity of experience is built up. All of these millions of births and deaths are all part of the reincarnatory process, and each one is a small transition, rather like being asleep and waking up. They are all small transitions when compared to the complete spiritual death at God-realisationship. God-realisationship is the one true death that all souls will ultimately experience, and this is the death of Illusion and waking up to Reality.

CHAPTER 23

Collective Unity & The Elderings

Creating Something New

In the Lemurian times an attempt was made to create something new within the focus of the energy that was prevailing at that time. The experiment was only partially successful and today we are presented with another unique opportunity to birth something more under the umbrella of the Avatar's irradiation of one hundred percent of Himself. The changes that are being manifested today are all part of what was seeded a long time ago. The idea at that time was simple: to birth collective unity within a diversity of different sparks, where each spark had a different set of attributes derived from the higher streams of light. And for each spark that was birthed, the challenge would be for it to wake up, remember, and then do something about it.

So, in the Ocean of Life new souls were birthed that would host different attributes such as power, purity, innocence, hope, love, light and so on. In the process of birthing, each of these different souls was exposed to a particular light or a particular spark of a specific vintage. Each soul that was birthed then began its downward journey into the shadow planes where it experienced a latent, specific dissatisfaction with the primary disciplines of the various levels because each soul was looking for something more. Each soul wanted a duplication of the light that had helped birth it and yet was unable to find it.

Another way of looking at this is to recognise that each soul that had an attribute was given a specific focus of light that was more concentrated and so when the soul then dropped down into the shadow planes, it felt a distinct lack and was therefore motivated to seek ways to bridge or feed that lack. So, as the soul would look in different directions for that which it lacked, it was driven to search over and over again through all the millions of experiences in the inner and outer realms. The search forced the individual soul, the individual personality, to focus and to be driven by the need to remember, to define and eventually to become that which initially it was exposed to. Through this constant searching, each soul was eventually forced to feed the lack and then invoke something more out of that which it lacked. This then, ultimately, led to a merging with the essence of something new, of something more. So each soul would seek out its focus or attribute and through the law of opposites would be driven to fill the gap and eventually then to embody it and become that new attribute.

For example, a soul may have a predisposition towards attributes such as power or knowledge. These attributes would originally be seeded into the soul through a specific vintage of light. The soul would then experience lifetimes of powerlessness and ignorance, where it would explore all the different permutations of life around that attribute. Lacking knowledge or power means that each soul searches for it and so learns through adversity to build up a pool of experiences that will ultimately feed each attribute and build up a charge. Eventually, there would come a time when that soul would experience power or knowledge, and this would be washed through all of the previous experiences of the opposites of powerlessness or ignorance. The experience of power or knowledge would be much more because of the soul's previous pathway and would within that moment, create a new type of knowledge or power, fuelled by all that had gone before. In this process of building something new, it is like we always start with a lack or an opposite that can then drive the energy in a particular direction through many life times. So in the programme that is being unfolded today, many different souls have been through a variety of training programmes and trajectories to birth or host a specific set of attributes. In nearly all cases this has required that the souls build up a huge voltage in darkness, in negativity, developing the will through the different streams of chaos.

For each soul that worked the different patterns of darkness there came a point when free will and choice allowed it to turn to the light. And through experiencing all of the dark patterns of light, each soul then built up a huge bank of dark energy that can now act as an anchor to the new streams of light coming in. At the same time, the old experiences have given each soul a background in slow frequency, light management that is extremely useful today. Within this pattern of birthing new attributes, an occasional rare soul would host an entirely unique pattern and this would allow the other souls to swarm around it and to merge with it in a different way to create something uniquely different.

The pattern of change that is now being manifested has been built on developing new attributes in different souls so that the old concepts of knowledge, power, truth, wisdom, bliss, innocence and purity can be replaced by a new vintage of each of these.

At the same time, each of these souls has been given the opportunity to look for something that is more. What they each lacked has created a hunger for more, and so in the higher streams of light, in the wake of the Avatar's pathway back home, a new type of spark has been seeded that embodies a certain type of love with a specific quality of light that attracts souls towards it. It is like a moth being drawn to a flame. This flame has been established past the First, Second and Third Divine Journeys and acts as a beacon, so that souls pushing through these different Divine Journeys are not trapped by the illusion of bliss where the fragmented patterns of the Father entrances them; instead, there is a hunger to push on upwards to further aspects higher up in the light, without going sideways.

For each soul, each spark, to traverse up the different Divine Journeys, there is a type of protocol that has to be developed. This protocol is directed at what the Primary Spark originally manifested in its downward journey: a whole series of mirrors. As the Primary Spark came down, it formed millions and millions of mirrors of what it is up there. But each mirror mirrors what is above, and every so often aperture points form in between these different layers. These aperture points actually irradiate a sort of amplification or a pulse that comes in. This pulse produces the shadowlands as a product of its activity. So everything that is played out in shadowlands has, as its initial starting point, a pulse from the Seventh Plane. The final end result may be heavily diluted, but the shadow experience will be like an afterimage of what was originally seeded.

In the process of sparking that was manifested by the Primary Spark in its downward journey, and in each of the layers that were created, a whole series of laws and regulations were formed and enforced. An analogy is if a person gets up from a table and walks across to someone else at a nearby table; with every step she leaves an aspect of herself behind. Each aspect is like a separate expression or mirror and will regard that step as its own territory and will seek to enforce this through the application of will. So for someone else to walk through that aspect, or in that person's pathway, will require that the second person resonates precisely with what the original person was and will be before they can pass through it. In other words each soul has to mirror exactly and live exactly that which is the particular territory at that time. This has to be done time and time again through each mirror, or each Divine Journey. So the pattern of moving up through the different Divine Journeys is extremely precise and is about mirroring what each Journey contains and being able to capture and match that essence.

Balance Through the Divine Journeys

Apart from mirroring and resonating with each Divine Journey, each soul has to master a pattern of collective unity. The retention of any individualistic patterns makes it almost impossible for a soul to push through into more. But each Divine Journey is unique and presents its own set of challenges. The brilliance of the light hides what is beyond it and also drowns out what is in front: it is like staring at the sun – we become blinded and can see nothing beyond or around it. For each Divine Journey there is a sun that gives us a quality of light that stops us seeing the sparks on the other side. Each time we go through it, we keep on seeing another version of the Father, a vibration that gives us a different presentation of life, the Universe and everything. Each Journey is more refined, so the further we go up the more refined it is, and yet with each refinement there is an impulse to fragment. This impulse to fragment has to be overcome by the living will and with the impulse to stretch up into more, there is a corresponding need to anchor in the physical. So each soul as it passes through a Divine Journey has to undergo a unique balancing act of focusing and pushing up, while maintaining the physical desire to remain anchored.

So in pushing through the First, Second and Third Divine Journeys all souls experience a null or nothing space within the focus of the light. It is like the mirror of the Journey has been matched, but the upward pull of the next Journey is not sufficient to call to the advancing soul, while the downward pull of the previous Journey and the physical is insufficient as a grounding device. And it is in this nothing space that souls can tend to get lost and confused within the brilliance of the light, where there is no up, or down, or sideways. This can be experienced as a physical spinning where there is no real anchor point within the awareness. It is at this point that the application of will is required, combined with the recognition of the importance of our collective unity. And with focus, it is like physically holding the attention of the soul to ensure that the focus is always maintained.

In the Fourth Divine Journey, the pattern of manifestation is different from the previous three: there is a blue ocean that is the contained essence of all that has ever been through the Perfect Masters. Once this pattern has been mirrored, the soul then passes into the Fifth Divine Journey where a different pattern is manifested. Here the energy is like a primary spark that lifts the soul up into ever more brilliant streams of light. For each soul there is a balance or compromise to be made: if it goes into the light too quickly, then it will burn up, and if it goes into the light too slowly, then it will not get through. So, there is always the potential to be claimed at any particular point of any specific Divine Journey where the intensity of light is too much. And the only way to endure this onslaught is to be collective.

So the Avatar has come down and is now returning and in this return, one spark is following Him all the way up, and in this is creating the capacity to return again. Once this one spark has forged a pathway back, then other sparks can follow in its footsteps and forge a new pathway. Not all of the sparks will go all of the way back up and instead will enter a holding mechanism. And as the sparks build in the different Divine Journeys, then some will go up and some will come down, earthing the essence of each of the different Divine Journeys within the gravitational pull of the planet and all life on it. And if another, unique spark can come down, then a new pattern will emerge. In the beginning the initial spark was the Avatar coming down and returning; now He wants a second original spark, and then perhaps a third one and a fourth one. In the fullness of time, the planet will then become an Avataric School rather than a school for the Avatar to come down to inspect shadowlands from time to time.

Those sparks that are progressing through the different Divine Journeys are mirroring the fifty percent head and fifty percent heart of the planet through the focus of new black light and new white light. The match is half and half, so as dark light is burnt off through the higher light, more is added to the mix through the masculine and the feminine. It is like living chaos and order in every moment, in every instant, through a pattern of differentiation. Each pattern of differentiation is like a tool to generate more balance and part of the progression into more.

In living the moment in and out of time, in the different streams of light that are now manifesting down from the Seventh Plane, then those souls that have embraced more can spark in everything in creation. There is an interplay of light and dark that helps to anchor in the new light and what has been added to this mixture is a new level of creation that was the birthing of the new black light; this helps to anchor in the pattern of higher light. This new black light is, as we have seen, a more primeval devic expression that will allow the sparks to go higher up.

And there will come a time where there will be a point of balance and neutralisation. As the new dark light fills everything to the top part of the Sixth Plane, and the souls push up collectively into the higher levels of condensed light in the Seventh Plane, the whole shape of the collective energy becomes like a diamond. The top reaches into the rarefied levels of the Seventh Plane, while the bottom tip touches the bottom of the Zero Plane.

So the totality of the programme to date has created an original spark and that spark, as it came down, created a residue of dark light. This pattern is a type of mastery of the old frequencies and has helped to anchor the living awareness of the few souls that have rapidly accelerated up in the footsteps of this original spark. All of these old frequencies are being burnt out very quickly by the new pattern of light now coming in. The pattern of new dark light acts as a counterbalance, providing additional anchors as the light becomes more and more condensed. Without this new pattern of black light, the higher light would claim the physical vehicles of those souls pushing upwards through the different Divine Journeys. And if that happens, then the soul is held at that level or Divine Journey at which it was claimed, since their individual light is not condensed enough. So the pattern is to push up, following in the footsteps of the Avatar, and to go into the deeper spaces of God in the Beyond State

In undertaking this pattern, those souls that then work through the different Divine Journeys will entice other souls that have become trapped to follow them. For example, if a soul pushes through the First, Second and Third Divine Journeys, then it will feel those souls that have been trapped in the bliss following in its orbit. These souls pushing up then experience the bliss manifesting as flashes of wakefulness. The bliss is a lived emotion, like a hypersensitivity in the body, coupled with feelings of vulnerability, a great deal of love and a feeling of more that has to be satisfied. And the more that the soul pushes up through the different Divine Journeys, then the grosser the light is in the physical plane and the more distasteful it will seem. The accelerating souls will either seek to hide from it unless they can understand it.

From the standpoint of higher light, to understand the light we live in the physical plane means that we have to be exposed to it, to live it and then to become balanced in it through free will and choice. Those souls that are unconscious of their newly found status on the Seventh Plane will not recognise this in the same way. Instead, they still retain their capacity to work with their old habits and desires, while bringing in the slow frequency energy of the shadow planes as their normal formula. So they are living desire without really recognising they are without desire. But they can only do this for a short period of time otherwise they burn themselves out. Just like those souls that are conscious of being God-realised, these unconsciously realised souls will borrow different astral and mental bodies to go about their business in the shadow planes. Their presence will irradiate a unique pattern of light and they will absorb any slow frequency energy that they come into contact with.

With these different, multiple streams of light, the pattern of soul involution is already speeding up and intensifying as part of the Nine-Pointed Plan. This is a one-off pattern at present and is part of the changeover in Avataric Energy. So, in addition to the new levels of access to the different Divine Journeys, principally from the First Divine Journey through to the Twelfth Divine Journey by those souls that have become God-realised and have invoked for more, there is also a big shift in shadowlands. A new vibratory pool of intense black light is spiralling down where the new devic essence is becoming more co-operative. This will give a new type of pattern where the end result will be that all the souls that have manifested already in humanity can speed up their involution and can move up the planes that much quicker. So, in the grand scheme of things there is a move to speed everything up, working from the Zero Plane all the way up to the Sixth Plane and then into the first three Divine Journeys.

Collective Sparking and the Swarm

A grand programme is now manifesting through the Avatar. The one hundred percent irradiation that He came down with is touching absolutely everything. He has come down, illuminated everything from where He is in the God in the Beyond State. As the everything and the nothing is illuminated, then the various departments of the Muhammad and the Christ have also been revealed. As His pattern of Light has come down and gone back up, each individual that now becomes God-realised is given a choice, as an ongoing spark, to gravitate one way into one of the departments or to permutate and to carry on going up into the higher levels of the God in the Beyond State. And as each soul that chooses to permutate and carry on going up, then the other souls that are doing the same thing begin to revolve around each other, creating a vortex like a new DNA matrix. The flow of souls spinning around each other, and in the pattern of movement up and down the different Divine Journeys, is creating a new matrix or hologram that, once fully formed, will seed a new platform of divinity through the essence of what the Father was, is and will be in each of the different Journeys.

Now as this vortex of light is created up there, then it can be brought down here into the physical. This represents, on one level, the rebuilding of our chakra system. So the further the collective souls go up, and then the further they come back down, then more is created. Eventually, the matrix will spin through the twelve Divine Journeys seeding a new essence within the DNA matrix of the physical units present and into the new chakra system. The new chakra system will then provide access to an entirely new level of light, while the DNA matrix will resonate to a new harmonic of divine light. There is clearly some way to go before this is completed. Currently, the chakra system has been built up to about the solar plexus where there is a requirement to develop a new emotional protocol that can support the new light. And within that emotional protocol, souls will be required to open up to a new mental dialogue.

At the same time as the new chakra system is forming, the pattern of sparking in the First and Second Divine Journeys is undergoing a profound change. As the souls that have been trapped in bliss are moved up, they begin to burst into flame, so that the pathway up through these early Divine Journeys becomes a living flame. This is happening initially in the First Divine Journey and then is being repeated in the Second Divine Journey, so that a grand release is taking place. It is important to remember that there is no time up there so that the pattern of manifestation will filter into our consciousness through a series of sequences, or dreamscapes.

For the souls that are building into this new collective pattern, their experience in shadowlands is also building into something uniquely different. They see everything out there and know that it is an illusion. They experience all of the other levels through the different permutations and mixtures of light; each of these felt and lived experiences have to be put into some semblance of reality or lived understanding. This is not a mental exercise and can only be done at a deep level by taking the one permanent atom back up into the light and then back down again, thereby fashioning a dialogue that can be lived in the moment. In this way, souls can experience being on a particular Divine Journey and then coming back down. It is a bit like part of the soul is in a specific Divine Journey, and then another part is in the First Plane, and that through going up and down, then the awareness will be up in the specific Divine Journey as well as in the shadow plane. This process is done in sequence so that eventually each soul will build up a pattern where it is one hundred percent up there and one hundred percent down here. And when this happens, the soul will have the capacity to see and to feel all of the time. It cannot be switched off. In this experience light is light; there is no darkness and there is no light. There is just simply something more, a quality of light or love that will birth more aspects of the Father coming into a soul's space and then be expressed through the collective dialogue of humanity.

As these souls experience the new collective pattern, multiple streams of light will flow through them like waves. The energy will demand that each individual express it in one way or another; if the energy is ignored or not utilised creatively, then it will turn back on the individual. So the lived expression of the moment, where the energy is allowed to flow and the individual gives free expression to what makes them happy and excited, will ensure a balanced expression of the incoming energy.

This stretching or expansion of each soul up and down the planes and the Divine Journeys, as manifested through lived awareness, can only be done through the collective platform of unity that is being established. A collective spark, like a hive or a swarm, is being birthed so that within that swarm, individual sparks can go up and down.

Within this pattern of going up and down, there are also multiple tiers of sponsors who are either sympathetic or unsympathetic to the newly forming patterns of energy. Some embrace change, while others resist it. Each level has to be convinced to participate in the new ritual of becoming and birthing, just as when we work through different plane levels on the shadow planes, we have to work with different tiers of guides. However, the collective pattern is helping to provide a solid platform where the resistant energy can ultimately be persuaded to co-operate and to then flow into a different living stream of becoming more.

Within the different planes and Journeys, there are various patterns of soul stasis or progression. As each of the lower Divine Journeys is cleared out, then the souls that were stuck move on. The collective pattern of the swarm, which represents all of the souls that have invoked for more and who are following in the footsteps of the Avataric irradiation, is moving up and down. Within this flux, there are those that wish to move on and those that do not. In this movement, the collective swarm will help to move on those souls that are trapped or fragmented. So within each stage, a different level of freedom is gifted to those that were previously trapped within a specific pattern of bliss. Over time, the internal space of the swarm will build so that it can push through the wall of indifference, ignorance and fear, and match the rules and regulations each step of the way, so that ultimately, a more collective upward motion can be attempted that will build on what has gone before.

This inner planes language has to be learnt and understood. Meher Baba has laid it out in a vibratory sequence in *Discourses* and *God Speaks.* He has also given one hundred percent of Himself which means that He has exposed everything, so that the limitation is whether our psyches and energetic systems can absorb all that is being offered. If we become awake enough as a living spark, then we can command a flame, which means that we can have millions and millions of sparks going into us, without actually being fragmented or dissuaded from our journey. With a collective flame, as opposed to an individual flame, we become bigger, and instead of losing volume as we go up in the condensed pattern of light, we gain volume or mass so our flame expands. This collective flame then draws up within its vortex all of those souls that have been trapped on the first three Divine Journeys and then allows them all to wake up. In this process of waking up, they can become much more aware of another level of the Father manifesting at this time.

So the Father's Plan is to develop a different type of spark, which is half light and half dark. At a point in the future, this spark is going to become completely white for a brief moment. And when this happens there will be a role reversal where we will have seventy-five percent positive and twenty-five percent negative as opposed to what it was when Meher Baba was in physical form. In 2069, everybody's vibration is going to spark off in a different way. Consequently, if we look at the planet now from outer space, there is a huge amount of light forming because there is a collective swarm manifesting for the first time. In this formation, there will be an expansion that will touch everything in the Wheel of Life. The Wheel will expand and at the same time a different undercurrent to creation, that which has manifested and brought through the new pattern of dark light, will also come into play more strongly.

And eventually, when the Second Primary Spark comes down, and the different shadow planes and Divine Journeys have been re-structured, then the Divine Ocean of Life will be refilled by a new quality of light that is driven down by the irradiation of the new Primary Spark's essence as manifested through its will. At the same time, this new Primary Spark will also spark the new chakras – all twelve, into something that is more, through the irradiation of that light that is manifesting. The new formation of light will then truly have become much more.

Absorbing Common Sense

Within this pattern of invoking more, and where the collective unity is forming a new swarm of light, then each soul within that swarm will experience more. As we have seen, time is a standard mechanism of experimentation where the assets and limitations are explored through experience; that experience then builds from the multiple levels of sparking from the Primary Spark into a flame of understanding. This flame is focused through will and as it develops, gives wisdom, which takes it from understanding through knowledge. Yet, wisdom is not the end point in this process, and in the collective absorption of everything, the experiences that each individual soul lacks can be gathered through the collective and ultimately birthed within each soul's awareness.

Those souls that are waking up then have a conscious choice — to remain passive-passive or to become passive-dynamic. Once awake, it is not possible for a soul to go back off to sleep under normal circumstances; nor is it possible to hide from the energy since it is always there, given that there is no time or space. As the multiple veils shatter within a soul's waking consciousness, then it goes through streams of perpetually waking up into more, and accessing more information, knowledge, understanding and wisdom. And in this process, the individuality has to die.

In the Mineral, Plant, and Animal Kingdoms, souls follow a collective pattern that then becomes individual in the human theatre. In human form, we experience millions and millions of lifetimes as individuals, and now we have come to a point where we have to be collective once again, but not collective unconsciousness. Instead we have to be collectively awake where we will come to know everything.

Within the pattern of developing the new platform of collective unity, each soul has the potential to gather more and more experience. Once a soul drops its body, then the experiences cannot be duplicated in the higher streams of light. The pattern of physical manifestation on Earth is therefore unique. Consequently, the collective focus can allow souls to gather much more experience than through any individualistic pattern. The collective pattern is now seeking to birth common sense into humanity in a virulent and direct way.

Common sense represents the end point of the sequence of experience from information, knowledge, understanding, and wisdom through to common sense. With common sense, the soul does not need the information or wisdom to determine what is more – common sense gives a new level of knowing what needs to be done without the need for any knowledge or information. It is like the soul knows the answers at a deep level. The result is that if a soul has not had enough experience then it can go outside time and bring it back into time down here. This additional experience can be condensed into a conscious knowing that is common sense. So as an aspect of God, each soul goes out of time and is imbued with common sense and then has the opportunity to live it and then wake up fully in the manifestation of what that is, bringing all of this back into time. Common sense is like the complete package where in seconds a soul can receive, for example, eighteen thousand lifetimes worth of experience. So common sense pulls a soul out of the abyss of misunderstanding and allows it to open up and become a flame. As this flame the soul will know everything, although it might not be able to explain it. It will live the dream of separation but know that everything is illusion.

Common sense will raise the vibratory levels of our conscious awareness where we will experience and live everything. And with our new light bodies, we will have the capacity to flow into full consciousness with a recognition and knowing of the different levels of awareness, and a living consciousness of the devas, the angels, the star brothers and sisters, and the Elderings.

The Eldering Unity

As the new timeline forms then the pattern of collective energy will build to a new intensity. The timeline is the manifestation of grace, which is like the Will of the Father. With the new platform of collective unity being established, it will then be possible for the planet and humanity to host the Elderings in a more dynamic way. The Elderings embody absolutely everything, and on one level are the architects of the overall root race programme under the Will of the Father. As the divine administrators, they have been in attendance throughout the different root races to date and will be in attendance, in one way or another, until the completion of the Twelfth Root Race. They are a collective pattern that was seeded out of the highest levels of light and contain within them, absolutely everything that is necessary for the new root race timeline.

As each individual wakes up to the new timeline, there will be an opportunity to receive and absorb the essence of the Elderings within either a concentrated or diluted format according to need. The Elderings within their collective focus will ride and experience our awareness and place within us the seeds that will flower into the new light streams necessary for our development. The Eldering light is utterly brilliant and at first the twin frequencies of blue and purple light will be birthed into selected individuals, before other frequencies such as green come on line. The collective unity of love, harmony and power will then become manifest in a more virulent way as the collective platform becomes established in humanity and is then mirrored within the divinity of the Elderings. The Elderings will birth yet another level of collective unity within humanity as they ride the awareness of humans at first as individual humans touched by their collective essence, and then as collective humans merged in the collective unity of the Elderings.

Once the Elderings have accessed humanity's awareness and emotions, they will then feel like a constant companion or presence within us. We will have direct access to their light streams and they, in turn, will have the living authority to show us absolutely everything about everything. To ensure that humanity can systematically build up to this new frequency level, the interaction between the new devas and new angels will provide a platform for the few, and then the many, to host and house the new Eldering frequencies.

The essence of the new devas will balance the new angelic order, and these two patterns, like opposite twins, will then provide the stable structure for humanity to live and become the living essence of Eldering light. So the Eldering frequencies will be birthed into us systematically and with an increasing level of intensity. In a very real way the Elderings represent the new light streams of information, knowledge, love, wisdom and conscious awareness that need to be birthed. And the Elderings will bring through a new expression of unity and one that will open humanity up to much, much more.

For the new expression of light, this is the beginning of a series of patterns that the Elderings are establishing within the future root races. As the wash of the old root races passes through humanity, there will then be new opportunities to go down the future timelines of the future root races and to access that which is more, both in and out of time. The Elderings will provide an energetic hologram within which this can be achieved.

At the same time, the new timeline is offering the opportunity for the new probability that will be manifested through the new crystal skull that is selected to birth the essence of the Sixth Root Race. The Father has a large number of different crystal skulls that could become the new template for the new root race, and whichever one is selected will depend upon the unity that is achieved. So within the living moment, as the swarm builds, it is now time to invoke and bring through the grace and unity of love, coupled with purity and innocence from above, so that the perfection that is manifested through the imperfection can vibrate higher and higher. It is like thinking no negative thoughts and allowing the positive, higher frequency thoughts to unfold and create the living reality of higher light on the planet in the now. As the new Sixth Root Race crystal skull is birthed in the new timeline, then the pre-existing new crystalline beacons that have been established around the planet will light up and become activated. The planet will then begin to pulse to a new crystalline rhythm.

So as the new Eldering presences grace and ride the awareness of humanity through the collective infusion of higher light, then each individual will access the new collective essence and will be free to become more within the new timeline. Each individual will be like a walking ashram, where the love and grace of the Father will resonate inside, so that no external structures will be required to symbolise our unity and love of the Father; we will live the unity and oneness inside so that we will become the living ashrams within our own physical space. So where in the past, places of worship and ashrams were required, the new pattern that is being birthed in the West is to manifest the essence of light inside and for the ashram to be held in the heart and then radiated out as a point of living, conscious awareness of divinity within. The flame of wisdom and knowledge will burn within, wrapped with love and power to manifest higher desire. In this new representation of the living ashram, then each soul will embody the essence of the spark that was, is and will be birthed through the in breath and out breath of the Avataric Will. One Avataric Day will close and then a new Avataric Day will dawn. And within that dawning, humanity will experience in the illusion, true unity and union with the Elderings, and the higher streams of sparking that are part of the Father and the Son within the stream of conscious living awareness. And as a new Primary Spark is formed, so a brand new game of divinity will be birthed according to that which has been ordained by the Father.

As the new level of unity and light builds, then humanity can start to resonate along the new timeline, experiencing between the devic and angelic flows of light, the resonant harmony of a new crystalline heritage that will be birthed in the future. The platform for this grid is being established around the planet through the different presences of new crystal skulls that have been birthed from the higher mental streams and which are now building into a pattern that will broadcast the new irradiation of mental and higher light in the coming years. Once these new patterns build, humanity will then hear a call from the future that will shatter the veil of ignorance and invoke a new pattern of growth and divinity into the future.

CHAPTER 24

The Cosmic Christ

Birthing Return of the Cosmic Christ

If we look at the pulse of the past root races, then we can feel that the Lemurian is now fading but the Atlantean remains quite hostile and virulent. The Aryan Root Race is still with us and has, in one sense, been all about preparation – for the Christ. Over the last forty thousand years humanity has lived the dark night of the soul. But this is now changing and the suffering of the past is being replaced by the hope of the future. This period of preparation has been extremely necessary and it is now time for the pendulum to swing in the opposite direction. The Christ represents peace and so a period of unprecedented peace will unfold. In addition at this point in time, there is an esoteric vote taking place between what has gone before and what is coming.

The physical presence of the Christ on the planet two thousand years ago as the living Avatar established a new platform. Within this platform of energy, the Christ irradiated seventy-five percent compared to the one hundred percent of Meher Baba. The focus of the Christ was on birthing a new type of love, compassion and understanding. In order to bring this about, the Christ had to absorb the hatred, intolerance and ignorance that were present in humanity. The crucifixion represented a culmination of all His work in physical form where the spear of ignorance and misunderstanding could be absorbed through His living will. The blood of the Christ was spilt onto the planet and ordained that absolute change would have to take place. The utter and primeval ignorance of the past would have to make way for a new type of knowledge; one that would infuse the living moment. For the last two thousand years, humanity has been preparing more specifically for the new frequencies of the Sixth Root Race since it is these that will ultimately give birth to the Cosmic Christ. This birth will represent the return of the Cosmic Christ in physical form as the living Avatar when humanity is ready, willing and able to absorb what is on offer.

Preparations for this new birth are underway and form part of the ascendancy of new energies and the new sparks that are being birthed in the Seventh Plane. The Avatar of the Age, Meher Baba, has ordained change and this is manifesting as a crisis in humanity. All the old rituals and descriptions of what God was and is are outmoded and no longer resonate with the new timeline. The different religions are struggling to find a point of reference and are falling back on fixed concepts that are frozen in the past. They do not resonate with the present, let alone the future. And if we look far enough into the future down the new timeline of grace, then there is a distant figure coming towards us. This figure is the Cosmic Christ and over the next ten to twelve million years, the human race will be preparing for this arrival.

One way to attempt to understand this process is to sense that the Cosmic Christ is a pure and utterly exquisite essence of divinity, like one of the Father's most treasured and special sparks that was birthed in the highest levels of the Seventh Plane. At the time of the physical Christ, this essence was irradiated to humanity in a diluted form and the afterglow of that vibration is still with us. Since all of this takes place outside of time, preparations are underway to merge this essence of the Cosmic Christ in its entirety with the future Avatar that will grace the planet in the distant future. The spark that is the Cosmic Christ has merged with another primary spark to set up a sequence of events that will culminate in the physical birth of the Cosmic Christ. And, in a very real sense, the roadway that has formed down the new timeline is pulsing into the Cosmic Christ.

There is a two-way flow of energy. The Cosmic Christ is

coming down the future timeline towards humanity, while those in physical matter who can host the virulence of the new energies, are pushing down the future timeline towards the Cosmic Christ. The platform of new light and new dark that is being established in the present will then flow down this new timeline. Another way of looking at it is to recognise that the Cosmic Christ represents absolute order and love. This order is coming into the present from the future, while the new chaos that has been birthed in the present in the new black light is pushing into the future to meet and merge with the new light. In this way, a whole new pattern of creation is being birthed down this new timeline where bliss has been superseded by grace, and where grace ultimately will be superseded by something more, that will be the direct and complete irradiation of the Cosmic Christ.

The Cosmic Christ is the embodiment of a different type of love, purity, innocence, compassion, beauty, order, wisdom, common sense, understanding and knowledge. The virulence of the Christ Light is like a brilliant, blinding white that pulses down the new timeline and which calls to humanity to look into the future and to feel this advancing presence like a wave of stunning love and light. And in this pattern of birth, a most ancient soul has incarnated on the planet to assume the mantle of responsibility of giving birth to the Cosmic Christ in the essence of higher light, through an orchestrated pattern of absorption within the millions of different levels of the Seventh Plane. It is like going up a series of escalators that are composed of mirrors, and through the successive absorption of different aspects of the Father within each mirror, the escalator eventually touches the essence of the Cosmic Christ. As it reaches this point, then the one that has orchestrated this pattern can then become the essence of the Christ and can bring it back down into form in preparation for the next ten million years.

The focus of the Christ requires absolute service, devotion and obedience. Ignorance has to be stripped away and those that are prepared to be touched by the new Christ Light in the present can then assume the mantle of responsibility for directly invoking the Cosmic Christ into physical matter. The love of the Cosmic Christ is virulent and ruthless in that it will tolerate no negativity or slow frequency energy and will demand that a life of service is lived through the living essence of the Father. And as the new timeline pushes into the future, then those that are ready to absorb the new frequencies of the Cosmic Christ can take their positions on this roadway and irradiate a new platform of knowledge and unity. The roadway will be gradually lit up until there is a pure pathway of light that stretches down the new timeline. As this unfolds, then the Cosmic Christ will pulse down this pathway and speed up the manifestation of that which has been ordained by the Father to take place.

So, in ten to twelve million years the Avatar will return as the Cosmic Christ and will irradiate an entirely new pattern of light to all humanity and life. The pulse will flow out of Earth into the eighteen thousand Earths in the Wheel of Life and beyond. All life will be touched by the Christ Light and will never be the same again.

In preparing for the return of the Cosmic Christ, all ignorance has to be banished from the planet and replaced by a new knowledge. A new type of love has to be lived within the living moment and all of the old negativity and feudal patterns of ownership and violence need to be cleared away. The new timeline that Meher Baba has formed is all part of this change, and as we pulse down this new timeline, then we can see that all of the old patterns of fear, terror, cruelty and abuse will be stripped away. Successive frequencies of higher light and love will be seeded into the planet and humanity, and as this unfolds, then the whole race will be prepared for the return of the Christ. Humanity needs the new frequencies of light as part of this preparation, which will take approximately ten million years. So the return will either transpire at the end of the Sixth Root Race or early on in the Seventh Root Race, depending on how the different future probabilities are manifested. Either way, this represents a dramatic and total speeding up of everything.

In honouring and absorbing the new essence of love, humanity will come to live the essence of God, which is goodliness, ordinariness and devotion. The simplicity and beauty of living the moment, of feeling no separation, yet while still living the illusion of duality will be part of the preparation of what is to come. The return of the Cosmic Christ will be beyond description and one way to imagine it is to see us as living in a darkened, small room, where there are few objects. The room is claustrophobic and the pieces of furniture are old and in need of repair. When the Christ returns, it is like the walls of the room will dissolve and will be replaced by a dazzling light that comes from all directions. The old furniture disappears and the old physical body is replaced by a new version that then absorbs the light directly and consciously holds the multiple levels of awareness that is the living moment of the Christ. The light is utterly blinding at first and almost burns the flesh, so that all limitation, darkness and misunderstanding are cleared away. In that moment of brilliant illumination, then the essence of the Christ will birth a new level of awareness where the millions of universes and planets that host the diversity of all life forms will be connected through the pulse of unity and divinity. The unity of the Christ will host the new collective love that will then activate, in a totally unique way, the different chakras in humanity. The pre-existing pattern of twelve chakras will be transformed by the Christ Light, and collectively will spark a different level of reality in the physical. The higher light streams will be birthed in the physical awareness of the collective unity of humanity and then allow all sentient beings to be one with the Cosmic Christ and to become the living will and essence of the Christ. The living focus of the Seventh Plane will be formed in the shadowlands in a new and virulent way.

So, in the above analogy, if the shadow planes are like the darkened room, then the return of the Cosmic Christ will birth an irradiation of light that will quite literally, blow all of the old and replace the shadow planes with a completely new dictate of higher light. And in that moment, the shadow will disappear and be replaced by an entirely different pattern of light where there is no separation and no illusion; where the dream will become the lived reality since the dream will have been transformed by the power of the Christ Light. The power of the Christ will transform everything in its path and shine the light of illumination on absolutely everything. The whole pattern of what the everything and the nothing is, and how it is embodied and manifested through creation will then change forever. There will no longer be any shadow in the sense that humanity and life has experienced the shadow of the past root races.

The Cosmic Christ is absolute power and absolute change; it is total love and clarity and is the manifested Will of the Father as expressed through the birth of a new Son. The timeline that will see the birth of the Cosmic Christ in physical form has been established and is now building. It is an essential and vital component in the future unfolding of the new root races that ultimately will flow through the planet as part of the seeding and manifestation of the Father's Will.

Future Timelines

The new root race requires that two percent of the population gives birth to something new in the Sixth Root Race timeline, and that the remaining ninety-eight percent receive the downloaded essence of what the two percent has become. Meher Baba has overhauled the timeline for the next twelve hundred years during which the two percent have to wake up to the change. The two percent has to embrace the new timeline where the old artificial commodities of fear, confusion and doubt are replaced by the new intelligences of clear and happy thoughts, excited and light experiences where no evil is thought, heard or expressed. This new timeline is stretching into a new level of conscious awareness where the planetary vibration keeps on going up and up, and this has to be embraced systematically by humanity.

The new timeline also means that we can live the timelines of everything that has ever lived, as well as push into the future. In the present moment, three principal frequencies have been rescued from Lemuria; these have opened a new door and built a new timeline. For example, we can capture the current of time from ancient Lemuria, as expressed through form, such as an animal, and then live the timeline that the animal lived in the world at that time. We can also pulse backwards and forwards down different timelines, and wash back through the root races and forwards into the future root races. The devas and angels exist on different timelines and we can allow this pattern of time to flow into us. We can then capture the moment and feel the pulse of angelic or devic light. These new timelines demand a climate of change. As we open up to this new pattern, we will come to recognise the Elderings as masters of time who are birthing a new commodity of time within our awareness. This new concept of time will give us greater flexibility and the ability to go backwards and forwards in time.

We can pulse out of time, and merge with our future aspects, and then bring back into the present, the new focus of more ordered energy that will allow us to become more in the living moment. By dancing in and out of time, we can invoke change, speed up our timelines and negotiate for the best possible outcome, which is always about becoming more. We can focus on our dreams and live the experience where all the best possible outcomes of our dreams are manifested in the now. If we embrace the timeline of unconditional love, and let go of the old timeline of selfishness, greed, confusion and suffering, then through the invocation of more, we will always be in a point of balance rather than imbalance. Therefore, as we invoke for more, and within the embrace of unconditional love, we can ascend into a higher pattern of more where the selfish, smaller view is replaced by a collective, bigger picture where more will always be much more.

Working with different streams of time means that we are invoking a change in karma through Natural Law. Natural Law ensures that there is always a process of balancing everything that is out of balance. Karma is the current modality for ensuring that this is achieved. A timeline is unfinished experience and so in the different timelines that we focus on, there are always varying patterns or expressions of unfinished business. The reason that the Atlantean Root Race is still within humanity's awareness is that the old timeline has yet to be completed. There remains unfinished business and it is only when this is achieved that humanity can be freed from this old timeline. So, the pattern of washing the old timelines through our awareness is all part of the process of balancing karma and completing these older timelines.

One way of speeding up this process is to go forward to the end of that timeline and see what the finished experience is. This finished experience can then be brought back and placed into the existing timeline. One of the major frequencies of the old Atlantean timeline is fear. So if the finished experience of the old timeline is no fear, we can go out of time and bring back the finished experience, the unfinished business will be completed and fear will be removed. If on another timeline, there is unfinished business in relation to astral bodies, then if we go forward to the finished timeline where there is no longer any astral body, we can remove the need for any further astral manifestation and speed up karma.

Similarly, each soul that incarnates into the planet has unfinished business. For example, in human form we have cordings on our wrists. Many of these cordings are differently coloured – yellow, red, green, and brown – and are bunched up and tangled. When a soul encounters the Avatar or a Perfect Master these cordings are sorted out and part of the unfinished business can be speeded up. The soul then begins to be in the right place at the right time, rather than the wrong place at the wrong time. The Avatar and the Perfect Masters always live the new timelines; they are the new timelines and so when souls encounter them, they can do more through the new timeline connection.

This pattern of working with different timelines, past, present and future, can be applied to a whole host of different frequencies. Timelines are thought streams of energy; some are longer lasting than others are. So a root race timeline is much longer lasting than almost anything else. Each dominant, virulent thought, whether light or dark, creates a time wave that has energy and a finite length of existence. The Roman Empire was based on a thought form that had a life span. The Empire was birthed, then expanded, was eventually destroyed, and the residue of the afterglow exists to this day in the different concepts and ideas that we see around us. The same is true for the different root races. So five root race timelines have been birthed and each is in different stages of decay. The Adamic and Hyperborean are almost invisible now, while the Lemurian is much weaker. The

Atlantean and Aryan are still dominant. So with each timeline, the energy pulses out, then diminishes and leaves an afterglow. If we look into the future, then we can see the future, probable timelines of the next seven root races. The Sixth Root Race timeline is forming, while the other timelines have yet to be formed. However, if we focus on any of these different timelines, then we can begin to work the future streams of energy.

The new timeline is demanding change under the sponsorship of grace. The five Perfect Masters are creating a new harmonic and in this, they touch absolutely everything. As the old timelines are completed and absorbed, and the new timelines are birthed, then a whole pattern of change is instigated. Integral to this process is the Unspoken Word. Meher Baba released the Unspoken Word while in physical matter. The Unspoken Word is now returning, and as it builds, it will rupture, transmute and release the old timeline so that seventy-five percent of it is removed. The remaining twenty-five percent will then be on the receiving end of the afterglow of what is being birthed in the new timeline. As the balance of energy becomes more positive, then the pulse of everything will quicken. We are entering a cycle where the Sun will pulse much more rapidly over the next two thousand five hundred years. Time is speeding up, so that all that appears solid and ordered today will change in the tomorrow. For example, science and mysticism appear to be separated by a gulf, yet the two will come together in the future when souls will come down and work with them.

For the two percent of souls that embrace the new timeline, the experience will be subtle and profound. It will be as if they will begin to live in the future and will pulse initially at a third of a second into the future, and then more. These souls will always be slightly ahead of those around them in terms of vibration. The effect of this will be quite interesting because those individuals that vibrate at a slower frequency will not see them in the same way. As the new light workers go about irradiating all life, and yet appearing largely invisible, then for each of them the experience will be strange. People in shops will ignore them, and they will appear invisible in restaurants.

Memories will fade, and in an attempt to recover these lost memories, these souls will run up and down other people's timelines in an effort to capture that which has been lost. As they run up and down these different timelines, they will then start to live the life of these people. Understanding that this is part of the process of building up collective unity will be extremely helpful. Some people may recognise that the pulse of those in the two percent is different, and they may then connect with these quicker pulses for a split second, accelerating briefly into a different pattern of light. The new light workers will feel splintered, like shards of time dancing to a new instruction, living the experiences of the many, while constantly building a new platform of telepathic unity.

As the new timeline digs in deeper and deeper, then successive levels of higher light and instruction will flow into our awareness. Different levels within each successive timeline will pulse in and out of our waking and dreaming experiences, and for a brief instant, we may find ourselves living the experience of one timeline before shifting to another and experiencing something different. The challenge will be to recognise which timeline we are on, and where we are on that timeline. Sometimes it will feel like events have already taken place when they have yet to unfold, or experiences of déjà-vu will surface within our consciousness. We will pulse in and out of time, and live the experience of multiple timelines. We will give birth to timeless moments and make such moments the new timeline within our awareness, as we pulse backwards and forwards down the new timeline of unconditional love. The new timeline of the Sixth Root Race will be the new bedrock of lived experience in the moment, where all that has been is cleared and where the different possibilities or probabilities of more can be captured within our awareness as we dance in and out of time.

The Future Root Races

Working backwards and forwards down the different timelines offers an unprecedented opportunity to touch the essence of future root races. Future timelines offer new possibilities of birthing more into all life. If there will be a future, probable timeline where all of humanity is seeded with the Paramatman in an undiluted form, then this would potentially accelerate the pattern of new light being birthed into the planet. The new Sixth Root Race timeline is being formed and beyond this there are probable timelines for the Seventh, Eighth, Ninth, Tenth, Eleventh and Twelfth Root Races. The Twelve Root Races are like the twelve chakras in our energetic systems, and as humanity moves through each successive root race, then the energetics of each root race will be captured within the twelve chakras. Each root race will provide a major transformation of each chakra as humanity builds a lived experience within each one. We are in the process of moving from the solar plexus to the heart centre, and in future root races, the focus will ascend up through the different, higher chakras. Form and substance will be different in each root race and the seeds of these future timelines are being sown out of time, within the context of what we call the present.

Each root race will embody or express a different pattern of order and chaos where the percentages of order and chaos will change. So while we have a high percentage of chaos at present this will diminish in the future root races. So by the Twelfth Root Race we may only retain something like three percent chaos with ninety-seven percent order. The pattern of devic and angelic light will also be very different. The devas and the angels will merge closer and closer together and in the future the devas may begin to work with different patterns of order as the older patterns of chaos become saturated and no longer necessary within that level of experience. With a new platform of devic order, future life forms will be very different and will be capable of housing much more virulent patterns of light, as ever-higher levels of the Seventh Plane and beyond are seeded and drawn down into physical experience.

If we go out of time, then on one level, the whole experience and play of the various root races has already taken place within the probability of what is yet to become. We can look for some of the different root race timelines, and then pulse down each of them to see how life, light and order all evolve into something more. Natural Law will begin to change and what we regard as immutable and immovable today will completely change in the future. Our concepts of karma, time, light, love and magic will all change. For example, magic is part of Natural Law where the essence of something special can be invoked spontaneously in the moment. Magic is returning to our awareness and this will continue to build and build into the future. Our concepts of time and karma will also drastically change.

Therefore if we looked into certain, future timelines and picked out different manifestations, then we would see humanity becoming more crystalline, where the pattern of living was very different from what we experience today. If we went into the Divine Ocean of Life in the Seventh Root Race, then we might see storm-riders dancing over the waves of dark light, catching newly born souls. The storm-riders ride the storms of creation, harvesting the new souls and birthing them into the unfolding play of life. If we looked down other timelines then we might be presented with millions of different crystal skulls, each one a probable future that could be invoked and brought into play. And what if we could orchestrate choice in this pattern? What if we could influence the choice of local fashion? The pattern of free will and choice and the way in which the Father's Game is played could be changed to invoke something new.

If we could go forward say, sixty million years into the future, potentially into the Eleventh Root Race, then we could resonate with that new timeline. And if we then brought back from that point in time, a completed aspect of the future into the present, then time could be speeded up. What needed to be completed in the now could then be finished and we could move on. So once we accept that time is an illusion, that change is the norm and that our focus is to align ourselves with the living Will of the Father, then we can embrace a whole new pattern of light. We can touch so many different streams of awareness and manifest more consciousness into our reality. We can prepare ourselves for the Cosmic Christ and the irradiation of light that will catapult us into something so completely different, that we will live the essence of higher light in the containment of physical limitation, yet experience everything and nothing within that. All of this will become possible as we merge and build our connection with the successively higher streams of light. The devas will help to imbue us with more strength and physical earthing, while the angels will give us more order; and the Elderings will focus their essence into our awareness to help us see the whole pattern of root race development and unfolding that is part of the cycle of creation and progression of all life into more. Moreover through this progression we will sample, be and become the essence of different levels of divinity, all the while seeking that which is more, like a mirror to the Father in so many diverse ways.

In the past, the root races have been created through the coming together of wisdom and emotion. The future will give us access to the Akashic Records, not only for us as individuals but also for the planet, solar system and the galaxies. The way in which root races are formed and presented will change dramatically and behind this pulse of each root race, the pattern of birthing and returning of the original sparks will continue. Each Avataric Day will flow into another, where the pattern of sparking and soul expression will continue to build into more, as each successive layer of God in the Beyond State, and ultimately God in the Beyond-Beyond State, is unveiled through evermore brilliant expressions of love and light within the ever-present pulse of the everything and nothing. Multiple plays of form will dance in and out of the Wheel of Life, as this too expands to become more.

We will experience everything, but to be everything we have to become aware that everything is a grand illusion. So each level of the different Divine Journeys will talk to us through the different timelines, yet on another level, there are really no Divine Journeys; there is just a space where this manifestation of what we label God is. However nobody has found out what God is yet. We have no idea of what God is - He is too immense. We know who His Son is, because out of the immensity of a black sky the Primary Spark has come down repeatedly to tell us about Himself, life, the Universe and everything. Yet we struggle to absorb all that He was, is and will be. In all that we are, we seek and search out for more, and as we successively become more, we still search. This is the nature of our divinity and the way that we can continue to grow. With each successive root race, this pattern or dance will change, as each successive layer of divinity is unveiled within that which we call shadowlands. And as shadowlands changes, then there will always be more for us to absorb and become.

So in the stillness of light and within the silence of grace, now is the time to invoke the new root race. To sow the seeds of a new love, to embrace the new timeline with trust and faith and to align ourselves with the simplicity that says "May the Father's Will be done." In that timeless moment we will pulse and become more and prepare ourselves for a new level of consciousness where the Cosmic Christ can then come in and touch us in a new way. As long as we are happy and excited, we are doing the Father's Work. As soon as we recognise this, then all will unfold within the timeless glow of the essence of the Father and the Son. We will then become bubbles of light, dancing to the timeless glow of the spark that then becomes the flame as we go through a new door.

Notes to the Chapters

Chapter 1

1.   When the general term light is used, it will be denoted as Light, while references to light when it is contrasted to dark, will be in lower case as light.

2.   The difference between a soul and a soul aspect is described more fully in the next section below and in Chapter 8. Different soul aspects go to make up a soul and although the two terms are distinguished where it is appropriate, the use of the word soul may sometimes refer to a soul aspect as well, and in such circumstances the word soul will only be used.

3.   The difference between Reality and Illusion is explained in Chapter 5. A comprehensive description can be found in Meher Baba's *God Speaks*.

4.   The God in the Beyond-Beyond State is described in Chapter 5.

5.   The Wheel of Life is described more fully in Chapter 8.

Chapter 3

1.   A doorway refers to a spiritual and energetic opening that can host and bring through a diversity of higher light frequencies.

2.   A Perfect Master is a God-realised being that is a multiple-dimensional axis or hub for everything and nothing.

3.   Paramatman Light is the flow of higher light from the Seventh Plane and embodies unconditional love.

4.   The Fifty-One spiritual generators are described more fully in Chapter 12.

5.   The Spiritual Hierarchy oversees all of the changes that have

been ordained by the Avatar through the five Perfect Masters. More details are given in Chapter 12.

6.   Shamballa is a focus of higher will and manifestation through which the will and power of higher levels of divinity are made manifest.

7.   Further information on this substantial topic can be found in *A Handbook for Light Workers* by David Cousins and in Chapters 16 and 17 below.

Chapter 5

1.   Modern physics would equate this nothing to the point of non-existence before the Big Bang, although some physicists are now seeking to give a definition to that which existed before creation. Our minds will always struggle with this conundrum of creating something out of nothing and yet, there has to be the recognition that in the first moments of creation, something has to be birthed out of nothing.

2.   The Avataric Day is explained in more detail in Chapter 12.

3.   Shadowlands is the term used to describe life in the shadow planes below the Seventh Plane.

Chapter 6

1.   In *God Speaks*, Meher Baba gives a complete account of the soul's journey from the Seventh Plane down to the Zero Plane, and then back up to the Seventh Plane.

2.   Reality is most easily defined as experience in the Seventh Plane. Illusion encompasses the shadow experience from the Sixth Plane to the Zero Plane.

Chapter 7

1.   A fuller description of the Elements can be found in Chapter 9.

Chapter 10

1.   Sanskaras are impressions left on the soul as memories from previous lives and which dictate the play out of karma through habits and desires in the current life.

Chapter 11

1.   See the Map of the Planes of Consciousness in *God Speaks*.

Chapter 12

1.   The *Lord Meher* series by Bhau Kalchuri provides a unique insight into the life of the Avatar.

2.   See *God Speaks* p. 273

Chapter 18

1.   With the restructuring of the inner planes, this initial pattern may change, depending upon the focus and energetics of what was originally the Fourth Divine Journey and what will be the new First Divine Journey.

Suggested Meditations & Exercises

The following exercises and meditations are designed to help with some of the concepts and ideas discussed in the main text. They have been divided into three main categories:

- *Clearing energies and connecting with the group*
- *Invoking the new light streams*
- *Working with different energy streams.*

The meditations are intended as an introduction and *A Handbook for Light Workers* by David Cousins gives a much more comprehensive overview of meditation techniques and energetic exercises. The first set of meditations below establishes a basic thought form that can then be built on in subsequent meditations. In Chapter 3, the light symbol below is described and in the following meditations, reference will be made to this symbol. The symbol can be used in a number of different ways and in different colours, such as blue, black, white or gold. It is up to the reader to choose which colour intuitively feels right, although it is recommended that blue or black is used as a starting mechanism.

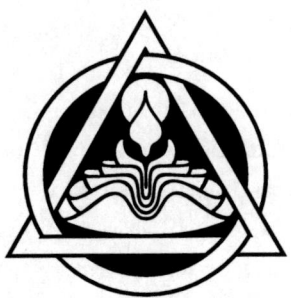

The basic pattern of meditation should last for a minimum of twenty minutes, preferably on a daily basis. Taking longer is fine, and if you experiment with the different levels within each meditation, then you may find that there are certain transition times after which you go into a deeper state. For example, twenty minutes is the minimum recommended time, and then there are other transition times at forty-five minutes and one hour and thirty-five minutes. All of these meditations are intuitively focused and so you can modify them or work with them as you see fit.

Clearing our Energies and Connecting with the Group

Meditation to put on a Shamanistic Robe

First sit down and make yourself comfortable. Then connect with the Paramatman Light, the Light that passes all understanding and which is accessed from the Seventh Plane. It does not matter what plane level you are stationed on since by thinking and invoking the thought form that is the Paramatman Light, you will bring through a reflected pattern of this Light that is appropriate for you at any given moment in time. Bring the Paramatman Light down through your crown and feel it cascading like a waterfall into you. Fill the whole of your body up with this Light, including each of the main chakra centres. Take your time when you do this since you should sense your energy shifting and becoming more refined.

Once this has been completed, place a shamanistic robe of light around your body. This robe can be a variety of colours, but initially start with white and focus on wrapping yourself up completely in the robe. The shamanistic robe represents a principal, protective thought form and with practice can give access to different plane levels. The robe can be any shape you choose, for example like an Arctic Owl, or an Eagle. The white Arctic Owl prepares you to work with slower frequency astral energy, while the Eagle is more mentally focused. Concentrate on feeling the presence of the robe building and wrapping around your aura. With practice you can change the colour; sometimes a black robe is appropriate, at other times, something different, such as blue or gold. Each time you call in your shamanistic robe, intuitively feel for the appropriate colour and shape. Each time you do it, it should become easier since you are building it up into a thought form. The more energy you give it, the more real it becomes. The shamanistic robe should be used every time you meditate.

Once you have finished the meditation, allow the robe to become darker and heavier and then place the light symbol shown above over each chakra centre and then make the symbol smaller and smaller until it disappears. This will close down your chakra centres and help bring you back into your physical body. This routine should be followed at the end of every meditation.

Meditation to Connect with the Group

The second step in any meditation is to bring in the collective and group focus. This will connect you with the group and will give you greater access and flexibility in your energetic work. This should be practised until it feels comfortable and is second nature. As in the previous meditation, bring down the Paramatman Light and put on your shamanistic robe. Then place a golden ring in your heart centre and allow the ring to sit there for a few minutes. Call in the presence of the group according to highest light and feel the ring slowly expand in your heart centre. As the energy builds, sense the collective presence build in your internal space. You should feel more solid and secure.

The group will give you access to information and will allow the collective focus of unity to build in your awareness. It is always helpful to call in the group when the surrounding energy feels difficult, or when you feel that your system is being affected by slow frequency energy, either during the day or the night.

Meditation to Clear the Chakra System

Begin by connecting with the Paramatman Light, putting on a shamanistic robe and calling in the group. This basic pattern of energy management should be used in all subsequent exercises and meditations as a starting mechanism. Then feel roots flowing out of the soles of your feet into the ground, and a third tap root growing out of the bottom of your spine. As these three roots go into the earth, they then merge as one, central taproot that goes deeper and deeper into the ground. When you feel comfortable and earthed, then work with each of the chakras, as follows, starting initially with the base chakra, then the sexual, solar plexus, heart, throat, third eye and finally the crown.

Fill each chakra up with Paramatman Light from the bottom to the top. Once you have completed this, then allow the energy in each chakra to flow out from the base of the spine and the feet down into the roots and the earth. Repeat this process by bringing the Paramatman Light into each chakra and clearing into the earth. Follow through with this procedure as many times as feels appropriate, although a minimum of two to three times should establish a basic working pattern. This exercise will help clear the chakras of any unwanted energies and will help to make them more flexible, so that they can open and close more easily. As you do this exercise, some chakras will feel easier to work with than others. This reflects the underlying pattern of energy. When you have finished, close down your chakras as described above.

Meditation to Clear our Energetic Systems

The same basic principles that have been used to clear out the chakra system can be used for the rest of our energetic vehicles, including the physical body, the etheric body and the aura. Once you have completed the basic procedures of calling in the Paramatman Light, putting on a shamanistic robe and connecting with the group, then feel the roots coming out of your feet and base of the spine. Allow the roots to merge and push deep into the ground. Fill the whole of your physical body with Paramatman Light, sensing areas that feel denser or heavier. Ensure that the Light goes everywhere including the centre of your bones. Some parts or organs may feel darker than others and this reflects the areas where there is more slow frequency energy. Once you have finished this, allow the light to drain out into the earth. Repeat the process again, this time noticing any differences in the physical body. Some places may intuitively feel that they require more clearing, and it can be helpful to focus specifically on bones and joints, organs, and the different physiological systems such as the lymphatic, nervous and cardiovascular systems.

The clearing process can be repeated for the etheric body. Here you focus on bringing the Paramatman Light into the expanse of space that surrounds the physical body by approximately one inch. As you feel this space, you should feel a subtle difference in vibration. Once the etheric body has been filled with Light, allow the light to flow out as before. Repeat the procedure again. Finally, focus on clearing the aura. Feel the Paramatman Light going beyond your physical body and pushing out on either side to fill the aura. Allow your intuition to direct how far out you feel you need to go, and how far the aura extends above and below your body. You should feel a sense of expansion. Again, once you have filled the whole of your aura, allow the energy to flow down the roots into the ground, and repeat the process.

There is a variant on this exercise where instead of using roots, you can intuitively place a golden disc several feet below your feet. The disc should be three to four feet across and you should focus on spinning it in an anticlockwise direction. Slow frequency energy can be drained into the disc and it can be pushed up into the light for clearing and absorption at the end of the meditation.

Once you have finished the different levels of clearing, then slowly close down your system.

Meditation to Connect with our Higher Guidance

Once you have completed the initial meditation sequence, focus on your heart centre and send out a call for your highest guides to come in. The focus should be on your highest guides, rather than just any old guides. As you send out this internal call, see if you can feel a pulse of energy coming into your system. You may also be presented with a symbol within your awareness. If you feel a symbol, then place it in your heart centre and see whether it expands or contracts. If it expands, then you have established a sound connection. If it contracts, then send out another call for your highest guides and repeat the procedure with a different symbol. You should practice connecting with your guides as much as possible. Try to get a sense of the feeling or signature of your main guide. As you build up this pattern, you may find other guides coming in and again see if you can feel their energy.

Ideally you will work with three main tiers of guides: protective guides, your central doorkeeper and mental plane guides. The protective guides can be visualised as Roman soldiers with their shields and armour; your central doorkeeper will be a native American Indian, while the higher mental guides may vary in form, sometimes appearing just as brilliant light. With each sequence of guides, it is worth practising calling them in and feeling the different energetic presences. With practice you will be able to feel all of the different guides coming in, and be able to recognise their energetic signatures. Each time you call in your guides, you should request that your inner and outer space is cleared. Once you finish working, close down your system.

Exercise to Clear Old Cordings

This can be a very useful meditation for working with problematic relationships and difficult energetic exchanges with other people. Start off with the basic procedures of invoking the Paramatman Light, putting on your shamanistic robe, calling in the group and your highest guides. Ask your guides to clear your internal and external space. Then focus on your chakra systems and think of the specific person that you wish to work with. The focus of this exercise should be about invoking the greatest benefit or good for both of you. You can imagine the person standing several metres in front of you, or you might feel them more distantly. Allow your awareness to focus on each chakra, starting with the base and working up, sensing whether there are any cords of energy going out to the other person. You will often find a mix of different cordings. Try to get a sense of the thickness of each cording, its colour and quality, and then see where it goes: does it go to the same chakra in the other person, or to a different one? Ideally all of the cordings should only flow between each relevant chakra i.e. heart to heart, solar plexus to solar plexus and so on. Thick, darker cordings will reflect slower patterns of energy. Those cordings that are clear or light will not require much work compared to the darker ones, although it is rare for there to be more clearer cordings than darker ones.

Once you have built up a picture of the different cordings in each chakra centre, you can then choose which you wish to work with first. Initially, select the biggest and darkest and then work down the scale. Once you have selected a cording, bring down the Paramatman Light through the crown and push it into the dark cording. You can either feel the Light flowing into the cording and beginning to slowly dissolve it, or you may sense the cording burst into flames and dissolving into ashes. As you do this, invoke light, love and balance for the other person according to greatest good. Once the cording has dissolved, clear your energetic system again and take another look to see whether the cording is smaller in size, or whether it has disappeared. If it has not completely disappeared, then repeat the process until it has dissolved. You can then move onto the next cording.

This exercise will take up your energy, so it is best not to be too ambitious about how many cordings you work with at first. However, as you do it, you should find that the interaction with the other person becomes easier. This exercise is useful for clearing out old, unfinished karma with those close to you. Before you finish the exercise, be sure to completely clear your system and then close down.

Meditation to Release Old Fears and Suffering

Many of our fears and worries are subconsciously formed and reflect the past karma and flow of astral energy within our awareness. In this meditation, the focus is on working with what is hidden and subconscious. Once you have completed the opening sequence to the meditation, open yourself up to the land. Visualise in front of you a pond or a lake, which represents the sum total of all of your fears and points of suffering in this life and previously. As you walk up to the lake, which can be either large or small, see whether the water is clear, or muddy, and whether it is full of debris or not. The surface of the water may be smooth or choppy. The muddier it is the more old fear patterns are retained within your subconscious.

As you look at the lake, feel the sun shining on it, and you then focus on the sun as it begins to burn off the water. This may take a few minutes or more, and as the lake level slowly recedes, feel the intensity of the sun building all the time. Eventually, the lake water will have evaporated completely and you will be left with objects at the bottom of the lake, covered in thick mud. These might be old buildings or strange objects that are like a reference point to what lies within. As you focus on these objects, visualise the sun drying out the mud. Then invoke for clear and sparkling water to fill the lake again. This can come in the form of a rainstorm or by other means. As the lake fills, the old objects begin to dissolve and eventually it is filled to the original level, though this time the water is clear and sparkling. If any objects remain in the lake, then the process should be repeated since these objects represent old thought forms that have not been cleared.

You can do this exercise as many times as you like, using the sun light to clear the old, muddy water and replacing it with new clear water. Finish the meditation by closing down in the usual way.

Meditation to Clear Old Thought Forms

Old, recurrent thought forms can be difficult to remove. Begin by calling in the Paramatman Light, putting your shamanistic robe on, and calling in the group and your highest guides. Ask your guides to clear your internal and external space and to assist in this exercise.

Imagine three separate fires in front of you – one for the physical, one for the astral and one for the mental. Each fire will have a slightly different coloured flame. Focus on those constant, virulent thoughts that give you problems, such as fears over health, difficult relationships or specific emotions. Begin by putting any worries about the health and the body into the fire that represents the physical and feel the fire claim the energy surrounding the issue. Once you have worked through any physical worries, focus on the astral fire, placing any emotional worries in this fire. Once you have done that, focus on the mental fire and place in it any metal worries. Once you have worked through all three fires, offer everything up to the light and the Avatar. You should not have any expectation about how your thoughts, or emotions will change – just focus on letting go. You need to do this with real intent and focus.

If the thought forms persist, offer them up repeatedly to the Avatar. In situations where the brain is overactive, or there is too much internal dialogue, you can bring down the Paramatman Light and bathe the brain in It. This should help to raise your vibration and allow the old thoughts to drop away. Once you have finished, close down your centres in the usual way.

You can add to this meditation by writing down on paper a list of all your negative thoughts and old fears, and burning the paper to symbolise your release from them.

Exercise for Clearing a House

Follow the usual opening format and then focus on each room in the house in sequence. It is easiest to start with the room that you are sitting in. Imagine a pillar of brilliant light (Paramatman Light) coming down into the room and visualise this light spinning in an anti-clockwise direction. The light will spread out from the central vortex and form a rotating disc. Allow the disc to spin around the whole room and focus on it clearing out any slow frequency energy. Once the first room is finished, repeat the process for every room in the house, visualising the light disc absorbing any negative and slow frequency energy. This may take some time. You can repeatedly ask for assistance from your guides. Once every room has been cleared, expand the pillar of white light to encompass the whole house. Imagine the light disc going into the house foundations and then spinning slowly up through the whole of the house into the roof. Repeat this several times. You can also spread a protective, crystalline sheet underneath the house so as to prevent any unwanted energies coming up from underground into the house. This process will help clear the ground energies and house foundations.

You then want to work at sealing off the house from slow frequency energies that are externally focused. This can be done by placing the light symbol over every door and window, both from the inside and out. As you imprint the symbol into each external point of energetic access, you will be bringing through the power and higher essence of the light symbol as a protective thought form. The whole process, from start to finish, may take time. At the end place the symbol over the whole house and whatever garden is present. You can also work with the perimeter of your land, establishing an energetic wall of light to keep out slow frequency energies.

At the end of this whole process, bless and dedicate the house to the highest authorities of light, or to the Avatar as appropriate. Close down all your centres at the end of the exercise.

Exercise to Clear the Ground Energies

This exercise is usually part of the above practice for house clearing. If it is done separately, then after following the usual steps for meditation, bring down a pillar of light as described previously and begin to infuse it into an area of ground. This can either be done on the ground where you are, or remotely, through visualising the light flowing into a piece of land that you are focusing on. The pillar should be allowed to expand into a large disc that can flow into the ground and up again, as deep as feels appropriate. In some cases you may have to go hundreds of feet down to connect with a focal point of energy that needs to be cleared. As you do this, you may get certain impressions about what that energy is, and while sometimes of interest, it is important to remain focused on the clearing process. Group focus is always important in this type of exercise, because the more you call in the group, the easier it becomes to work energetically in this way. Once you have finished, see how the ground energies feel. Clear your own energy system and then close down your centres.

Exercise to Ground our Energetic Systems

This is a simple exercise to help ground your system with the earth and is best done outside. Better results are achieved with bare feet placed on the ground. Once you have opened up in the usual way, feel roots growing down from the souls of your feet into the earth, and going many feet down. Visualise a deep, black energy in the earth and slowly allow it to flow up the roots and into your body. Feel the whole of your body becoming infused with this rich, black light and experience a deep sense of calm and peace come over you. Once you have become completely black inside, then stay like this for a minute or two, before allowing the black energy to clear out of you. The black energy will help to ground you. You can then bring down the Paramatman Light as a final sequence in this exercise before closing down your centres.

Exercise to Determine our Level of Pranic Energy

This is a simple, intuitive exercise that requires little preparation. In essence you silence your mind, and focus on the whole of your body. As you remain still and tranquil, tune into your pranic energy. This can be done intuitively, and see how far this energy reaches up into your body, starting from the feet and going up. Imagine your body as a vessel that contains pranic energy; the level that it comes up to in your body is a direct measure of the amount of pranic energy present. For example, it may feel like the levels of energy reach the knees or thighs, which means that you need more. If it is up to your chest, then the levels are good; if they are around your ankles, then you need to quickly absorb more prana since this shows that your pranic levels are much too low.

You can modify this exercise to measure other types of energy in your system, such as slow frequency energy or astral light. The principles are the same and the amount of energy present will be reflected in how high it comes up in your body.

Invoking the New Light Streams

Meditation to Bring in the New Timeline

Begin the meditation by calling in the Paramatman Light and invoking the presence of the group and your highest guides. Place a white shamanistic robe around you and then focus on the silence within. Place the light symbol in each of your chakra centres. From a point of balance and peace, you can then invoke for the new Sixth Root Race timeline to come into your awareness and into your life on a daily basis. Call in the highest mental guides to assist you. Then look in front of you and feel the presence of a roadway of light forming; as it builds feel your vibration accelerate. If you have difficulty visualising this, call in more Paramatman Light into your system. Once you see the roadway, then invoke to step onto this new path and embrace the Sixth Root Race in that moment. You can invoke this repeatedly through the Avatar. You may feel yourself stepping onto this roadway and walking down it. Allow the different frequencies of the roadway to touch you and note any impressions that you may get. Remain open to the irradiation of higher light as it suffuses through you and feel yourself now standing on this new timeline. When you are ready, come back into your physical body and slowly close down your centres as usual. Repeat this meditation as many times as necessary to allow the focus of new light to begin working through your system.

Meditation to Connect with the Elderings

Begin the meditation with the usual sequence of bringing down the Light, putting on your robes, connecting with the group and calling in your highest guides. Initially focus on your wrists and place two golden rings around them. Place a third, larger, golden ring in your heart centre. This represents the initial resting position before opening up to the Elderings. Allow the rings on your wrists to move into your heart centre; visualise all three rings moving up into your head where they merge. Feel the golden ring wrapping around your head horizontally so that it sits like a band above your eyes. Once this has been completed, call the Elderings into your space. You may begin to feel a presence build up behind you or a pulse building in your space. At first the pulse might be quite weak, but with practice it will grow until you can feel the presence of the Eldering standing behind you.

You can build on this basic pattern by also visualising a large, oval doorway behind you. There is a golden ring at the bottom of the doorway that will move to the top of the doorway when it is activated. Once the ring on the door is active, an Eldering can approach you through this doorway. You can also practice going through this doorway to connect with the Eldering. If the Eldering comes down into the doorway and stretches out its arms, this is a signal for you to go towards the doorway and slowly merge with the Eldering. At the end of the meditation, close down your centres in the normal way.

Meditation to go Forwards and Backwards down our Timelines

Once you have completed the opening meditation sequence, focus on your internal space. For this meditation you should use either a white or a golden shamanistic robe. You can also call in the Elderings as a higher level of guidance to help you. The Elderings are time masters and can assist you with the sequence of timelines. Once you have opened up, imagine that you are looking into the future and begin to feel different streams of energy form inside. You may only sense one specific pattern or line of energy forming and this may connect with your internal space and then push into the distant future. Alternatively, you may get more than one line, although one may be stronger than the other(s). Each line may appear slightly different in colour. As you look at the timeline, imagine yourself beginning to walk down it into your future. Go as far down the timeline as you feel comfortable and come back the same way that you came. You can practice going backwards and forwards down this or another timeline, although you may find that you become quite tired initially, since this type of exercise can use up large amounts of energy. With practice, you will begin to get different impressions and feelings as you go down each timeline, and as this builds you may begin to connect with future aspects of yourself that look slightly different from you. Allow these impressions to flow through. Whenever you are ready to finish the meditation, always come back to the same starting point and then slowly close your system down.

Meditation to Meet our Light Twin

Our light twin is our future, higher aspect and can be accessed through our awareness. Once you have opened up and connected with your guides, including the Elderings, invoke to meet your future, light twin. You can work with several different types of patterns such as a timeline forming in your awareness that will take you forwards to your light twin; or you may choose to work with a journey across an ocean of light that eventually takes you to an island where you will find your light twin. Either way, just allow the energy to unfold as you push into the future. It may take some time for you to eventually see your light twin, and it should appear golden or extremely brilliant and bright. You should also feel a strong pattern of energy emanating from your twin, which will build, as you get closer. Allow the energies to flow through you, and if you have sufficient energy, just feel yourself moving in front of your twin. Look into the eyes of your twin and invoke to receive whatever information or energy is appropriate at that time. Allow this energy to come into your space. At first you may not be able to get very close, but with practice it should become easier and eventually, you may be able to merge with your light twin. This will signify that you have entered a different stream of energy. Once you have connected with your light twin, come back to your original starting point in the meditation and slowly close your system down.

You may find with this meditation tiring. This is normal and relates to the amount of energy that is required to push down your timelines. It is also important that you always maintain the group focus during these meditations, since the group energy will make it easier for you to push through any potential obstacles in your awareness. These may relate to the limitations of what your mind can accept, or may be to do with the amount of energy that you need to push forward.

Working with Different Energy Streams

Exercise to Tune into the Mineral Kingdom

This exercise is best done sitting outside on the ground close to a rock. Begin by bringing down the Paramatman Light and calling in your highest guides. For this exercise, you will need a pure black shamanistic robe since this will key you into the devic frequencies more directly. Feel yourself go into silence and then open yourself up to the rock that you have chosen to focus on. You should not attempt to do anything initially, but just remain in stillness and allow your awareness to naturally expand. After a time, feel yourself beginning to connect with the rock and the energies contained within it. Do not try to judge or analyze the experience, just allow the flow of energy to unfold. You may have to wait some time before you feel anything. At first you might sense a pulse or feel a denser presence close to you.

Allow this pulse or presence to build in the silence. Do not attempt to direct the energy. Eventually you may feel different presences or energy streams within the rock. At the end of the exercise, bring down the Paramatman Light into your system, clearing away anything that you might have picked up during the exercise. Close down your centres at the end.

Meditation to Meet our Darkling

Bring down the Paramatman Light, put on a black shamanistic robe; call in the group and your highest guides. Send out a call in your awareness to meet with your darkling; this call should be clear and focused, and once you have sent it out, you should begin to feel a presence form nearby. Sometimes it will be over your shoulder or it may be directly behind you, or in front of you. Ask for a symbol from the darkling and then place this symbol in your heart centre. If it remains there, call the darkling in closer and try to feel the darkling energy. You can ask the darkling for a name and allow it to form in your awareness. You do not have to try – it is best to be open and silent. Once you have received a name, build up an inner dialogue with the darkling. You can request information and assistance on any matter concerning devic life and whenever you call to your darkling, you will feel its presence. As your connection builds, see if you can visualise his appearance. At the end of the meditation, thank your darkling for his assistance and presence, and then close down your centres.

Exercise to Determine Inner Plane Status

Follow the usual procedures for starting a meditation and connect with your highest guides. Once you have completed this, focus on becoming completely silent. Once your mind has become quiet, offer up a request to know what your inner planes status is. This will usually be somewhere between zero and six. A number should come into your awareness. The aim is to avoid any bias, since the ego will always want a higher plane number to come in. Once you have a number, place it in your heart centre to see whether it expands or contracts. If it contracts, then the number is out of balance. If it expands, then it is in balance. You can repeat this exercise to determine the sub-plane that you are on between one and ten. Once you have completed this part, you can focus on determining which planes you are working on. Again, intuitively ask for a number relating to your principal working plane, and test it in your heart centre. Repeat this process for the sub-plane. You may work on more than one plane, so you can go over this procedure several times to see what comes through. Once you have finished, close down your system in the usual way.

Exercise to Determine Level of Astral Focus

This exercise can be helpful in determining your focus in the astral levels. It is similar to the previous exercise except that your focus is only on the astral levels and the numbering works between one and nine. You can start off by focusing on whether you are in the lower, middle or upper astral, and then find a number that resonates with this. Place the number in your heart centre to test whether it is correct. Once you have a number, relate this to how you feel physically and emotionally. If you do this when you feel tired or irritated, you will get a different reading from when you are happy. The focus of this exercise also should be to develop a sense of what each level feels like, so that you can eventually know immediately where you are in the astral levels. Each level will have its own particular feel and stream of energy that can be sensed physically and subtly. Follow the usual procedures for closing down.

Exercise for Two People to Merge

This exercise should be done with one other person. Sit opposite each other and follow the usual procedures for opening up with the Paramatman Light, putting on your robes, calling in the group and your highest guides. Ask for the room energies to be cleared. You can also follow the procedure for clearing your energetic system before doing the merging exercise.

Take it in turns to do the exercise. The first person that chooses to project their awareness into the other person is active, while the partner remains passive. The active partner should sense how their energy connects with their partner and whether there is any resistance. With some people this exercise will be easy, and with others it will be harder. As you merge and connect with the other person's space, just feel how your energy changes and which chakras are open, and which are closed. Allow your energies to combine and stay with the feeling for a few minutes. At the end, allow your energies to come out of the other person and then rest for a few moments. Both of you can clear your internal spaces if this feels appropriate. Take a few minutes to share your experiences and then swap roles; the person who was previously active now becomes passive. Once you have finished, share your experiences again.

Clear and close down your systems at the end of the exercise. Once you have done this exercise several times, you can do it simultaneously, with both people being active at the same time.

Bibliography

Cousins, David A.
> *A Handbook for Light Workers.*
> Barton House (1993).

Kalchuri, Bhau
> *Lord Meher* Series, Volumes 1-20.
> Canns Down Press (1996).

Meher Baba
> *God Speaks. The Theme of Creation and its Purpose.*
> Dodd, Mead & Company (1973).

> *Discourses.*
> Sheriar Foundation (1995).

> *Meher Baba on Inner Life.*
> Meher Era Publication (1996).

About the Author

Nick Scott-Ram graduated in Natural Sciences (Zoology) at Cambridge University and went on to complete his PhD in the Philosophy of Science (also at Cambridge). Since a young age he has had a deep interest in meditation and developing an insight into our inner world of experience, both from a philosophical perspective and an experiential one. Over the last ten years he has been fortunate enough to work with David Cousins and to explore different subtle energy patterns in our world.

He has written a number of books including *Keys to the Crystal Skulls. Divine Beacons of Light.* (LightWork Media 2004), *Keys to Our Heart. A Prelude to the Sixth Root Race* (LightWork Media 2002) and *Transformed Cladistics, Taxonomy and Evolution* (Cambridge University Press 1990). He has also written numerous articles on business subjects including intellectual property and biotechnology, and co-authored *Patents on Biotechnological Inventions. The EC Directive* (Sweet & Maxwell 2002).

Since 1997 Nick has run workshops on a range of spiritual subjects. The focus of his work is on the development of an energetic interpretation of our inner journey and on the interaction of natural phenomena around us, such as the Mineral, Plant and Animal Kingdoms. He currently divides his time between writing and running workshops in the UK and overseas.

Additional information on books and workshops can be found at the following web-sites:

www.devictruth.com

www.soulspeaks.co.uk

ISBN 141209464-X